Contraception: An Evidence-Based Approach

Contraception: An Evidence-Based Approach

Editor: Emerson Burton

AMERICAN
MEDICAL PUBLISHERS
www.americanmedicalpublishers.com

AMERICAN
MEDICAL PUBLISHERS
www.americanmedicalpublishers.com

Cataloging-in-Publication Data

Contraception : an evidence-based approach / edited by Emerson Burton.
p. cm.
Includes bibliographical references and index.
ISBN 979-8-88740-022-8
1. Contraception. 2. Conception. 3. Human reproduction. 4. Fertility, Human.
5. Birth control. I. Burton, Emerson.
RG136 .C66 2023
613.94--dc23

American Medical Publishers,
41 Flatbush Avenue,
1st Floor, New York,
NY 11217, USA

ISBN 979-8-88740-022-8 (Hardback)

Contents

Preface

Over the recent decade, advancements and applications have progressed exponentially. This has led to the increased interest in this field and projects are being conducted to enhance knowledge. The main objective of this book is to present some of the critical challenges and provide insights into possible solutions. This book will answer the varied questions that arise in the field and also provide an increased scope for furthering studies.

Contraception refers to various methods, medicines or devices used for birth control. There are a number of factors like effectiveness, safety, availability, affordability and accessibility, and acceptability that must be considered while choosing the appropriate method of contraception. Measures of contraception that are widely utilized include female and male sterilization, long-acting reversible contraceptives or LARC methods, short-acting hormonal methods, barrier methods, and natural rhythm methods. Among these methods female sterilization and male sterilization are permanent contraception methods. Female sterilization is a surgical procedure in which the fallopian tubes are tied or closed to prevent the sperm and eggs to fuse for fertilization. The commonly used barrier methods are condoms, diaphragms, cervical caps, and contraceptive sponges. Intrauterine contraception devices include levonorgestrel intrauterine system (LNG IUS) and copper T intrauterine device (IUD), which are implanted into the uterus to prevent pregnancy. This book provides an evidence based approach to contraception. From research to practical applications, case studies and examples related to all contemporary topics of relevance to this field have been included herein.

I hope that this book, with its visionary approach, will be a valuable addition and will promote interest among readers. Each of the authors has provided their extraordinary competence in their specific fields by providing different perspectives as they come from diverse nations and regions. I thank them for their contributions.

Editor

Pregnant or recently pregnant opioid users: Contraception decisions, perceptions and preferences

Rebecca L. Fischbein[1*], Bethany G. Lanese[2], Lynn Falletta[2], Kelsey Hamilton[2], Jennifer A. King[3] and Deric R. Kenne[2]

Abstract

Background: Multiple factors are linked to extremely high unintended pregnancy rates among women who use opioids, including various barriers to contraception adherence. These include patient level barriers such as lack of knowledge and education about highly effective contraception, and potential provider barriers. Using a mixed-methods framework to examine the contraception-related perceptions and preferences of opioid using women is a necessary next step to understanding this phenomenon.

Methods: A mixed-method study was conducted which included both self-report questionnaires along with a semi-structured qualitative interview of opioid-using pregnant or recently pregnant women in two drug treatment facilities in Ohio.

Results: Forty-two women completed the study. The majority of recent (75%) and total pregnancies were unintended. Male condoms were reported as the highest form of lifetime contraception used within the present sample (69%). Participants reported low lifetime use of long acting reversible contraception (LARC) (ranging from 5 to 12%). Participants preferred hormonal injections first (40%), followed by IUDs (17%). Reasons for preferences of injections and LARC were similar: not needing to remember, side effects, and long-term effectiveness.

Conclusions: Most of the study population participants stated they would utilize contraception, particularly Tier 1 LARC methods, if freely available; however, high rates of unintended pregnancy were observed in this sample. This indicates the need for contraception education, and addressing the procedural, logistical and economic barriers that may be preventing the use of LARC among this population.

Keywords: Contraception, Pregnancy, Opioid Drug Use

Background

Women who misuse or abuse opioids are at great risk for unintended pregnancy with nearly eight out of every ten pregnancies unintended [1, 2]. Drug use during pregnancy can cause complications and potential adverse outcomes, including pre-term delivery, low-birth weight, microcephaly, and miscarriage [3]. Further, studies show that pregnant women with a substance use disorder (SUD) are less inclined to seek prenatal care, and often have higher rates of HIV, hepatitis, and other STIs [4]. Use of opioids during pregnancy and the number of newborns delivered with Neonatal Abstinence Syndrome (NAS) have been increasing rapidly in the United States [5]. Newborns suffering from NAS require special medical attention and other services [6] and are likely at-risk for future developmental delays, disabilities, and chronic medical conditions [7].

Increasing the use of contraception could reduce unintended pregnancy and associated health care problems among drug-using populations. While many of the available methods of contraception are effective when used correctly and consistently, in typical use among this population [8–11], pregnancy rates are much higher than

* Correspondence: rfischbein@neomed.edu
[1]Department of Family and Community Medicine, Northeast Ohio Medical University, 4209 St. Rt. 44, PO Box 95, Rootstown, OH 44272, USA

for the general public, except for intrauterine devices (IUDs) and subdermal implants. In part, in real-world settings, this may be due to reduced adherence relative to non-drug using populations [12, 13]. Women in drug-using settings may face challenges and barriers that magnify their likelihood of unintended pregnancy [12, 14]. Because they have very low failure rates in both perfect and typical use, IUDs and subdermal implants are categorized as Tier 1 (defined as "very effective") by the World Health Organization [15]. These long acting reversible contraceptive (LARC) methods are proven to be safe, effective, cost-effective, high in patient satisfaction and convenient (e.g., no daily or weekly requirements) [16–20]. Recently, LARC usage rates have increased in the United States with approximately 11% of contraception using women choosing LARC methods [17]. By improving contraception adherence, it is possible LARC methods also reduce the likelihood of unintended pregnancy among opioid using populations. However, while these products are safe and effective [20], there may be a gap in patient knowledge about LARC methods and/or patient and provider barriers to accessing LARC methods that may limit use among women in this population [21–23]. Most fundamentally, it is not known what women who use opioids think about these contraception options.

Women who use opioids may comprise a population who feel targeted to use these effective methods of contraception [2]. Investigating perceptions regarding contraception methods is crucial to ensure that effective methods are available for women to use in accordance with their preferences rather than because they feel pressured or coerced. However, decisions, preferences and perceptions regarding contraceptive methods are understudied among this complex group [24]. Previous research with this population strongly supports the inclusion of a qualitative component to better understand and eventually address their reproductive healthcare needs [25]. To date, only a few studies have examined the issue using qualitative methodology [26–28]. Semi-structured interviews conducted with seven women at a methadone clinic in rural New South Wales found that the participants were aware of contraception methods, but tended to use less effective methods [26]. In Australia, a qualitative study among 90 current or former injection drug-using women found that the reasons for contraceptive use differed among women. These participants also revealed varying concerns and barriers to different contraception methods [27]. One California study of substance-abusing pregnant women found that participants held misperceptions such as the belief that they were unable to become pregnant while using drugs due to the amenorrhea that is often associated with substance abuse [28].

To our knowledge, no mixed methods study has been conducted that examined decisions, preferences and perceptions related to contraceptive methods among opioid-using pregnant or recently pregnant women in the United States with a mixed methods approach. Given the dramatic increase in opioid use, including opioid use during pregnancy in the United States, this complex topic requires further investigation. Consequently, we asked pregnant or recently pregnant women who misuse or abuse opioids to share their thoughts on these topics.

Methods

A comprehensive mixed-method study was conducted which included both self-report and interviewer-guided questions along with a semi-structured qualitative interview. The project was conducted in two stages with stage 1 interviews serving as a pilot study. Questions were exploratory and derived from the literature. Stage 2 expanded and replicated stage 1 with minor adjustments to the questions based on the evolution of the literature and newly emerging drug trends.

Interviews were conducted at two treatment facilities in Ohio. Treatment location 1 provided only non-residential services and treatment location 2 provided both residential and non-residential patient services. Using convenience sampling, participants were identified as eligible by program staff at the facilities. Participants were then recruited for the study by research staff. Individuals were eligible to participate if they met the following criteria: 1) currently or recently (within past 12 months) pregnant including miscarried or terminated pregnancies, 2) current or recent (within past 12 months) abuse/dependence of pharmaceutical opioids, 3) not actively psychotic, 4) English-speaking, 5) no current or past diagnosis of schizophrenia, 6) not currently suicidal, 7) not intellectually disabled, and 8) at least 18 years of age. Participants received $10 compensation for their participation. The final sample size reflects all women who agreed to participate and completed the study.

Stage 1 interviews were conducted in-person while stage 2 interviews were conducted remotely. The interviews were recorded with a digital recorder and each lasted approximately 90 min. A full board human subjects review was conducted due to the participants' complex status. The participant population was identified as having multiple layers of vulnerability due to their status as pregnant, with substance use disorders, and further some may have had status as "prisoners" due to court-ordered residential treatment. The IRB approved this study and all protections were in place to protect this vulnerable population in this minimal risk study. Informed consent was obtained from all individual participants included in the study. The project was approved by the Kent State University institutional review board under protocol numbers: 12–277 and 13–063.

The questionnaires and semi-structured interview included the following domains: participant characteristics, pregnancy history, contraceptive utilization history, preferences and opinions, and perceptions of contraception effectiveness and dangers/side effects.

Participant characteristics

Demographic questions reported in the current research include: age, race and marital status. Additional questions included lifetime use of means-tested programs including unemployment, cash assistance, food stamps, Medicaid and Woman, Infants and Children (WIC).

Pregnancy history

Pregnancy history included questions about number of pregnancies, pregnancy outcome, whether each pregnancy was intended, and custody status for delivered pregnancies.

Sexual history

Participants were asked about sexual history including the number of partners in the past year and whether they had ever traded sex for money, food, or drugs. Participants were also asked to indicate their STI history.

Contraception use

Participants from treatment location 1 were asked an open-ended question "What kind(s) of birth control do you or have you used?" and participants from treatment location 2 were asked "What kind(s) of birth control do you currently use or have you used in the past?" The options for participants at Site 2 included: "the pill", diaphragm, Vaginal Ring (NuvaRing), IUD, condom (male), female condom, the patch, sterilization/tubes tied, implant/Norplant, family planning (rhythm/pulling out), spermicides, Depo-Provera injection (3-month shot), Plan B/emergency contraceptives. These two questions were combined to represent contraception type lifetime use. Participants were asked about contraception access, including whether they had difficulty obtaining or purchasing contraception and how birth control was obtained. Participants were also asked decisions regarding contraception use, including reasons for contraception use and whether they primarily used contraception to prevent pregnancy, sexually transmitted infections (STI), or both. Women in treatment location 1 were asked about the situations in which they would or would not use condoms, while women in treatment location 2 were asked about the situations in which they would or would not use birth control.

Contraception types and preferences

Questions about contraception type included what method they preferred to use, and if participants had access to free contraception 1) if they would use it, and 2) what method they would prefer and why.

Perceptions of contraception effectiveness and dangers/side effects

Participants recruited from treatment location 2 were asked additional questions about their perceptions of effectiveness and dangers/side effects of different contraceptive methods. Participants were asked to respond to the following question "What percentage (or number of women out of 100) do you think would get pregnant in a year?" Possible responses included: < 1, 1–5, 6–10, > 10%, I don't know. Participants were then asked to report "How bothered are you or would you be by the dangers or side effects of [contraception method]". Possible responses included: not at all, a little, a lot, extremely, or I don't know.

Data were analyzed using quantitative and qualitative methods. Quantitative data analyses included descriptive statistics which were conducted using SPSS Version 21. Qualitative data were coded for themes.

Results

Table 1 reports participant characteristics. Forty-two participants provided complete information during the two-year study period 2012–2014; four individuals who enrolled did not and were not included in the analysis. Participants were predominantly white (81%) and single (74%), with an average age of 27.6 years. In addition, most women reported lifetime use of means-tested

Table 1 Participant Characteristics ($n = 42$)

Variable	Statistic
Age, Mean (SD)	27.6 (5.14)
Race	
African American	4 (9.5%)
Caucasian	34 (81.0%)
Multi-racial	3 (7.1%)
Missing	1 (2.4%)
Marital Status	
Divorced/Separated	5 (11.9%)
Married	5 (11.9%)
Single	31 (73.8%)
Missing	1 (2.4%)
Lifetime Use of Means-tests Programs	
Woman Infants and Children (WIC)	29 (69.0%)
Medicaid	31 (72.1%)
Unemployment	2 (4.8%)
Food Stamps	37 (88.1%)
Cash Assistance	10 (23.8%)
Treatment Location	
Site 1	17 (40.5%)
Site 2	25 (59.5%)

programs. The majority of participants indicated use of food stamps (88%), Medicaid (72%) and WIC (69%).

Pregnancy history

The participants reported a total of 137 pregnancies in the lifetime, of which 24 were ongoing (see Table 2). Subjects reported having custody of slightly less than half ($n = 31$) of the 74 children who had been delivered. Overall 75% of the 137 pregnancies were unintended. The average number of pregnancies was 3.3 per individual, ranging from one to nine.

Sexual history

The majority of participants ($n = 25$, 60%) indicated they had two or fewer sexual partners in the past year (see Table 3). Twenty-one participants (50%) reported having ever traded sex for money, drugs, or food. Nearly 62% ($n = 26$) of participants reported ever having been diagnosed with an STI, with chlamydia ($n = 15$, 36%) as the most frequently occurring.

Contraception decisions and access

Decisions About Contraception Use. Most women reported using birth control to prevent pregnancy ($n = 33$, 79%) and fewer responded that birth control was only used to prevent STIs ($n = 17$, 41%), but 16 (38%) reported they used contraception for both reasons. One participant reported that she used condoms as a contraceptive method because of its protection against both pregnancy and STI:

Table 2 Pregnancy History

Variable	Statistic
Total Pregnancies	137
Pregnancy Outcomes (n = 137)	
Terminated	15 (11.0%)
Miscarried	23 (16.8%)
Delivered	74 (54.0%)
Currently Pregnant	24 (17.5%)
Missing	1 (0.7%)
Pregnancies Per Individual, Mean (Range)	3.3 (1,9)
Custody of Delivered Children (n = 74)	
Has Custody	31 (41.9%)
Does not have Custody	43 (58.1%)
Intended Status of All Pregnancies (n = 137)	
Intended	18 (13.1%)
Unintended	103 (75.2%)
Missing	16 (11.6%)
Intended Status of Current/Recent Pregnancy (n = 42)	
Intended	5 (11.9%)
Unintended	31 (73.8%)
Missing	6 (14.3%)

Table 3 Sexual History

Variable	Statistic
Number of Sexual Partners in Past Year	
1	15 (35.7%)
2	10 (23.8%)
3	2 (4.8%)
4	3 (7.1%)
5	4 (9.5%)
6–10	2 (4.8%)
Over 50	1 (2.4%)
1 don't know	1 (2.4%)
Missing	4 (9.5%)
Ever Traded Sex for:	
Food.	6 (14.3%)
Money	8 (19.0%)
Drugs	10 (23.8%)
Ever Diagnosed with STI	
Yes	26 (61.9%)
Missing	1 (2.4%)
Ever Diagnosed with:	
Chlamydia	15 (35.7%)
Gonorrhea	3 (7.1%)
Hepatitis C	1 (2.4%)
Herpes	5 (11.9%)
HIV	2 (4.8%)
HPV	5 (11.9%)
Syphilis	1 (2.4%)
Trichomoniasis	5 (11.9%)

> "I think that's the safest. From almost, you know, higher chance of preventing a pregnancy and STDs and birth control is just you know getting pregnant but there's always that chance that you can get something."

Condom Use (treatment location 1). Participants from treatment location 1 provided insights into reasons for using male condoms. Partner newness was an important factor, but uptake was low. Fewer than 20% said they would use male condoms with a new ($n = 3$) or different ($n = 3$) partner.

> "I have only been with one guy since I was 19, which is my kid's dad. If it was somebody else, I would. Like I used a condom even when we first met but once we got serious we didn't. So if it was somebody I was seeing casually then yes [a condom would be used]."

Birth control use (treatment location 2). Experience with one's partner also influenced the decision to use birth control among participants at treatment location 2. Just over 21% of participants ($n = 4$, 21.1%) stated that they would not use birth control with a monogamous partner. Two participants (10.5%) reported they would use birth control with a new partner.

Contraception Access. Only one participant reported ever having difficulty obtaining birth control covered by insurance including Medicaid. Many participants ($n = 18$, 43%) reported birth control prescriptions were obtained through an OB/GYN or healthcare provider. Seven participants (17%) indicated obtaining birth control directly from Planned Parenthood or a clinic.

Contraceptive preferences and perceptions

Lifetime use of contraception types are reported in Table 4. The majority of participants had used male condoms (69%) and oral contraceptives (60%). Slightly over 40 % reported using hormonal injections. Seventeen percent indicated ever having used a LARC method, with most indicating use of IUDs (12%).

Participant responses regarding preferred and preferred if free contraceptive types are reported in Table 4. When asked about preferred methods of contraception, Tier 1 and Tier 2 methods were preferred. Specifically, 40% of participants indicated a preference for injections, followed by IUDs (17%). Participants were also asked "If you could receive free birth control, would you use it? What type of free birth control would you use and why?" Approximately 90% of participants stated they would use free birth control. Injections were the most frequently reported method participants would use if freely provided, with 41% of women indicating they would choose this type. Implants, IUDs, and oral contraception were the next most frequently reported preferred types of contraception if freely provided.

Eighteen participants indicated a total of 24 reasons why they would use a specific type of contraception if free. Most of these responses centered around not needing to remember to take the contraception ($n = 10$, 56%), side effects with other types of methods ($n = 5$, 28%), and long-term effectiveness ($n = 4$, 10%). Among those who listed not needing to remember to take the contraception, most preferred injections ($n = 6$), followed by the implant ($n = 3$). Of the five women who were concerned about side effects with other types of methods, three preferred LARC methods. For example, one participant cited concerns about problems with oral contraception as the reason she might consider getting an implant:

> "The pill was [my preferred method]. . .I hear all these horror stories and something messes up. I wasn't thinking about getting the thing in my arm. Now maybe I would get the thing in my arm."

Table 4 Contraceptive Methods: Typically Used, Preferred, and Preferred if Freely Provided

		Lifetime Use n (%)	Preferred Method[a] n (%)	Preferred Method if Freely Provided[a] n
Contraceptive Method[b]		([a]42)	($n = 35$)	(%) ($n = 37$)
None				
	None	1 (2.4%)	–	1 (2.7%)
Tier 1 (Very Effective)				
	IUD	5 (11.9%)	6 (17.1%)	6 (16.2%)
	Implant	2 (4.8%)	1 (2.9%)	7 (18.9%)
	Tubal Ligation	–	1 (2.9%)	1 (2.7%)
Tier 2 (Effective)				
	Oral Contraception	25 (59.5%)	5 (14.3%)	6 (16.2%)
	Nuvaring	3 (7.1%)	–	1 (2.7%)
	Injection	17 (40.5%)	14 (40.0%)	15 (40.5%)
	Hormonal Patch	5 (11.9%)	–	–
Tier 3 (Moderately Effective)				
	Male Condom	29 (69.0%)	1 (2.9%)	1 (2.7%)
	Diaphragm	1 (2.4%)		
Tier 4 Less Effective				
	Spermicide	2 (4.8%)	1 (2.9%)	–
Other				
	Unsure	–	–	2 (4.5%)
	Plan B	5 (11.9%)	1 (2.9%)	–
Missing		–	7 (20.0%)	4 (11.0%)

[a]Percentages may total greater than 100% as some participants provided more than preferred or preferred if freely available contraception method
[b]Tier rating based on World Health Organization's (WHO) four-tiered rating of contraceptive effectiveness

Four participants indicated they preferred their reported choice due to the method's long-term effectiveness. The methods preferred by these women were LARC. For example, one woman reported her preference for an implant due to its long-term effectiveness. This participant also indicated concerns about problems as a reason for her preference of the implant over the IUD:

> "Just cause it lasts. Well, I know the IUD lasts for 5 years and the implant lasts for 3, but I've heard, like I know a few people that have a lot of problems with the IUD and I haven't heard of a lot of issues with the implant."

Participants at treatment location 2 were also asked about perceived effectiveness of contraceptive methods; participants indicated the percentage or number of women out of 100 who would get pregnant in a year using different methods (Table 5). Tubal ligation, followed by injections and implants were perceived to be the most effective methods with 68%, 40% and 36% of participants, respectively, indicating that less than one woman out of 100 would get pregnant after the procedure. Participants were the least certain about diaphragms, spermicides, the ring, and the patch with regards to the percentage of women who would get pregnant in a year using those methods.

Participants at location 2 also reported how much they were bothered by the different the dangers/side effects of the different contraceptive methods (Table 6). The most common response was "I don't know" for IUDs, implants, vaginal rings and diaphragms. For tubal ligation, oral contraception, injection, hormonal patch, condom, family planning, and spermicide the most frequent response was "Not at all" or "A little".

Discussion

The current research confirms and expands upon prior work examining contraception decisions, preferences and perceptions with a sample of current or recently pregnant in-treatment women in the United States who use opioids.

Table 5 Frequency of Responses to the Question "What Percentage (or number of women out of 100) do you think would get pregnant in a year using the following methods?" ($n = 25$)

	< 1%	1–5%	6–10%	> 10%	Don't Know
Contraceptive Method[a]	n (%)	n (%)	n (%)	n (%)	n (%)
Tier 1 (Very Effective)					
IUD	5 (20.0%)	8 (32.0%)	5 (20.0%)	1 (4.0%)	6 (24.0%)
Implant	8 (36.0%)	4 (16.0%)	4 (16.0%)	–	9 (36.0%)
Tubal Ligation	17 (68.0%)	5 (20.0%)		1 (4.0%)	2 (8.0%)
Tier 2 (Effective)					
Oral Contraception	1 (4.0%)	7 (28.0%)	10(40.0%)	4 (16.0%)	3 (12.0%)
Vaginal Ring	3 (12.0%)	6 (24.0%)	5 (20.0%)	–	11 (44.0%)
Injection	10 (40.0%)	7 (28.0%)	3 (12.0%)	–	5 (20.0%)
Hormonal Patch	1 (4.0%)	10 (40.0%)	1 (4.0%)	3 (12.0%)	10 (40.0%)
Tier 3 (Moderately Effective)					
Condom (male or female)	–	7 (28.0%)	10 (40.0%)	7 (28.0%)	1 (4.0%)
Diaphragm	2 (8.0%)	6 (24.0%)	2 (8.0%)	1 (4.0%)	14 (56.0%)
Tier 4 Less Effective					
Spermicide	4 (16.0%)	5 (20.0%)	3 (12.0%)	1 (4.0%)	12 (48.0%)
None					
No method	1 (4.0%)	1 (4.0%)	–	22 (88.0%)	1 (4.0%)

[a]Tier rating based on World Health Organization's (WHO) 4 tiered rating of contraceptive effectiveness

Table 6 Frequency of Responses for the Question "How bothered are you or would you be by the dangers or side effects" ($n = 25$)

	"Not at all" & "A Little"	"A lot" & "Extremely"	"I Don't Know"
Contraceptive Method[a]	n (%)	n (%)	n (%)
Tier 1 (Very Effective)			
IUD	10 (40.0%)	3 (12.0%)	12 (48.0%)
Implant	9 (36.0%)	4 (16.0%)	12 (48.0%)
Tubal Ligation	13 (52.0%)	6 (24.0%)	6 (24.0%)
Tier 2 (Effective)			
Oral Contraception	17 (68.0%)	1 (4.0%)	7 (28.0%)
Vaginal Ring	10 (40.0%)	3 (12.0%)	12 (48.0%)
Injection	18 (72.0%)	2 (8.0%)	5 (20.0%)
Hormonal Patch	13 (52.0%)	1 (4.0%)	11 (44.0%)
Tier 3 (Moderately Effective)			
Condom (male or female)	20 (80.0%)	2 (8.0%)	3 (12.0%)
Diaphragm	11 (44.0%)	1 (4.0%)	13 (52.0%)
Tier 4 Less Effective			
Spermicide	13 (52.0%)	1 (4.0%)	11 (44.0%)

[a]Tier rating based on World Health Organization's (WHO) 4 tiered rating of contraceptive effectiveness

Decisions to use contraception

Nearly all our participants reported easy access to birth control. Most participants indicated past or present use of Medicaid, which has historically covered family planning services and also mandates recipients be entitled to choose a method of contraception [29]. However, despite reporting easy contraception access, similar to other drug using populations [1], our sample had an unintended pregnancy rate of 75%. Further, only five of the most recent pregnancies were intended, suggesting low contraception use rates and/or use of less effective means of contraception. Correspondingly, Terplan et al. [30] reported that contraceptive use among opioid and other drug-using women ranged from 6% to 74% with the median rate of 55%.

Comparable to research conducted by Olsen et al. [27], participants provided a diversity of situations in which they would or would not use contraception. However, familiarity with one's current partner was the most cited reason for why a participant would or would not use contraception with nearly a third of participants reporting they would not use contraception with a monogamous partner. Conversely, nearly 30% of participants stated they would use contraception if with someone they did not know very well or with someone other than their monogamous partner. Likewise, prior research has found that, among female teenagers who are intravenous drug users, being engaged in a longer-term sexual relationship significantly decreased the likelihood of using contraception [31].

Contraception method preferences and perceptions

In our sample, LARC and injections shared comparable perceived benefits, yet injections were much more highly preferred. The opioid-using women in our study demonstrate similar perceptions as non-drug-using women in the United States about LARC contraception methods. This includes concerns and lack of knowledge about side effects, overestimation of efficacy of all forms of Tier 2 and Tier 3 methods, and overreliance on verbal testimonies of other women's experiences with LARC methods [32–34]. Substance abusing women have been demonstrated to hold additional perceptions that may impact LARC preferences including: misperception of fertility; underestimation of the benefits of LARC; overestimation of the costs and risks associated with LARC; intimate partner violence; fear of losing custody of children; and denial or embarrassment of their substance use [21–23]. Understanding the factors that may make women hesitant about LARC methods relative to injections is important because injections have not been demonstrated to have high rates of use among drug-using women [25] and at least one study has demonstrated reduced injection adherence among an opioid using sample [12]. Sinha et al. reported that of 14 postpartum opioid-using women who received injectable contraception post pregnancy, none continued with injections beyond their initial administration. However, of the 20 women who received implants, 95% continued with this method of contraception [12].

Educational programs for women that accurately explain the side effects, effectiveness and safety associated with Tier 1 LARC products may be an effective way to help opioid-using women decide which product is correct for them and thus increase adherence and decrease unwanted pregnancies. Similar projects have been found to be effective in informing women about their contraceptive decisions [35, 36].

Contraceptive CHOICE provided contraception counseling to over 9200 women and teenagers recruited from abortion clinics in St. Louis, Missouri [37]. Participants were educated about all reversible contraception choices with the benefits of long-acting reversible contraception highlighted. Participants selected the freely provided contraceptive method of their choice. Relative to national levels, the researchers found significantly lower rates of teenage pregnancy and abortions within their cohort. Another study that provided patient education, The Family Planning Initiative, provided approximately three hours of contraception education to 681 pregnant or recently post-partum substance abusing women [36]. Participants were offered freely available contraception of their choice. Participants chose LARC, particularly implants, at slightly relatively higher levels (14% among postpartum women) in comparison to general public utilization [38]. These findings hold promising implications for the benefits of patient education on LARC methods; however, further research is needed to warrant the effectiveness of specific approaches to patient education, including how providers interact with patients when helping them choose a method of contraception [39, 40].

Limitations and future research

There are several limitations to the current study that merit discussion. First, generalizability is limited due to our relatively small and geographically limited sample. Second, several limitations are related to measurement methods. Because the measures were self-report, the possibility exists for inaccurate or biased recall and/or socially desirable responses. Further, some questions differed between treatment locations preventing the compilation of data across both sites. Additionally, our study would have benefited from greater precision when assessing perceptions of effectiveness and the dangers or side effects of different contraception methods. For example, other research has defined efficacy as 100 minus the "method's first year failure rate in typical use". Correspondingly, when estimating efficacy, participants are asked to indicate which of the following choices represent the effectiveness for each method: 99, 95, 91, 83, and 70% [33]. It would have been helpful if our study had qualified efficacy as applying to either perfect or typical use and also used similar response options.

Third, in addition to limited generalizability and measurement weaknesses, collection of additional relevant data would have assisted with the interpretation of results. While we focused on decision making, preferences and perceptions, assessing which women were currently sexually active, planning on a future pregnancy, and/or not currently using contraception would have been useful. Further, despite our finding that 79% of the women used contraception to prevent pregnancy, our survey did not ask the women what priority they assigned to contraception—either its initiation or continuation of use. Consequently, we do not know whether unintended pregnancy was a sufficiently negative event to motivate the use of contraception among our sample. Recent findings indicate that many women do not think a woman should plan for pregnancy [41], and this would be important to assess among opioid-using women. Additionally, while we addressed lifetime utilization of Medicaid, it would have been informative to measure participants' access to Medicaid during pregnancy-only versus time periods outside of pregnancy. Lastly, women in this study stated that they would use free contraception if it were available. However, this study does not assess actual uptake of specific modes of contraception under those circumstances.

Despite limitations, this study provides additional insight into the contraception decision-making, perceptions and preferences of pregnant and recently pregnant opioid-using women, a complex and understudied population, particularly in the United States. Future research that operationalizes key concepts, such as conditions under which contraception is used, as well as inquires about the acceptability of specific contraceptive methods, is warranted among a larger sample of opioid-dependent women. For example, the current research was conducted in a treatment facility that included both residential and non-residential treatment services. It would be important to understand how contraception choices are impacted by stage of recovery and setting.

Additionally, it is necessary to investigate how or whether healthcare providers are presenting and discussing contraception options with this population. For example, to what extent are the safety and effectiveness of LARC methods such as IUDs and implants being discussed with patients and misconceptions remedied? Likewise, given the high rates of STIs in drug using populations [42, 43], providers may be focused on promoting condom use as a means to prevent STIs, despite only moderate effectiveness in preventing pregnancy.

Conclusion

Nearly all participants stated they would utilize contraception if freely available, yet high rates of unintended pregnancy were measured in our study population. However, despite participant reported ease of access to contraceptives, and participants reported perceived benefits of LARC, very few had ever used these methods. This indicates the need to address potential patient-level barriers, such as LARC misperceptions, through research on the impact of patient education for both opioid-using and non-opioid using women. Further, we must continue to listen to the voices of women, whose feedback in recent literature has consistently stressed the importance of education on effective methods of contraception and education on the risks and benefits associated with them.

Abbreviations

IUD: Intrauterine Device; LARC: Long-Acting Reversible Contraception; NAS: Neonatal Abstinence Syndrome; STI: Sexually Transmitted Infections

Acknowledgments

We wish to thank the participants who shared their stories with us for this research. We also wish to thank the treatment centers and staff for their assistance with this project.

Authors' contributions

RF conducted the analysis and drafted the manuscript. BL helped draft the manuscript. LF helped draft the manuscript. KH helped revise and draft the manuscript. JK assisted in data collection and participated in manuscript drafting. DK conceived of the study and participated in drafting the manuscript. All authors read and approved the final manuscript.

Author details

[1]Department of Family and Community Medicine, Northeast Ohio Medical University, 4209 St. Rt. 44, PO Box 95, Rootstown, OH 44272, USA. [2]College of Public Health, Department of Health Policy and Management, Kent State University, 750 Hilltop Drive, 322 Lowry Hall, P.O. Box 5190, Kent, OH 44242, USA. [3]Old Brooklyn Community Development Corporation, Cleveland, OH, USA.

References

1. Heil SH, Jones HE, Arria A, Kaltenbach K, Coyle M, Fischer G, et al. Unintended pregnancy in opioid-abusing women. J Subst Abus Treat. 2011;40:199–202.
2. Black KI, Haber PS, Lintzeris N. Offering incentives to drug-using women to take up contraception: the ethical and clinical issues. Addiction. 2012:1361–2.
3. Forray A. Substance use during pregnancy. F1000 Res. 2016;5:1–9. Available from: https://www.ncbi.nlm.nih.gov/pmc/articles/PMC4870985/.
4. Vucinovic M, Roje D, Vucinovic Z, Capkun V, Bucat M, Banovic I. Maternal and neonatal effects of substance abuse during pregnancy: our ten-year experience. Yonsei Med J. 2008;49:705–13. Available from: http://www.pubmedcentral.nih.gov/articlerender.fcgi?artid=2615365&tool=pmcentrez&rendertype=abstract.
5. Ko JY, Patrick SW, Tong VT, Patel R, Lind JN, Barfield WD. Incidence of Neonatal Abstinence Syndrome — 28 States, 1999–2013. MMWR Morb Mortal Wkly Rep. 2016;65:799–802. Available from: http://www.cdc.gov/mmwr/volumes/65/wr/mm6531a2.htm.
6. Jansson LM, Velez M, Harrow C. The opioid exposed newborn: assessment and pharmacologic management. J Opioid Manag. 2009;5:47–55.
7. Ross EJ, Graham DL, Money KM, Stanwood GD. Developmental consequences of fetal exposure to drugs: what we know and what we still must learn. Neuropsychopharmacology. 2015;40:61–87. Available from: https://www.nature.com/articles/npp2014147.
8. Cleland J, Ali MM. Reproductive consequences of contraceptive failure in 19 developing countries. Obstet Gynecol. 2004;104:314–20.
9. Vaughan B, Trussell J, Kost K, Singh S, Jones R. Discontinuation and resumption of contraceptive use: results from the 2002 National Survey of Family Growth. Contraception. 2008;78:271–83. Available from: https://www.ncbi.nlm.nih.gov/pmc/articles/PMC2800035/.
10. Trussell J. Contraceptive failure in the United States. Contraception. 2011; 85(3):397–404. Available from: https://www.ncbi.nlm.nih.gov/pmc/articles/PMC3638209/.
11. Curtis KM, Tepper NK, Jatlaoui TC, Berry-Bibee E, Horton LG, Zapata LB, et al. U.S. Medical Eligibility Criteria for Contraceptive Use, 2016. In: MMWR. Recomm. Reports; 2016. Available from: http://www.cdc.gov/mmwr/volumes/65/rr/rr6503a1.htm.
12. Sinha C, Guthrie KA, Lindow SW. A survey of postnatal contraception in opiate-using women. J Fam Plann Reprod Health Care. 2007;33:31–4.
13. Freeman S, Shulman LP. Considerations for the use of progestin-only contraceptives. J Am an Acad Nurse Pract. 2010;22:81–91.
14. Finer LB, Henshaw K. Disparities in Rates of Unintended Pregnancy In the United States , 1994 and 2001. Perspect Sex Reprod Health. 2006;38:90–6.
15. CCP and WHO. World Health Organization (WHO) Family Planning: A Global Handbook for Providers. Baltimore, MD and Geneva: World Health Organization Department of Reproductive Health and Research (WHO/RHR) and Johns Hopkins Bloomberg School of Public Health/ Center for Communication Programs (CCP), INFO Project; 2007.
16. Diedrich J, Zhao Q, Madden T, Secura G, Piepert J. Three-year Continuation of Reversible Contraception. Am J Obstet Gynecol. 2015;213:662.e1–8.
17. Daniels K, Daugherty J, Jones J, Mosher W. Current Contraceptive Use and Variation by Selected Characteristics Among Women Aged 15-44: United States, 2011-2013. Natl Health Stat Report. 2015;1:–14. Available from: https://www.cdc.gov/nchs/data/nhsr/nhsr086.pdf.
18. Stoddard A, McNicholas C, Peipart J. Efficacy and Safety of Long-Acting Reversible Contraception. Drugs. 2011;71:969–80.
19. Finer LB, Zolna MR. Declines in Unintended Pregnancy in the United States, 2008-2011. N Engl J Med. 2016;374:843–52. Available from: https://www.ncbi.nlm.nih.gov/pmc/articles/PMC4861155/.
20. Shoupe D. LARC methods: entering a new age of contraception and reproductive health. Contracept Reprod Med. 2016;2:4. Available from: https://contraceptionmedicine.biomedcentral.com/articles/10.1186/s40834-016-0011-8.
21. Black K, Day C. Improving Access to Long-Acting Contraceptive Methods and Reducing Unplanned Pregnancy Among Women with Substance Use Disorders. Subst Abus Res Treat. 2016;10:27–33. Available from: http://www.ncbi.nlm.nih.gov/pmc/articles/PMC4869602/.

22. Matusiewicz AK, Melbostad HS, Heil SH. Barriers to long-acting reversible contraceptive use among opioid-maintained women. Drug Alcohol Depend. 2017;171:e133.
23. Griffith G, Kumaraswami T, Chrysanthopoulou SA, Mattocks KM, Clark RE. Prescription contraception use and adherence by women with substance use disorders. Addiction. 2017;112:1638–46.
24. Schwartz SR, Baral S. Fertility-related research needs among women at the margins. Reprod Health Matters. 2015;23:30–46.
25. Cornford CS, Close HJ, Bray R, Beere D, Mason JM. Contraceptive use and pregnancy outcomes among opioid drug-using women: A retrospective cohort study. PLoS One. 2015;10(3): e0116231. Available from: https://doi.org/10.1371/journal.pone.0116231.
26. Harding C, Ritchie J. Contraceptive practice of women with opiate addiction in a rural centre. Aust J Rural Health. 2003;11:2–6.
27. Olsen A, Banwell C, Madden A. Contraception, punishment and women who use drugs. BMC Womens Health. 2014;14:5.
28. Jessup MA, Brindis CD. Issues in reproductive health and empowerment in perinatal women with substance use disorders. J Addict Nurs. 2005;16:97–105.
29. Department of Health and Human Services Centers for Medicare & Medicaid Services. Frequently Asked Questions (FAQs) Medicaid Family Planning Services and Supplies. 2017 [cited 2017 Oct 26]. Available from: https://www.medicaid.gov/federal-policy-guidance/downloads/faq11117.pdf
30. Terplan M, Hand DJ, Hutchinson M, Salisbury-Afshar E, Heil SH. Contraceptive use and method choice among women with opioid and other substance use disorders: A systematic review. Prev Med. 2015;80:23–31.
31. Harvey M, Bird S, Johnson De Rosa C, Montgomery S, Rohrbach L. Sexual Decision Making and Safer Sex Behavior Among Young Female Injection Drug Users and Female Partners of IDUs. J Sex Res. 2003;40:50–60.
32. Madden T, Secura G, Nease R, Politi M, Piepert J. The Role of Contraceptive Attributes in Women's Contraceptive Decision Making. Am J Obstet Gynecol. 2015;213:46.e1–6.
33. Kakaiya R, Lopez LL, Nelson AL. Women's perceptions of contraceptive efficacy and safety. Contracept Reprod Med. 2017;2:19. Available from: http://contraceptionmedicine.biomedcentral.com/articles/10.1186/s40834-017-0046-5
34. Okpo E, Allerton L, Brechin S. "But you can"t reverse a hysterectomy!' Perceptions of long acting reversible contraception (LARC) among young women aged 16-24 years: A qualitative study. Public Health. 2014;128:934–9.
35. Secura GM, Allsworth JE, Madden T, Mullersman JL, Peipert JF. The Contraceptive CHOICE Project: Reducing barriers to long-acting reversible contraception. Am J Obstet Gynecol. 2010;203
36. Elko A, Jansson M. L. Contraception in Drug-Dependent Women: A Novel Approach. Soc Work Ment Health. 2011;9:445–55.
37. Peipert JF, Madden T, Allsworth JE, Secura GM. Preventing Unintended Pregnancies by Providing No-Cost Contraception. Obstet Gynecol. 2012;120:1. Available from: http://www.pubmedcentral.nih.gov/articlerender.fcgi?artid=4000282&tool=pmcentrez&rendertype=abstract.
38. Stern LF, Simons HR, Kohn JE, Debevec EJ, Morfesis JM, Patel AA. Differences in contraceptive use between family planning providers and the U.S. population: Results of a nationwide survey. Contraception. 2015;91:464–9. Available from:. https://doi.org/10.1016/j.contraception.2015.02.005.
39. Hathaway M, Torres L, Vollett-Krech J, Wohltjen H. Increasing LARC Utilization : Any Woman, Any Place. Any Time Clin Obstet Gynecol. 2014;57:718–30.
40. Jacobs Institute of Women's Health. Current Research and Policy on Long-Acting Reversible Contraception (LARC): Key Points for Policymakers. 2016.
41. Mazza D, Chapman A. Improving the uptake of preconception care and periconceptional folate supplementation : what do women think ? BMC Public Health. 2010;10:786. Available from: http://www.biomedcentral.com/1471-2458/10/786.
42. Mathers BM, Degenhardt L, Phillips B, Wiessing L, Hickman M, Strathdee SA, et al. Global epidemiology of injecting drug use and HIV among people who inject drugs: a systematic review. Lancet. 2008;372:1733–45.
43. Jones A, Striley C, Cottler L. Prescription opioid use, illicit drug use, and sexually transmitted infections among participants from a community engagement program in North Central Florida. J Subst Use. 2016;22:90–5.

2

Subfascial-located contraceptive devices requiring surgical removal

Justin E. Hellwinkel[1*], Matthew W. Konigsberg[1], Johana Oviedo[2], Paula M. Castaño[3] and R. Kumar Kadiyala[1]

Abstract

Background: Subdermal etonogestrel implants are highly effective contraceptive methods. Despite standardization of insertion technique by the manufacturer, some implants are inadvertently placed too deeply within or below the plane of the biceps brachii fascia. Placement of these implants in a deep tissue plane results in more difficult removal, which is not always possible in the office setting. In rare cases, surgical removal by an upper extremity surgeon is warranted.

Case presentation: Here we present 6 cases of etonogestrel implants located in a subfascial plane requiring removal by an upper extremity surgeon. Implants were all localized with plain radiography and ultrasound prior to surgical removal. All cases had implants located in the subfascial plane and one was identified intramuscularly. The average age was 28 years (19–33) and BMI was 24.0 kg/m^2 (19.1–36.5), with the most common reason for removal being irregular bleeding. The majority of cases (5/6) were performed under monitored anesthesia care with local anesthetic and one case utilized regional anesthesia. All implants were surgically removed without complication.

Conclusions: Insertion of etonogestrel contraceptive implants deep to the biceps brachii fascia is a rare, but dangerous complication. Removal of these implants is not always successful in the office setting and referral to an upper extremity surgeon is necessary to avoid damage to delicate neurovascular structures for safe removal.

Keywords: Contraceptive implant removal, Etonogestrel complication, Subdermal etonogestrel, Subfascial implant removal

Background

Subdermal etonogestrel implants are highly effective contraceptive methods [1]. The manufacturer recommends subdermal placement of the implant overlying the triceps muscle in the medial upper arm using a preloaded insertion implant [2]. All healthcare practitioners providing insertions are trained in proper placement techniques, including immediate palpation to confirm subdermal location, and in-office removal techniques. Deep placement can make removal particularly challenging.

* Correspondence: jh4034@cumc.columbia.edu
[1]Department of Orthopedics, Columbia University Irving Medical Center, 622 W 168th St PH 11 – Center, NY 10032 New York, USA

Our institution is a referral center for complex implant removals. After review of plain radiographs (XR) to confirm upper-arm location of non-palpable implants, evaluation and in-office high-frequency ultrasonography (US), we refer patients with deeply-located implants not amenable to in-office removal to a single upper extremity orthopaedic surgeon for operative removal.

Case Series

After IRB approval, we identified 6 cases of etonogestrel implants referred for surgical removal from 2018 to 2020 (Table 1). All patients had Nexplanon® implants placed within the preceding three years. The average age was 28 years (19–33) and BMI was 24.0 kg/m^2 (19.1–36.5). The most common reason for removal was

Table 1 Characteristics of 6 patients undergoing removal of subfascial etonogestrel contraceptive implant by orthopaedic surgeons, including the length of time each patient had their implants, any attempts at in-office removal and surgical duration. One patient with prior implant transitioned to an alternative form of contraception before receiving her second implant and the other patient had her implant removed at the time of replacement of the most recent one. (BMI: Body mass index reported in kilogram/meters^2; MAC: Monitored Anesthesia Care)

AGE	BMI	Subfascial/ Intramuscular	Duration (years)	First implant or prior?	Removal Attempts	Anesthesia	Procedure Duration (minutes)
31	19.1	Subfascial	2.96	First	Once	MAC/local	15
26	22.0	Subfascial	2.68	First	None	MAC/local	12
28	24.6	Subfascial	0.76	One prior (ipsilateral), removed in office	None	MAC/local	18
31	20.5	Subfascial	2.88	First	Once	MAC/local	11
33	36.5	Subfascial	1.02	First	None	Regional	10
19	21.5	Intramuscular	0.92	One prior (ipsilateral), removed in office	None	MAC/local	20
28	24.0						14.3 average

irregular bleeding. We localized implants with XR (Fig. 1 a) and in-office high-frequency US to confirm deep location prior to referral to orthopaedic surgeon. Each implant was identified through physical examination by a qualified provider through palpation, XR and US guidance to determine the location within the soft tissue. For removal, a small incision and dissection clamp were utilized in attempt to retrieve the implants. Reasons for failure of in-office removal included close proximity to neurovascular structures, excessive pain with palpation concerning for neurologic irritation, and failure to adequately visualize the implants. Surgeons obtained informed consent after discussing the risks of medial upper arm exploration. Surgeons positioned patients supine with an arm table to allow adequate visualization of the upper extremity. Surgeons utilized conscious sedation and local anesthesia for all cases except one, where the patient preferred regional anesthesia. Intraoperative fluoroscopic guidance aided localization of the implant by its relative radiodensity within the soft tissue. Surgeons made a 2 to 7 centimeter incision longitudinally over the implant placement scar (Fig. 1b). Careful dissection was carried down through planes to expose the distal end of the implant. Implants were all located deep to the biceps brachii fascia or within the muscle belly itself (Fig. 1 c, d). The fascia and overlying soft tissue were then closed using suture. No intraoperative or postoperative complications occurred. The average procedure time from skin incision to closure was 14.3 min (Table 1).

Discussion/conclusion

This series presents 6 cases of etonogestrel implants located in a subfascial location requiring complex surgical removal by an upper extremity orthopaedic surgeon. Other series have identified subfascial location of contraceptive implants; very few described surgical extraction [3–5]. In our series, none of the implants were able to be retrieved in the office, despite subfascial exploration. Although not noted in this series, removal from subfascial planes has the potential for significant morbidity from larger incisions, anesthetic risk, and damage to nearby neurovascular structures [6, 7]. Rare cases describe migration of implants to the axilla and pulmonary vasculature, requiring more invasive surgical interventions [8–12].

The rarity of this condition precludes identification of specific risk factors for deep location. We noted no trends in prior implant use or removal attempts but 5 of 6 patients had normal BMI. Researchers theorize that low BMI may confer risk due to smaller distance between tissue planes in the upper arm [3]. Whether subfascial location alters contraceptive efficacy, side effects (e.g., bleeding profile) or duration of use warrants future study.

Incorrect placement of etonogestrel implants occurs in 12.6 per 1000 cases [13]. Alternate insertion sites in the skin overlying the scapula have been described [14]. The Food and Drug Administration requires a training session before providers can order implants; this training allows for as many placement and removal attempts as desired on a simulation arm. It is impossible to quantify whether providers do not complete training or are informally trained and how closely training mimics placement in a real arm. Adherence to recommendations to elevate the skin and perform placement at eye level may help avoid deep placement. All certified implant providers underwent mandatory retraining by June 1, 2019, to ensure placement in the ideal site 8–10 cm proximal to medial epicondyle and 3–5 cm posterior to the sulcus to avoid possible neurovascular injury [15]. All of the

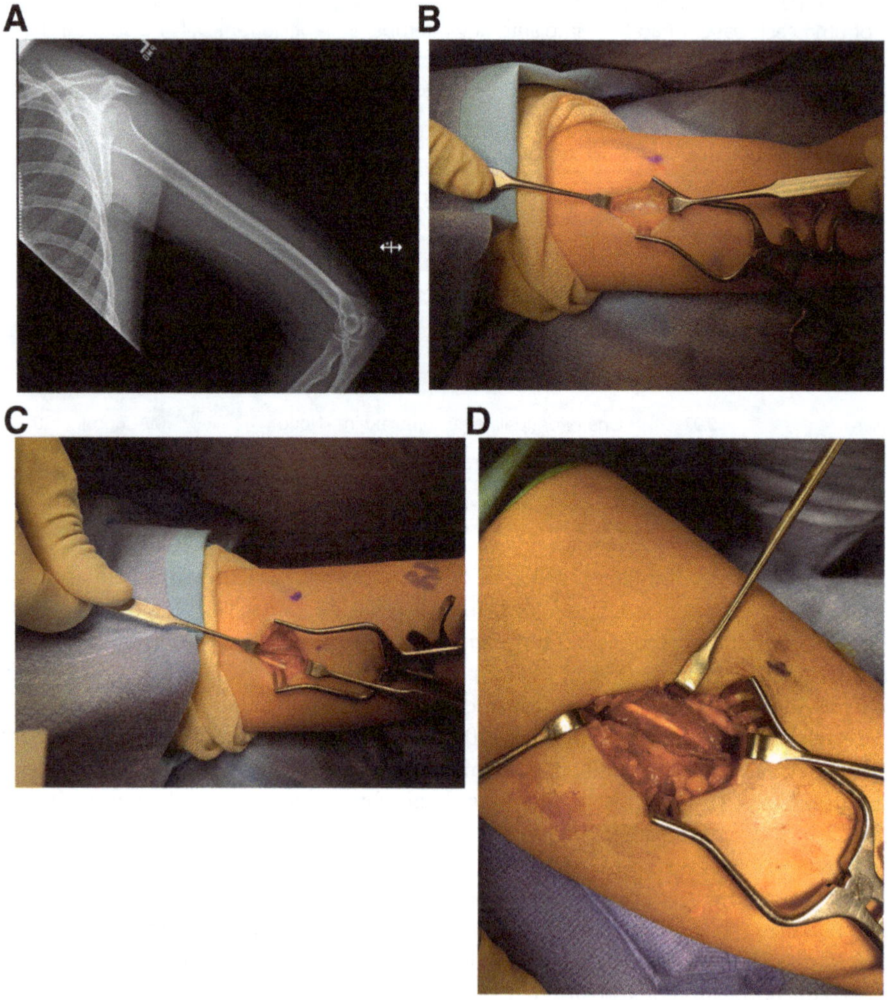

Fig. 1 Radiographic identification of implanted contraceptive implant prior to incision in operating room (**a**). Incision and blunt dissection carried down to the fascial layer of the biceps brachii, which must be incised to retrieve the implant (**b**). Etonogestrel implant located deep to the biceps brachii fascia (**c**). Etonogestrel implant located within the muscle belly of the biceps brachii, surrounded by muscle fibers (**d**)

implants reported in this series were placed prior to this change in placement recommendation; future series should explore whether these new guidelines have minimized complications in placement.

Even with perfect technique, it is possible to insert the implant too deeply and the clinician or patient may not know until implant removal [9]. Informed consent at time of placement should include discussion of these rare complications. Initial attempt to remove the implant in the office setting is most optimized with plain radiography and ultrasound guidance, along with manual palpation to identify the location of the implant. Local anesthesia with lidocaine with epinephrine is typically adequate for this procedure, but providers may select a longer acting form of anesthesia if needed. If the implant is found to be within close proximity to neurovascular structures or deep within the soft tissue, there is considerable risk for injury to delicate structures due to poor visualization. These include superficial and deep sensory nerves, motor branches to muscles of the forearm and delicate vascular structures that can be difficult to visualize and control in a minimally invasive setting. Complex in-office removal and concern for neurovascular injury or inability to adequately localize the implant benefit from co-management with an upper extremity surgeon to safely remove intra-/subfascial implants.

Abbreviations

XR: X-ray; US: Ultrasound; BMI: Body Mass Index

Acknowledgements

Not applicable.

Authors' contributions

JEH contributed to data gathering, figure generation and manuscript preparation; MWK contributed to data analysis and manuscript preparation; JO contributed to manuscript preparation and editing; PMC contributed in care for each patient in the office prior to referral to the surgeon; RKK was the primary surgeon responsible for safe removal of the contraceptive

Background

Abortion is intentional or unintentional termination of pregnancy [1] Worldwide about 205 million female become pregnant annually, and an estimated 40–50 million women undergo abortions, 20 million of which are considered unsafe and of all unsafe abortions 95% take place in developing countries From this 43% occurred in Africa and this accounts for an estimated 14% of maternal death in the region [2]. In most African countries abortion has been illegal and associated with unsafe abortion and high maternal morbidity and mortality rate [3]. In developed countries the recent policy reforms towards abortion law have reduced the problem associated with illegal and usafe abortion significantly [4]. Some Sub-Saharan African countries including Ethiopia have formulated abortion laws that allow safe abortion [5]. This law states that abortion can be performed legally based on woman's request in cases of rape or incest, if the woman has physical or mental disabilities, if there is serious fetal deformity and observed needed to preserve the woman's life or health, or if the pregnant girl is physically or mentally unprepared for childbearing because of her age [6]. Lack of awareness of this abortion law forces female youths to seek unsafe abortion in a secret place [7]. Research in several countries found that public knowledge about abortion law is often minimal [8–10]. The Ethiopian case is not different from other countries and that is why this study was conducted to assess the knowledge of regular female student on the abortion law and factors affecting. Abortion laws have a spectrum of restrictiveness. Evidence indicates that there is an association between unsafe abortion and restrictive abortion laws. The median rate of unsafe abortions in the 82 countries with the most restrictive abortion laws is up to 23 of 1000 women compared with 2 of 1000 in nations that allow abortions [11]. The impact of abortion law on women's health and survival is high and abortion related deaths are more frequent in countries with more restrictive abortion laws [12].

The same correlation appears when a given country tightens or relaxes its abortion law, for example in Romania where abortion was available upon request until 1966; the abortion mortality ratio was 20 per 100,000 live births in 1960. But when new legal restrictions were imposed in 1966, and by 1989 the ratio reached 148 deaths per 100,000 live births. The restrictions were reversed in 1989, and within a year the ratio dropped to 68 of 100,000 live births; by 2002 it was as low as 9 deaths per 100,000 births [13]. Similarly, in South Africa, after abortion became legal and avail available on request in 1997, abortion related infection decreased by 52%, and the abortion mortality ratio from 1998 to 2001 dropped by 91% from its 1994 level [14]..

One of the primary methods for preventing unsafe abortion is providing less restrictive abortion laws particularly in developing nations, where most unsafe abortions (97%) occur. Less restrictive abortion laws do not appear to entail more abortions overall. Even where these laws were availed by the government to its people, women s need to be educated and a warred about the availability of legal and safe abortion, and women need better access to safe abortion and post abortion services. Otherwise, women in a great need of it, will continue to risk their lives by undergoing unsafe abortions [13]. In Ethiopia there is no research findings that showed change came as a result of abortion law implementation. Therefore this study was to assess knowledge on abortion law and associated factors among female regular undergraduate students of Ambo University.

Methodology

Study area and period

The institutional based cross sectional study was conducted in Ambo University which is located 114 km West of Addis Ababa the capital city of Ethiopian from March, 28-May, 18, 2018. Ambo University has 9 colleges/institutes, 38 academic departments and a total of 15,433 regular students of which 9675 were males and the rest 5758 were females [12]. A sample size of 795 was calculated by a single proportion formula, taking $P = 50\%$, 95% confidence interval, $\alpha = 0.05$ margin of error, d = 5% degree of precision, design effect of 2 and considering 10% non- response rate Stratified multistage sampling was implemented. In the first step the university stratified based on campus i'e main, technology and Guder campus. Then the campuses were stratified into colleges, departments and year of study These campus were further stratified in to as, colleges, departments and year of study and the study participants were calculated from each stratum using probability proportional to their size. Finally the study participants were selected using systematic random sampling technique using the student identification number as sampling frame.

The data were collected using structured questionnaire adapted from previous similar literature. The questionnaire includes socio-demographic and economic characteristics, questions that measure respondent's knowledge on abortion law, source of acquiring information, and exposure of abortion and contraceptive related factors of the respondents. The question part that used to measure the respondent's knowledge of abortion has skip pattern i'e if they answered 'No'. The data entry was done with Epi Data version 3.1 and transported to Statistical package for social sciences (SPSS) version 21. Both descriptive statistics and logistic regression analysis were done. To have more candidate variables for multivariate logistic regression analysis a p-value of < 0.25 were considered as cut of point on bivariate logistic regression analysis. The abortion law knowledge part of the questionnaire contains eight items on yes or no score to which the respondents gave their response. The study participants level of knowledge on abortion law then measured using these eight abortion knowledge questions and respondents who score above or equal to the mean abortion knowledge was considered as having good knowledge and those who score less than the mean score was classified as poor knowledge for abortion law. Ethical approval to conduct the study was obtained from Ambo University, College of Medical and health sciences research and ethical review committee. The data was also collected after full informed verbal consent is obtained from the study participants.

Result

All of the 795 undergraduate female students' participated in the survey making the response rate of 100%. Majority of the respondents were in the age of between 18 and 24 with the mean ages of 21. About 62.5% of respondents' age was above mean age while 37.4% were below mean age. About 47% of the study participants were protestant Christian followed by Orthodox (33.8%), Majority (86.4%) were single in marital status and 44.7% of them came from the rural areas of the country. Regarding current living arrangement, almost all respondents (91.4%) were living in campus and only 8.6% live out of the campus. The study participants distribution by year of study indicated that (29.5%) of them were first year, 61 30.8.0% second year, 25.0% third year, 11.1% fourth year, and 3.5% fifth year (Table 1).

Knowledge on abortion law

Regarding abortion law, 58.9% of the study participants hear about the existence of abortion legislation in Ethiopia of which the majority (55%) heard from clubs in school/University and followed by relatives / someone who had an abortion (48.1%). Among the respondents, 55.1% of them hear that the law in Ethiopia allows for legal abortion while 44.9% didn't. Among those who knew that abortion is legal, 57.4% of them knew as abortion is permitted under all circumstances while 42.6% said abortion is only permitted under certain circumstances. Of the total respondents who reported abortion is legal under certain circumstances, 37.2% mentioned abortion is legal for pregnant mothers who have mental or physical disability followed by 36.0% for serious fetal deformity and 34.9% if pregnancy is as a results of rape, 33.3% if the pregnancy threaten the life of mother while the least 26.7% is if pregnancy is from incest.

In this study, 79% of the study participants were not knowledgeable about abortion law while 21% were knowledgeable (Table 2).

Pregnancy, abortion and contraceptive utilization

From all respondents, 9.9% of them had a previous history of pregnancy and about 72.2% of those ever pregnant were reported that their pregnancy is not intended. Those who

Table 1 Socio-demographic characteristics of under graduate female students of Ambo University, West Shoa Zone, Ethiopia, 2018

Variables	N(%)
Age	
Below median age (21 years)	298 (37.4%)
Above median age (21 years)	497 (62.5%)
Religion	
Orthodox	269 (33.8%)
Muslim	103 (13%)
Protestant	374 (47%)
Wakefata	49 (6.2%)
Marital status	
Single	687 (86.4%)
Married	83 (10.4%)
Widowed	13 (1.6%)
Divorced	12 (1.5%)
College or faculty	
Natural science and computational	100 (12.6%)
medicine and health sciences	50 (6.3%)
Social science and Humanities	174 (21.9%)
Institute of cooperative	12 (1.5%)
College of business and Economics	40 (5%)
Institute of technology	260 (32.7%)
Mother educational level	
No formal education	244 (30.7%)
primary school	231 (29.1%)
High school	148 (18.6%)
College and above	172 (21.6%)
Father educational level	
No of formal education	135 (17.0%)
Primary school	234 (29.4%)
High school	178 (22.4%)
College and above	248 (31.2%)
Previous Residence area	
Urban	277 (34.8%)
Semi-urban	163 (20.5%)
Current residence	
In Campus	727 (91.4%)
Outside campus	68(8.6%)
Pocket money per month	
< 300	180 (22.6%)
Above 300	61(77.4%0
Estimated family income	
< 4500 or below	389 (48.9%)
Above 4500	406 (51.1%)

Table 2 Sources of information and knowledge on abortion legislation among female under graduate students of Ambo University, West Shoa Zone, Ethiopia 2018

Variables	N(%)
Heard about abortion legislation	
Yes	468 (58.9%)
No	327 (41.1%)
Sources of information on abortion legislation	
Received health education, on abortion legislation	180 (38.2%)
From TV/Radio	130 (27.8%)
From relatives / Someone who had an abortion	225 (48.1%)
From clubs in school/University	260 (55.6%)
The Current abortion law allow a women to have abortion	
Yes	258 (55.1%)
No	210(44.9%)
If yes,	
Under all circumstances	148 (57.4%)
Under some circumstances	148 (57.4%)
The current law on Abortion allows the woman on rape to run abortion	
Yes	90 (34.9%)
No	144 (55.8%)
The current law on Abortion allow the woman on incest to run abortion	
Yes	69 (26.7%)
No	163(63.2%)
The current law on Abortion allow the woman if the pregnancy threaten the life of mother.	
Yes	86(33.3%)
No	160(62%)
The current law on Abortion allow the woman if the mother has physically or mentally problem.	
Yes	96(37.2%)
No	142(55%)
Does the current law on Abortion allow the woman if serious fetal deformity	
Yes	93(36%)
No	133 (51.6%)
Over all abortion legislation knowledge	
Knowledgeable	98 (21%)
Not knowledgeable	370 (79%)

ever had pregnant, the majority had history of induced abortion of whom 21% of them aborted at health institution, 40.3% at traditional healers\ and 30% in their own house. Reasons were given why they had induced abortion. The majority, 40.3% of them reported to continue schooling and 2 of the girls reported for they had suffered rape. The methods used to induce abortion were roots and leaves 61.2%, plastics tube 18%, and oral drugs 9%. Among exposed to abortion 86.6% of the participants visited health facility due to problems related to induced abortion. Among all respondents, 81.3% of them heard about emergency contraceptive of which nearly half of the respondents 48.7% described they are currently using contraceptives among which condoms are the highest percentage (32.0%) (Table 3).

Predictors of abortion law knowledge

In this study all socio-demographic variables did not have an association with kowlege of abortion law. Study participants who were involved in the health club in the university, knew the place where induced abortion can be done and received health education on the abortion law were identified as the predictor of abortion law knowledge. Among those who know that abortion is legal under certain circumstances, 50.9% were being member of health club in school. The odds of having good knowledge of abortion law are 2.09 times more likely among students who were member of health club when compared with those who were not a member of health club (AOR = 2.09, 95% CI: (1.256–3.484)). Students knowing the place where abortion can be conducted have 3.12 times the odds of having good knowledge of abortion law than those who did not know where abortion can be done (AOR = 3.12, 95% CI: (1.854–5.239)). In addition, students received health educations on the abortion law are 7.38 times more likely to have good knowledge of Abortion Law compared to those who did not get health education on Abortion law (AOR = 7.38, 95% CI: (1.118–48.761)) (Table 4).

Discussion

The study revealed that 21% of the respondents have good knowledge on abortion legislation while 79% have poor knowledge. This result is higher than the study reported from Ghana, which only 3% of women reported as having knowledge on abortion legalization [15]. This difference is probably due to the difference in study design in which the study conducted in Ghana is a community-based survey which included all reproductive age women while this study is institutional based.

On the other hand the finding of this study is much lower compared to a study from South Africa, which revealed that 68% of the study participants knew that abortion is legal [10]. This difference is probably due to the difference in circumstance of the existing abortion law in South Africa is more applied better than the study setting. In addition the difference is probable due to the study design in which the study in South Africa is community based which involved reproductive age groups. The finding of this study is also lower when compared to the result of the study done at Harari region Eastern Ethiopia in which 35.7% of female students reported as

Table 3 Pregnancy and Abortion related frequency distribution among female under graduate students of Ambo University, West Shoa Zone,Ethiopia, 2018

Variables	N(%)
Ever been pregnant	
Yes	79 (9.9%)
No	716 (90.1%)
Intended pregnancy	
Yes	22 (17.8%)
No	57 (72.2%)
Reason for not intended	
Faced Physical violence	27 (47.4%)
Faced Sexual violence	26 (45.6%)
Rape	4 (7%)
Ever undertaken abortion	
Yes	67 (85%)
No	12 (15.2%)
The place where induced abortion done.	
Health facility	14 (21%)
Abortionists houses	27 (40.3%)
Your house	20 (30%)
Others	6 (9%)
Method which used for induced abortion	
Plastic	12 (18%)
Oral drugs	6 (9%)
Roots and leaves	41 (61.2%)
currently using contraceptive method	
Yes	387 (48.7%)
No	408 (50.9%)
Method of contraceptive used	
Pills	55 (6.9%)
Condom	255 (32%)
Inject able	70 (8.8%)
Other	34 (4.3%)
Ever heard about emergency contraceptive	
Yes	646 (81.3%)
No	149 (18.7%)

having good awareness to legalization of safe abortion [16]. This difference could be due to poor information dissemination to the target population about their reproductive health issues in the study setting .

This finding is also lower than the studies from Ethiopia among reproductive age women at Yirgachefe town, where (48.9%) of them know abortion is legal in Ethiopia under certain circumstances [17]. The difference might be due to the socio-cultural difference between the two populations. Since this study was conducted in university, the respondents came from different corners of the country having different cultural, religious and ethnic backgrounds. But the study from Yirgachefie includes all women in the reproductive age group who have similar backgrounds.

The result of this finding is also lower when compared to study done among preparatory students at Dabat District of Ahmara region, where 62.8% students know that the law in Ethiopia allows safe and legal Abortion under certain circumstances [18]. This difference might be due to study setting difference and health facility coverage at Dabat district which works with stakeholder like Engender to expand safe abortion service and gives information about Abortion legality.

The result of our study also shows that nearly 79% of students did not know that abortion is allowed under certain circumstances in Ethiopia. This is somewhat close to the finding of the study done in Wolayita Sodo University (61%) of women reported that they don't know abortion is legal [19]. This is due to similar socio-economic and educational status of the study population, similar study setting. This result is lower than study done at Ghana which shows 92% of the women are not aware that abortion was permitted by law under certain circumstances in Ghana [20]. This difference is may be due to population difference, study setting and focus of MOH for Abortion service and education between two countries and socioeconomic difference.

In addition, this study also shows that 79(9.9%) of the students had a previous history of pregnancy and 67(85%) had history induced abortion. The magnitude of induced abortion in this study is much higher than the related study from Ethiopia, Ahmara region, Dabat district 10 (43.5%) [21]. this difference is may be because of different study population and place of residence since the preparatory students in Dabat District are living with their family and monitored. About 40.3% of the abortions reported in this study were carried out at the illegal and unlicensed abortion houses. That means nearly half of the induced abortions reported in this study were unsafe. This implies that unsafe abortion is still a major maternal health problem affecting young female students. This is much higher with the finding reported from Arba Minch University students, 17% of the abortions conducted were reported to be unsafe abortion [22]. Knowledge about abortion law has significant implications for accessing legal and safe induced abortion services. Larger proportions of the abortions were not conducted through legal and safe procedures while abortion is legal under certain circumstances. Another finding of this study is respondents' use of roots and leaves to induce abortion, this might cause further complications. One possible reason that leads women to practice unsafe abortion might be the lack of knowledge of the abortion law. This is strongly supported by various studies [18, 22].

Table 4 Binary and multiple Logistic regression analysis factors associated with knowledge of Abortion legislation, among under graduate female students of Ambo University, West Shoa Zone, Ethiopia, 2018

Variables	Knowledge of legal abortion		COR (95% C. I)	AOR(95% C.I)	*p*-value
	Poor (N)	Good (N)			
Year of study					
Year I	140	30	1	1	
Year II	105	22	.98(.534–1.792)	1.16(.598–2.250)	.661
Year III	78	25	1.496(.822–2.722	1.55(.811–2.965)	.184
Year IV	39	14	1.675(.810–3.465)	2.00(.914–4.373)	.083
Year V	8	7	4.083 (1.375–12.125)	3.20(.950–10.772)	.061
Know the place where safely induced abortion performed					
Yes	137	66	3.51 (2.188–5.624)	3.12 (1.854–5.239)	0.000[a]
No	233	32	1	1	
Know some-one who had Abortion					
Yes	118	46	2.25 (1.429–3.542)	1.46(.880–2.426)	.143
No	252	52	1	1	
Ever visited health institution					
Yes	214	71	1.92 (1.176–3.125)	1.59(.927–2.725)	.092
No	156	27	1	1	
Received health education on abortion legislation					
Yes	117	43	1.69 (1.072–2.665)	7.38 (1.118–48.761)	0.038 [a]
No	253	55	1	1	
Being member of health club in schools					
Yes	145	58	1.89 (1.201–2.972)	2.09 (1.256–3.484)	0.01 [a]
No	225	40	1	1	
Currently using contraceptive					
Yes	164	59	1.87 (1.189–2.948)	1.44(.858–2.403)	0.169
No	203	39	1	1	

[a]indicate factors that showed association with outcome variable
*Statistically significant at 95% confidence interval.at *p*-value 0.05

This study showed that there is a significant association between knowledge of abortion law and received health educations on the abortion legislation, knowing places where abortion is conducted and Being member of health club in school. Students received health educations on the abortion legislation are 7.38times more likely to have good knowledge of abortion legislation. The possible explanation might be due to their better Awareness they got from health education regarding revised abortion law, increased exposure to maternal health and abortion-related information.

Respondents' awareness of where safe abortion can be performed is significantly associated with knowledge of abortion legislation. Students knowing the place where abortion can be conducted have 3.116 times the odds of having good knowledge of abortion legislation than those who did not know where abortion can be done. This finding is in line with findings from Dabat District among female preparatory students [19]. This might be due to their improved information exposure and health facility access. Students who were member of health club are 2.092 times more likely to have knowledge of Abortion legislation when compared with those who were not a member of health club. This might be due to the reason that those who were member of health club can expose to health information related to different issues including Abortion.

Conclusion

Overall, this finding indicates that Ambo University female regular students had limited knowledge on the existence of legal abortion in Ethiopia. Participants who received health education about abortion law, who knew where abortion can safely be performed and those who involved in health club were found to be predictors of abortion law knowledge

Therefore ministry of health had better to work and encourage stakeholders on dissemination of information regarding the existing abortion law.

Strength of the study

One of the strength of this study was able to achieve 100% response rate. This could be true as the data were collected by interview methods and the interview was done by well trained professionals.

Limitation of the study

The data from this study may not represent all reproductive age groups because the study respondents were limited to only university female students.

In addition, there is lack of data and literature for the comparative analysis of the result.

In addition to these the limitation of this study was the smallness of the sample size.

Abbreviations

AOR: Adjusted odds ratio; CAC: Compressive abortion care; CI: Confidence interval; COR: Crude odds ratio; FMOH: Federal Minister of Health; GA: Gestation age; ICPD: International Conference on Population and Development; SDG: Sustainable development goal; WHO: World Health Organization

Acknowledgements

The Authors would like to thank AU for allocating fund to conduct the study. We would also like to express our deepest appreciation to all individuals who supported us during this research work for their indispensable contributions. Last but absolutely not the least, the contribution of the study participants is greatly appreciated.

Authors' contributions

MM contributed to the conception, design and conduct of the study, analyzed and interpreted the data, and prepared the manuscript. DD contributed to the conception, design and conduct of the study, analyzed and interpreted the data, and prepared the manuscript. TG contributed to the conception, design and conduct of the study, analyzed and interpreted the data, and prepared the manuscript. AB contributed to the design and conduct of the study, analyzed and interpreted the data, and prepared the manuscript. All authors read and approved the final manuscript.

Authors' information

MM has Master of Public Health in Health Service Management and currently working as a lecturer in Ambo University college of medicine and health science, department of Public health.
TG has Master of Public Health and currently working as a lecturer in Ambo University College of medicine and health science, department of Public health,
DD has Master of Public Health and currently working in West Shoa health office.
AB has Master of Science in Psychiatry and currently working as a lecturer in Ambo University, college of medicine and health science, Department of Psychiatry.

Author details

[1]Department of Public health, Ambo University College of Medicine and Health Science, Po Box 19, Ambo, Ethiopia. [2]West Shoa Health office, West Shewa, Ethiopia. [3]Department of Psychiatry, Ambo University College of Medicine and Health Science, Ambo, Ethiopia.

References

1. WHO. Global and regional estimates of the incidence of unsafe abortion and associated mortality in 2008.
2. Ganatra B, Tunçalp Ö, Johnston HB, Johnson BR Jr, Gülmezoglu AM, et al. From concept to measurement: operationalizing WHO's definition of unsafe abortion. Bull World Health Organ. 2014;92(3):155.
3. World Health Organization (1998b). Unsafe abortion. Safe motherhood fact Sheet: 2000.
4. WHO. Unsafe abortion: global and regional estimates of incidence of unsafe abortion and associated mortality in 2003. Geneva: WHO; 2007.
5. Institute, G. Making abortion services accessible in the wake of legal reforms: a framework and six case studies. New York: Guttmacher Institute; 2012.
6. FDRE, editor. In section II (ed FDRE) 219–221. Addis Ababa; 2004.
7. Berer M. Making abortions safe: a matter of good public health policy and practice. Geneva: Bull World Health Organ; 2000.
8. WHO. Knowledge and Opinions about Abortion Law among Mexican Youth. Int Fam Plan Perspect. 2012;28:205–7.
9. Teixeira A, Andersen, et al. Marital status and abortion among young women in Rupandehi, Nepal. BMC Womens Health. 2015.
10. Morroni C, Myer L, Tibazarwa K. Knowledge of the abortion legislation among South African women: a cross-sectional study. Reprod Health. 2006; 3(7):29.
11. Grimes DA, Benson J, Singh S, et al. Unsafe abortion: the preventable pandemic. Lancet. 2006;368:1908–19.
12. World Health Organization. Unsafe abortion: global and regional estimates of the incidence of unsafe abortion and associated mortality in 2003. 5th ed. Geneva: World Health Organization; 2007.
13. Lisa B, Nour NM. Unsafe abortion: Unnecessary maternal mortality: women's health in the developing world. Rev Obstet Gynecol. 2009;2(2):122–6.
14. Jewkes R, Rees H, Dickson K, et al. The impact of age on the epidemiology of incomplete abortion in South Africa after legislative change. BJOG. 2005; 112:355–9.
15. R.A.S Morhee, E.S.K. Morhee. Overview of the law and availability of abortion services in Ghana. Ghana Med J. 2006;40(3):80–6.
16. Davida B, Sandra GG, Ulla L. Knowledge and opinions about abortion law among Mexican youth. 2002;28(4):205–13.
17. Geleto A, Markos J. Awareness of female students attending higher educational institutions toward legalization of safe abortion and associated factors. Reprod Health. 2015.
18. Bitew S, Ketema S, Worku M, Hamu M, Loha E. Knowledge and attitude of women of childbearing age towards the legalization of abortion, Ethiopia. J Sci Innovative Res. 2013.
19. Mihiretu M. Kebede, knowledge of abortion legislation among female preparatory school students in Dabat District, Ethiopia. Afr J Reprod Health. 2016;20(4):13–21.
20. Gelaye A, Taye K, Mekonen T. Magnitude and risk factors of abortion among regular female students in Wolaita Sodo University, Ethiopia. BMC Womens Health. 2014;14:1–9.
21. Pathfinder International. Improving Abortion and Post abortion Care Services Using Community Survey Data in Ghana 2009. www.pathfind.org/site/PageServer?pagename=Pubs Abortion. Accessed 13 Jan 2018.
22. UNFPA, Making Reproductive Rights and Sexual And Reproductive Health, 2008.

4

Counseling on family planning during ANC service increases the likelihood of postpartum family planning use in Bahir Dar City Administration, Northwest Ethiopia

Tadese Ejigu Tafere[1,2*], Mesganaw Fanthahun Afework[3] and Alemayehu Worku Yalew[3]

Abstract

Background: Closely spaced pregnancies within the first year postpartum increases the risk of death for both the mother and baby. Many countries recommend providing pregnant women with post-partum family planning counselling during antenatal care visits. However, data on the extent to which providers utilize these opportunities and the role of family planning counseling during antenatal care in promoting the use of postpartum modern family planning remain limited especially in developing countries. Therefore, this study was aimed at investigating the role of family planning counseling during antenatal care in promoting postpartum modern family planning use within 6 weeks after birth.

Methods: Nine hundred seventy pregnant women with gestational age ≤ 16 weeks who came for their first Antenatal Care (ANC) visit were enrolled and followed until 6 weeks after delivery. Longitudinal data was collected during consultation with ANC providers using structured observation checklist to assess whether or not the providers counsel pregnant women on post-partum family planning use during their four focused ANC visits. Exit interview was also conducted at 6 weeks after they gave birth when they came to immunize their child to assess whether they were starting to use postpartum modern family planning. Completed data were obtained from 823 women. Generalized Estimating Equation was carried out to identify predictors of postpartum modern family planning use by controlling the cluster effect among women who received ANC services in the same health facility.

(Continued on next page)

* Correspondence: tade_et@yahoo.com
[1]School of Public Health (SPH), College of Health Sciences, Addis Ababa University, Addis Ababa, Ethiopia
[2]School of Public Health, College of Medicine and Health Sciences, Bahir Dar University, Bahir Dar, Ethiopia

(Continued from previous page)

Results: Postpartum modern family planning use within 6 weeks after delivery among the study women was 157(19. 1%) with 95%CI (16.4, 21.9); Among 187 pregnant women who were counseled at least once, 72(38.5%) of them used post-partum modern family planning compared to 13.4% of post-partum women who were not counseled at all ($p < 0.001$). Counseling about postpartum family planning during antenatal care, satisfaction on the antenatal care services women received while they were pregnant, counseling on birth preparedness and complication readiness plan, counseling on breast feeding and post-natal care use were independent predictors for postpartum modern family planning use.

Conclusion: Less than one in five post-partum women were using postpartum family planning within 6 weeks after birth. Family planning counseling during ANC services had a significant effect on promoting postpartum modern family planning use. Therefore, health providers need to ensure continuity of care through strengthening integration of family planning counseling services during ANC and referral linkages between community and health workers.

Keywords: Postpartum family planning use, Unmet need for family planning, Postpartum period

Plain English summary

Immediate post-partum family planning use helps women to space their pregnancies, lowering their risk for low birth weight and premature birth, both linked with infant mortality. In Ethiopia, nearly half (47%) of all pregnancies occurred within < 24 months after preceding birth; To what extent providers utilize opportunities of ANC visits for family planning counseling to promote the use of postpartum modern family planning remain limited especially in developing countries.

Pregnant women with gestational age ≤ 16 weeks who came for their first ANC visit were enrolled and followed until 6 weeks after delivery. Longitudinal data was collected during consultation with ANC providers to assess whether or not the providers counsel pregnant women on postpartum family planning use during their four focused ANC visits. Exit interview was also conducted at 6 weeks after they gave birth when they came to immunize their child to assess whether they were starting to use postpartum modern family planning.

Among 823 pregnant women, 187(22.7%) were counseled about post-partum family planning at least once during their four ANC visits and postpartum modern family planning use within 6 weeks after delivery was 157(19.1%). Injectable and implants were the most common adopted modern post-partum family planning methods.

A fraction of pregnant women was provided with family planning counselling during antenatal care that led to lower level of adoption of post-partum family planning within six weeks after delivery which implied a need to ensure integrity of maternal health services during antenatal care.

Background

Family planning counselling during the antepartum period provides a crucial window of opportunity to address unmet need for family planning during the post-partum period. Rates of maternal and infant mortality and morbidity could be substantially decreased if unplanned and unwanted pregnancies were prevented and if all new pregnancies could be spaced at least two years after a birth [1].

Family planning can avert more than 30% of maternal deaths and 10% of child mortality if couples space their pregnancies more than two years apart [2, 3]. On the contrary, closely spaced pregnancies within the first year postpartum increase the risk of death for both the mother and baby, resulting in increased risks for adverse outcomes, such as preterm birth, low birth weight and small for gestational age [4].

The period after delivery is complex and challenging, during which a woman has to care for her newborn child as well as cope with psychological and physical changes. Focused antenatal family planning counseling increased the possibility postpartum family planning use [5].

The service delivery guidelines for antenatal care services in many countries recommend providing pregnant women with counseling concerning post-partum family planning, breastfeeding, danger signs birth preparedness and complication readiness plan and other topics. However, only a fraction of clients in Sub-Saharan Africa(SSA) receive information on any of these topics during their antenatal care visits [6].

In five countries of Latin America and the Caribbean, about half of pregnant women receive some family planning information during antenatal care visits [7]. In Sub-Saharan Africa, the proportion of postpartum women who are exposed to the risk of pregnancy by having sex while using no family planning method within two years after childbirth was nearly one third [8, 9].

In Ethiopia, evidence has been found that nearly half (47%) of all pregnancies occurred within a short birth interval of less than 24 months after the preceding birth and 86% of post-partum women within six months have unmet need for family planning [10].

Postpartum women are an important target groups because they may not realize that they are at risk of pregnancy even if they are breastfeeding [11]. However, 37% of sexually active women are at risk of pregnancy during the first six months postpartum, this risk increases to 64% among women 6–11 months postpartum [10].Therefore, concentrating efforts on increasing postpartum family planning use among these women could have a proportionally greater impact than focusing attention on other populations.

A very limited number of studies examined the role of ANC as a facilitator for post-partum modern family planning use (short/long acting hormonal contraceptives, permanent family planning techniques or barrier methods like male or female condom use). Those studies were cross sectional focused on the assessment of the relationship between the frequency of ANC visits rather than the antenatal care family planning counseling and post-partum family planning use. In addition those who assessed the association between provision of antenatal care family planning counseling during any of their ANC visits and postpartum family planning use were based on the women's' self-report and they also assessed post-partum family planning use within one or two years after birth rather than within the six weeks postpartum which is the WHO recommendation [12, 13].

Therefore, this follow up study was intended to bring an insight about the role of family planning counseling during the four focused antenatal care visits in promoting the use of modern family planning use within 6 weeks after birth. More over to explore the relationship between other contents of antenatal care services (like counselling on birth preparedness and complication readiness plan, counselling on breast feeding, satisfaction on ANC) and the use of post-natal care with post-partum modern family planning use. The findings of this study will provide credible evidence for maternal and child health program implementers and policy makers to reduce maternal and child mortality.

Methods

Study design, settings and population

A facility based prospective follow up study was conducted from October 2015 to August 2016 in seven public health facilities; one hospital and six health centers of Bahir Dar City Administration, Amhara National Regional State, which is located in the North West part of Ethiopia. According to the Amhara National Regional State Bureau of Finance and Economic Development report, the projected population by 2015/16 was 297,775 (80.5% urban Vs 19.5% rural), of these 156,515 (52.6%) were females and there were 10,035 eligible pregnant women in the same year [14]. All first visit pregnant women with gestational age ≤ 16 weeks attending antenatal care services during data collection period who were selected by systematic random sampling (k = 3) and voluntary to participate in the study were included. Pregnant women were followed from their first to fourth antenatal care visits while they received their antenatal care services to investigate whether health professionals provide them with postpartum family planning counseling. Exit interview was also conducted just after their fourth ANC visit to measure their satisfaction on the ANC service they received and at 6 weeks after birth when they came to immunize their child to assess whether or not they started to use postpartum modern family planning and to identify the type of postpartum modern family planning. The satisfaction scores were included to provide insight on whether satisfactory scores influenced postpartum family planning use. The detail of the method is described elsewhere.

Sample size and sampling technique

The current study is part of a follow up study with multiple objectives. The detail of the sample size calculation to address all objectives (considering the maximum adequate sample size which was 970) and the sampling procedure is described elsewhere [15]. For the current study a sample size was calculated with 2.8% postpartum modern family planning use among women who had no ANC (considering these women as they were not counseled on postpartum family planning during ANC) [16] and 5% difference in post-partum modern family planning use among women who were counseled, 80% power, 5% level of significance and 10% non-response rate. The final calculated sample size was 777. However, to increase the power of the study, all 823 women who completed the follow up period were included in the analysis.

Data collection process

Seven female diploma midwives and two female Bachelor of Science midwives who were not the staffs in the study health facilities were recruited as data collectors and supervisors respectively to observe whether or not the ANC provider counsels a woman about postpartum family planning during each of the four ANC visits and provide other contents of ANC services.

To measure the satisfaction of pregnant women on ANC services they received during their pregnancy period an exit interview was conducted just after their fourth ANC visit using eight items. Each item has five point Likert scales from strongly disagree (1) to strongly agree (5).

In addition, there was also another exit interview with women at 6 weeks after birth when they came to the health facility to immunize their child to assess whether or not they were using a modern family planning. If a woman doesn't come to the health facility for immunization, the data collectors were expected to trace her at home based on her address registered during the first visit.

Dependent

Post-partum modern family planning use (yes/no).

Independent

Counseling on postpartum modern family planning during each of the four ANC visits was the main exposure variable and the other independent variables include: satisfaction on the ANC services that women received while they were pregnant, counseling services given about birth preparedness and complication readiness plan, breast feeding and immunization; postnatal care use and place of delivery.

The satisfaction score of pregnant women on the ANC services they received was computed from the eight items aimed to assess privacy, confidentiality, costs related to ANC service, client-provider interaction, their perception about ANC services provided and whether they recommend the health facility for others or not. The items had internal reliability (Cronbach's α of 0.74). A respondent had a minimum of 8 and a maximum of 40 points on ANC satisfaction score. The satisfaction score was converted to percentage satisfaction score to make it standardized [17]. The percentage mean satisfaction score for client satisfaction on the ANC services received was 73.2. Clients were categorized as satisfied (if they score above the percentage mean satisfaction score) otherwise not satisfied.

Data analysis

Data were coded and entered into EPI data version3.1 and exported to SPSS version 20 for analysis. Descriptive statistics were used to describe the data. Generalized Estimating Equation logistic regression analysis with robust estimator and exchangeable working correlation matrix was carried out to control the cluster effect of women who received ANC services within the same health facility and to identify the predictor variables for postpartum modern family planning use at 6 weeks after birth. A p-value < 0.2 was considered to retain variables for the multivariable Generalized Estimating Equation logistic regression analysis. And P-value < 0.05 was considered to identify statistically significant predictors for postpartum modern family planning use.

Results

Characteristics of study participants

Among 970 pregnant women who were enrolled to the larger study 823(84.8%) completed the follow up period. The reasons for 15.2% loss to follow up were abortion, self-referral to other health facilities permanent change in work place and the long distance to reach health facilities especially when the gestational age increases. There was no statistically significant difference in family planning counseling service during ANC between those women who completed the follow up and those who were loss to follow up. The mean age (±standard deviation) of 823 women who completed the follow up period was 25.46 ± 4.37 years. Nearly 90 % of women were urban residents (88.5%) and Orthodox Christian (90.9%). With regard to their educational status, 21.0% of women had no formal education while 57.5% of women had completed secondary school and above (Table 1).

Family planning counselling during antenatal care and post-partum modern family planning use

Among 823 pregnant women, 187(22.7%) of pregnant women were counseled about postpartum family planning at least once during their four ANC visits. All pregnant women were not counseled about postpartum family planning during their first and second ANC visits; however, 60(7.3%) and 186(22.6%) of pregnant women were counseled about postpartum modern family planning during their third and fourth visits respectively.

The magnitude of postpartum modern family planning use within 6 weeks after delivery among the study women was 157 (19.1%) with 95%CI (16.4, 21.9) though the contraceptive methods like IUCD were provided in the immediate post-partum period before discharge in the same room. Injectable, Implanon, pills and IUCD were used by 111(13.5%), 34 (4.1%), 10(1.2%) and 2(0.2%) post-partum women respectively.

Among 187 pregnant women who were counseled at least once during their ANC visits, 72(38.5%) of them used postpartum modern family planning compared to 13.4% of postpartum women who were not counseled at all during their four ANC visits ($p < 0.001$).

With regard to satisfaction on the ANC service provision, among 376(45.7%) women who were satisfied with their ANC service, 111(29.5%) were using postpartum family planning. However, among 447(54.3%) who were not satisfied by the service, only 46(10.3%) were using postpartum modern family planning ($p < 0.001$) in their postpartum period within 6 weeks after delivery.

Factors associated with postpartum modern family planning use

In a Generalized Estimating Equation binary logistic regression analysis, there was a positive association

Table 1 Socio-demographic characteristics and postpartum family planning counseling (PPFP) of ANC attendants at public health facilities of Bahir Dar City administration (*N* = 823), October 2015 to August 2016

Variables	PPFP counseling at least once during ANC		Total frequency
	Yes (%)	No (%)	
Age			
15–24 years	81(22.9)	273 (77.1)	354 (100.0)
25-34 years	101 (23.5)	328 (76.5)	429 (100.0)
≥ 35 years	5 (12.5)	35 (87.5	40 (100.
Residence			
Urban	174 (23.9)	554 (76.1)	728 (100.0)
Rural	13 (13.7)	82 (86.3)	95 (100.0)
Educational status			
No formal education	36 (20.8)	137 (79.2)	173 (100.0)
Primary	37 (20.7)	140 (79.1)	177 (100.0)
Secondary and above	114 (24.1)	359 (75.9)	473 (100.0)
Occupation			
Farmer	11 (12.4)	78 (87.6)	89 (100.0)
House wife	108 (25.5)	315 (74.5)	423 (100.0)
Employee[a]	68 (21.9)	243 (78.1)	311 (100.0)
Religion			
Orthodox	175 (23.4)	573 (76.6)	748 (100.0)
Muslim	12 (16.4)	61 (83.6)	73 (100.0)
Protestant	0 (0.0)	2 (100.0)	2 (100.0)
Marital status			
Married	184 (22.7)	627 (77.3)	811 (100.0)
Divorced	2 (20.0)	8 (80.0)	10 (100.0)
Widowed	1 (5.0)	1 (50.0)	2 (100.0)
Ethnicity			
Amhara	179 (22.7)	609 (77.3)	788 (100.0)
Tigre	6 (24.0)	19 (26.0)	25 (100.0)
Awi	2 (28.6)	5 (71.4)	7 (100.0)
Oromo	0 (0.0)	3 (100.0)	3 (100.0)
Grand total	187 (22.7)	636 (77.3)	823 (100.0)

[a]governmental employees, nongovernmental employees,daily laborers and waiters

between postpartum modern family planning use and family planning counselling during ANC, satisfaction on the ANC service, birth preparedness and complication readiness plan, place of delivery, post-natal care service utilization, counselling on breast feeding, residence, educational status and occupation of the mother.

In multivariable Generalized Estimating Equation logistic regression analysis, since post-natal care use and place of delivery showed co linearity effect, place of delivery was not fitted in the final model. Family planning counselling during antenatal care, birth preparedness and complication readiness plan, counselling on breast feeding at least once during ANC visits, satisfaction on the antenatal care service while she was pregnant and post-natal care visit remained to have statistically significant association with postpartum modern family planning use.

The odds of postpartum modern family planning use within 6 weeks after birth among women who were counseled about postpartum family planning at their third or fourth visit were 3.5 times higher compared to those who were not counselled at any of their visits (AOR = 3.5; 95% CI:2.19,5.49). The odds of postpartum modern family planning use within 6 weeks after birth among women who were counseled about birth preparedness and complication readiness plan at their third or fourth ANC visit were 2.2 times higher compared to those who were not counselled at all (AOR = 2.2; 95% CI:1.32,3.55). The odds of postpartum modern family planning use within 6 weeks after birth among women who were counseled about breast feeding at least once during their ANC visits were 1.8 times higher compared to those women who were not counselled during their ANC visits (AOR = 1.8; 95% CI:1.15,2.82). The odds of postpartum modern family planning use within 6 weeks after birth among women who had at least one post-natal care visit during their postpartum period were 13.5 times higher compared to those who had no any post-natal care visit ((AOR = 13.5; 95% CI:8.24,22.07). In addition, the odds of partum modern family planning use within 6 weeks after birth among women who were satisfied by the ANC service they received for their recent pregnancy were 4.1 times higher compared to their counter parts (AOR = 4.12; 95% CI:2.55,6.66) (Table 2).

Discussion

Based on the 2016 Ethiopian Demographic and Health Survey (EDHS) report, with only 35% modern family planning use, and high unmet need (22%) [18], investigating the effectiveness of providing postpartum family planning information through antenatal care services on postpartum family planning use, and the extent to which providers utilize these opportunities, are increasingly important. For women who are not breastfeeding, pregnancy can occur within 45 days of giving birth [19].

The current study found that less than one out of five postpartum women were using modern family planning at 6 weeks of after birth. The finding is consistent with a study done in Adigrat Northern Ethiopia 24.6% [20] but is higher than a study done including different countries

Table 2 Multivariable GEE logistic regression results to assess the association between counseling on postpartum family planning (PPFP) during ANC and PPFP use at public health facilities of Bahir- Dar City Administration ($N = 823$), October 2015 to August 2016

Variables	Postpartum modern family planning use		COR(95%CI)	AOR(95%CI)
	Yes (%)	No (%)		
PPFP counselling during ANC				
Counselled at least in one visit	72 (38.5)	115 (61.5)	4.06 (2.80,5.89)	3.47 (2.19,5.49)*
Not counselled at all	85 (13.4)	551 (86.6)	1.00	1.00
Residence				
Urban	154 (21.2)	574 (78.8)	8.23 (2.57,26.34)	1,02 (0.33,3.12)
Rural	3 (3.2)	92 (96.8)	1.00	1.00
Educational status				
Secondary school and above	118 (24.9)	355 (75.1)	3.78 (2.10,6.77)	1.47 (0,67,3.25)
Primary school	25 (14.1)	152 (85.9)	1.87 (0.936,3.73)	1.12 (0.47,2.71)
No formal education	14 (8.1)	159 (91.9)	1.00	1.00
Occupation				
Employee [a]	84 (27.0)	227 (73.0)	10.61 (3.27,34.46)	1.93 (0.50,7.48)
House wife	70 (16.5)	353 (83.5)	5.67 (1.75,18.49)	1.47 (0.41,5.32)
Farmer	3 (3.4)	86 (96.6)	1.00	1.00
Counselling on BPRCP				
Counselled at least in one visit	116 (26.9)	315 (73.1)	3.15 (2.14,4.64)	2.16 (1.32,3.55)*
Not counselled at all	41 (10.5)	351 (89.5)	1.00	1.00
Counselling on breast feeding				
Counselled at least in one visit	72 (32.6)	149 (67.4)	2.94 (2.04,4.23)	1.80 (1.15,2.82)*
Not counselled at all	85 (14.1)	517 (85.9)	1.00	1.00
At least one PNC visit				
yes	96 (60.4)	63 (39.6)	15.06 (9.97,22.80)	13.49 (8.24,22.07)*
no	61 (9.2)	603 (90.8)	1.00	1.00
Satisfaction on ANC service during pregnancy				
Satisfied	111 (29.5)	265 (70.5)	3.65 (2.50,5.32)	4.12 (2.55,6.66)*
Not satisfied	46 (10.3)	401 (89.7)	1.00	1.00

*Indicates significant difference at $p < 0.05$

[a]Government, private and Nongovernmental organization employees

using their respective most recent (2008–2012 DHS data); Ethiopia (8%), Comoros(6.4%) and Burundi (5.8%) [21].

The possible explanations for higher postpartum family planning use compared to studies done in some of the afore mentioned countries could be attributed to the time gap between the current study and Demographic Health Survey (DHS) data collected in different countries; all participants of the current study had four ANC visits that might increase their tendency to use postpartum family planning and the difference in background characteristics of study participants, for instance most (88.5%) of the participants of this study were urban dwellers so that they might have better awareness and access to family planning methods compared to DHS studies that includes both rural and urban population groups. In addition, efforts by the Ethiopian government to strengthen strategies for maternal and child health mortality reduction like the different community based reproductive health services and health education being given on house to house basis by health extension workers might also have an effect for the increase in postpartum modern family planning use.

Among postpartum women who adopted postpartum modern family planning, Injectable and implants were the most common methods reported by the current study and this is also in line with the analysis done to assess method mix among PPFP users from DHS 2011 data [22] except that there is improvement in utilization of Implanon compared to EDHS 2011 report (21.7% Vs 10%). Similarly, studies done on the general population in Gondar and 2016 EDHS report also reported that the most commonly used PPFP methods are injectable and implants [16, 18] .

This implied method mix in Ethiopia relies heavily on short-acting methods, with the majority of women using injectable and only a fraction of postpartum family planning users using long-acting methods (implants and IUDs).

This study also revealed that even if less than one–fourth of the women were given counseling on postpartum family planning; information on family planning during antenatal care had significant effect on improving the use of postpartum modern family planning. This finding is also supported by studies done in Mexico [23], Uttar Pradesh [24] and systematic review published in 2014 that reported integration of family planning into antenatal care services showed increased modern family planning use where the demand is high [25].

This might be due to the reason that frequent exposure of pregnant women to health professionals during antenatal care offers ample opportunity to discuss about family planning when couples are not distracted by a new baby and when they have time to consider all the options.

Satisfaction by the ANC services during pregnancy was significant in predicting the likelihood of using postpartum modern family planning within 6 weeks by the current study. The study in Mexico among low-income women also supported this finding as it reported women living in communities with high quality care were more likely to use a family planning method than those in communities with lower quality of care [23].

This might be attributed to high quality care increases the confidence of women on the health system there by comply with the advice given by health professionals and might have a positive effect to use the continuum of care (antenatal care to post-natal care including postpartum family planning use).

The use of modern family planning is significantly associated with the use of post-natal care in this study. This relationship is also evidenced by other studies findings conducted in North West Ethiopia [16],India [26] and Mexico [23].

The present study showed women who were counseled about birth preparedness and complication readiness plan during antenatal care were more likely to use post-partum modern family planning compared to their counter parts. This might be due to the reason that when health professionals discuss about birth preparedness and complication readiness plan they are more likely to discuss with the danger signs of pregnancy and the probability of their occurrence in closely spaced pregnancy; which might have an influence on the decision of women to use postpartum family planning. Similarly, this study also reported women who were counseled about breast feeding were more likely to use postpartum modern family planning.

As the data collection was done by direct observation while women received antenatal care services using observation checklist adapted from WHO Basic Emergency Obstetric and Newborn Care (BEmONC) guideline, the study might not be affected by self-report bias.

However, ANC providers might maximize their effect due to the presence of data collectors (hawthorn effect) though its effect will decrease as the providers familiarize their presence since the data collection period was long (1 year). Since the focus of this study investigating the presence or absence of family planning counseling during ANC rather than about the standard/ quality of the counseling session, it might also have a limitation.

In addition, this study might also have selection bias as it was a facility based study and women who came to health facilities might have different characteristics from those who didn't come.

Conclusion and recommendation

A fraction (less than one-fourth) of pregnant women was provided with family planning counselling during antenatal care. Family planning counseling during antenatal care services had a significant effect on postpartum modern family planning use. Counseling about postpartum family planning during antenatal care, satisfaction on the antenatal care services women received while they were pregnant, counseling on birth preparedness and complication readiness plan, counseling on breast feeding and post-natal care use were independent predictors for postpartum modern family planning use.

Therefore, programme managers and health providers need to ensure continuity of care through coordination within the health system such as integrating family planning counseling services during antenatal care and providing referral linkages between community and health facility for antenatal care, postnatal care and postpartum modern family planning use to reach postpartum women when their demand for family planning is high.

Abbreviations

ANC: Antenatal Care; AOR: Adjusted Odds Ratio; BPRCP: Birth preparedness and Complication Readiness Plan; CI: Confidence Interval; COR: Crude Odds Ratio; FANC: Focused Antenatal Care; GEE: Generalized Estimating Equation; PNC: Post-natal Care

Acknowledgements

The authors would like to thank Addis Ababa and Bahir Dar Universities for covering the transportation and Perdiem cost of data collectors and supervisors during the data collection process of the study. They also sincerely thank the study participants for their participation and the data collectors and supervisors for their unreserved effort to realize this study.

Authors' contributions

TET was involved in the conception, and design of the research project proposal; analysis, interpretation, report and manuscript writing. MFA had been involved in the conception and design of the research project proposal and AWY was involved in the conception, design of research project, analysis, interpretation and approval of manuscript writing. All authors read and approved the final manuscript.

Author details

[1]School of Public Health (SPH), College of Health Sciences, Addis Ababa University, Addis Ababa, Ethiopia. [2]School of Public Health, College of Medicine and Health Sciences, Bahir Dar University, Bahir Dar, Ethiopia. [3]School of Public Health, College of Health Sciences, Addis Ababa University, Addis Ababa, Ethiopia.

References

1. Rutstein SO. Further Evidence of the Effects of Preceding Birth Intervals on Neonatal, Infant, and Under-Five-Years Mortality and Nutritional Status in Developing Countries: Evidence from the Demographic and Health Surveys. DHS Working Papers, No. 41: Demographic and Health Research Division, Macro International Inc; 2008.
2. Campbell OMaWJG. Strategies for re ducing maternal mortality: Getting on with what works. Lancet. 2006;368(9,543):1,284–281,299.
3. Cleland JBS, Ezeh A, Faundes A, Glasier A, Innis J. Family planning: the unfinished agenda. Lancet. 2006;368(9549):1810–27.
4. DaVanzo JHH, Razzaque A, Rahman M. Effects of interpregnancy interval and outcome of the preceding pregnancy on pregnancy outcomes in Matlab, Bangladesh. BJOG. 2007;114(9):1079–87.
5. Yee LSM. Urban minority women's perceptions and of preferences for postpartum contraceptive counseling. J Midwifery Womens Heal. 2011;56: 54–60.
6. Abdel-Tawab N, Youssef H, Loza S, Zaki A, Farag S. "Helping Egyptian women achieve optimal birth spacing intervals through maximizing opportunities in antenatal and postpartum care." FRONTIERS research update No. 9. Cairo: Population Council; 2006.
7. Solis F, Rojas AC, Gadea A, Rivero-Fuentes E, Vernon R. "Situational analysis of the use of contraception in postpartum, post abortion and prevention of mother to child transmission (PMTCT) programs, Nicaragua." FRONTIERS final report. Washington, DC: Population Council; 2007.
8. Clements SMN. Who is being served least by family planning providers? A study of modern contraceptive use in Ghana, Tanzania and Zimbabwe. Afr J Reprod Health. 2004;8(2):124–36.
9. Ndugwa RPCJ, Madise NJ, Fotso J-C, Zulu EM. Menstrual pattern: menstrual pattern,Sexual behaviors, and contraceptive use among postpartum women in Nairobi urban slums. J Urban Health. 2010;88(2):341–55.
10. United States Agency for International Development: Family planning needs during the first two years postpartum in the Ethiopia. 2011.
11. World Health Organiozation: Statement for collective action for postpartum family planning. . 2013.
12. Do MHD. Relationships between antenatal and postnatal care and post-partum modern contraceptive use: evidence from population surveys in Kenya and Zambia. BMC Health Serv Res. 2013;13:6.
13. Hernandez LE, Sappenfield WM, Goodman D, Pooler J. Is effective contraceptive use conceived prenatally in Florida? The association between prenatal contraceptive counseling and postpartum contraceptive use. Matern Child Health J. 2012;16:423–9.
14. Amhara National Regional State Bureau of Finance and Economic Development: Population projection report 2015.
15. Ejigu Tafere T, Afework MF, Yalew AW. Antenatal care service quality increases the odds of utilizing institutional delivery in Bahir Dar city administration, North Western Ethiopia: a prospective follow up study. PLoS One. 2018;13(2):e0192428. https://doi.org/10.1371/journal. pone.0192428.
16. Mengesha ZBWA, Feleke SM. Contraceptive adoption in the extended postpartum period is low in Northwest Ethiopia. BMC Pregnancy Childbirth. 2015;15:160.
17. Legesse MTSW, Walle AA. Adult Patient Satisfaction with In-patient Nursing Care in a Referral and Teaching Hospital in Southern Nations Nationalities and Peoples' Region (SNNPR), Ethiopia. J Nurs Care. 2016;5:334. https://doi. org/10.4172/2167-1168.1000334.
18. Ethiopian Centeral StatisticsAgency: Ethiopian Demography and Health Survey Report. 2016.
19. Jackson E, Glasier A. Return of ovulation and menses in postpartum nonlactating women: a systematic review. Obstet Gynecol. 2011;117(3):657–62. https://doi.org/10.1097/AOG.0b013e31820ce18c.
20. Teferra AS, Abraha TH, Gelagay AA. Postpartum modern contraceptive use and associated factors. Epidemiol Health. 2017;39:e2017012.
21. Winfrey W, Rakesh K. Use of Family Planning in the Postpartum Period. DHS Comparative Report No. 36. Rockville: ICF International; 2014.
22. Program(MCHI). MaChI: Family planning needs during the first two years postpartum in Ethiopia, a report based on 2011 data. 2013.
23. Barber SL. Family planning advice and postpartum contraceptive use among low-income women in Mexico. Int Fam Plan Perspect. 2007;33(1):6–12.
24. Ma AP, Montana L, Sengupta R, calhoun LM, Nanda P. Integration of family planning with maternal health services: an opportunity to increase postpartum modern contraceptive use in urban Uttar Pradesh, India. J Fam Plann Reprod Health Care. 2016;42:107–15.
25. Sonalkar SMS, Gaffield ME. Outreach and integration programs to promote family planning in the extended postpartum period. Int J Gynaecol Obstet. 2014;124(3):193–7.
26. Mahmood SESA, Shrotriya VP, Shaifali I. Mishra5 P: postpartum contraceptive use in rural Bareilly. Indian J Community Health. 2011;23:56–67.

5

Peripheral nerve injury with Nexplanon removal

Rachel Lefebvre[1*], Marianne Hom[2], Hyuma Leland[3] and Milan Stevanovic[1]

Abstract

Background: Implantable devices offer convenient, long-acting, and reversible contraception. Injury to the peripheral nerves and blood vessels have been reported as rare complications of implantation and extraction.

Case presentation: We present a case of ulnar nerve injury in a 21-year-old woman from attempted in-office removal of a deeply implanted Nexplanon® device. The injury resulted in an ulnar nerve palsy requiring surgical exploration, neuroma excision, and sural nerve cable grafting.

Conclusions: In-office attempts to remove contraceptive implants that are deep or have migrated can cause iatrogenic nerve injury. Devices that are non-palpable, deep, or migrated should be imaged before formal surgical exploration and removal. Any patient with neurologic symptoms after placement or after attempted removal requires prompt diagnosis and referral to a peripheral nerve surgeon.

Keywords: Contraception complications, Iatrogenic peripheral nerve injury, Implant migration, Neuroma

Background

Subdermal contraceptive implants, such as the Nexplanon® (Merck, Kenilworth, NJ), are a popular form of long-acting, reversible contraception. Insertion and removal procedures are designed to be safely performed in the outpatient setting with local anesthetic. However, serious complications, including neurovascular injury, can occur [1–6]. These complications were more commonly reported with older devices, especially if they were placed deeply or if they migrated proximally. Multiple case reports have described implant-related injuries to the median [2, 3], ulnar [4, 5], and medial antebrachial cutaneous nerves [6]. These reports prompted device modifications and technique adjustments.

Due to safety concerns, the Food and Drug Administration mandated that healthcare providers undergo training and certification before using the Nexplanon® in practice [7, 8]. Current training recommends the Nexplanon® be placed subdermal and "at the inner side of the non-dominant upper arm about 8-10 cm (3-4 inches) above the medial epicondyle of the humerus, avoiding the sulcus (groove) between the biceps and triceps muscles" [9, 10]. Some providers use a different placement site, over the triceps muscle, to place the implant even further away from neurovascular structures of the medial arm, located between the triceps and biceps [11]. To help guard against deep placement, the proper technique involves insertion at an angle of less than 30° [10]. Furthermore, the newly added plastic barrier over the insertion needle is designed to guide the Nexplanon® into the superficial layer below the dermis [12, 13].

Proper removal technique is also important in avoiding complications. The safest method of extraction involves definitive palpation of the device immediately before attempting in-office removal [10]. Devices may be non-palpable because they were placed deeply or because they have migrated. Contraceptive devices placed in the arm have migrated as far as the shoulder, axilla, chest wall, and even the pulmonary arteries [9]. From the hand surgeon's perspective, implant migration is a well-documented complication and is known to occur even when an implant is originally placed into solid bone [14]. Merck acknowledges that Nexplanon® migration is

* Correspondence: Rachel.Lefebvre@med.usc.edu
[1]Department of Orthopaedic Surgery, Division of Hand Surgery, University of Southern California, 1200 N State Street A7-CT, Los Angeles, CA 90033, USA

a risk and recommends that if the device is not palpable at the time of planned removal, X-ray, computed tomography (CT), ultrasound, or even magnetic resonance imaging (MRI) can be used to aid location [10].

Even with the mandated training, technique guidelines, and design improvements, serious complications can still arise. Merck maintains a database of deep implants and complex removals [15]. The complication we present is the first case reported of ulnar nerve injury during attempted in-office removal of a deep Nexplanon®. The patient required formal surgical exploration for implant removal, resection of an ulnar nerve traumatic neuroma, and reconstruction of the ulnar nerve.

Case report

A 21-year-old woman presented to our hand and peripheral nerve clinic 4 months after attempted Nexplanon® removal from her left arm. The patient reported that neither she, nor her nurse practitioner (NP), was confidently able to feel the Nexplanon® before the attempted removal. Imaging studies to confirm location of the Nexplanon® were not performed. The patient remembered a small incision being made at the site of insertion after local anesthetic was injected. The provider was not immediately able to find the Nexplanon®, but after exploring the local area, did grasp another structure in her arm. The patient felt an "electric shock" sensation that radiated down to her medial elbow as the NP pulled. No further attempts to remove the Nexplanon® were undertaken.

Immediately after the removal attempt, the patient had complete numbness in her small and ring fingers. She returned for follow up to her NP. As months progressed, the numbness did not improve, and she began to notice wasting of her hand muscles and weakness in her grip. At almost 4 months after the attempted removal, her NP ordered a nerve conduction study which showed 50% loss of ulnar nerve function.

On presentation to the office, she had classic signs of severe, chronic ulnar nerve injury: wasting of the ulnar nerve-innervated intrinsic muscles of the hand, a claw position of the ring and small fingers, and dense numbness in an ulnar sensory nerve distribution (Fig. 1). On examination of her arm, there was a well-healed incision with surrounding scar tissue from the extraction attempt. The Nexplanon® was not palpable. X-rays showed the radio-opaque Nexplanon® at the junction of the proximal and middle thirds of the humeral shaft with the most distal end 16.5 cm proximal to the medial epicondyle (Fig. 2).

Given the patient's history, physical exam, and nerve tests, timely surgical intervention was recommended. In the OR, the upper extremity surgery team used fluoroscopy to mark the location of the Nexplanon® (Fig. 3). On surgical exploration, the Nexplanon® was found deep to the brachial fascia of the arm and in direct contact with the ulnar nerve. Less than five millimeters away was the undamaged brachial artery–the main blood supply to the arm, forearm, and hand. The Nexplanon® was removed using microsurgical instruments.

Because of the patient's dense ulnar nerve palsy, the ulnar nerve at the level of the attempted extraction was also explored. Dissection showed that the ulnar nerve had been severely damaged at this level (Fig. 4). Nerve injury can take many forms; this patient's injury was a neuroma-in-continuity whereby the ulnar nerve was still

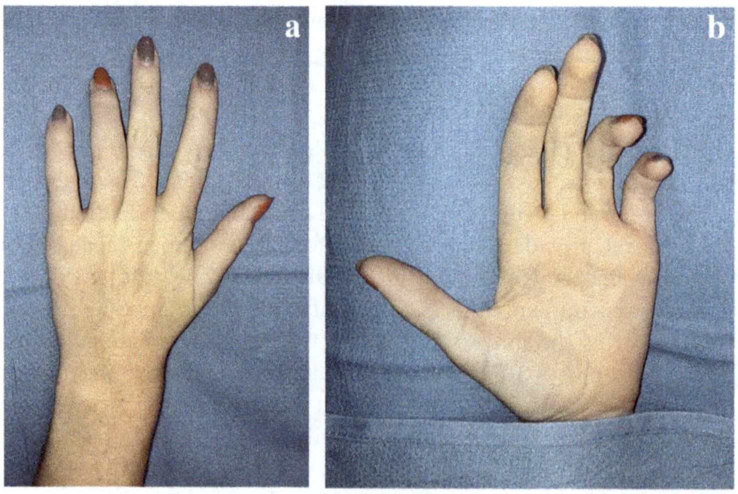

Fig. 1 Clinical appearance on initial presentation to the hand surgery service The patient had wasting of the ulnar innervated intrinsic muscles of the hand between the metacarpals. **a** The patient also had an ulnar claw hand deformity. When the ulnar innervated intrinsic muscles cannot fire, there is extension at the metacarpalphalangeal (MCP) joints and flexion at both the proximal and distal interphalangeal (IP) joints in the ring and small fingers (**b**)

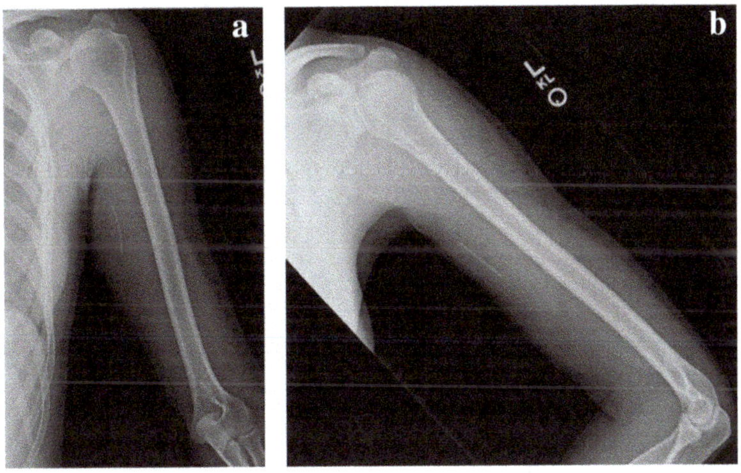

Fig. 2 AP (**a**) and lateral (**b**) radiograph views of the left humerus show the radio-opaque implant located at the level of the proximal to mid humeral shaft, 16.5 cm proximal to the medial epicondyle

one solid, longitudinal structure, but contained an abnormal portion, filled with scar tissue and damaged nerve fascicles that could not conduct electrical signal. The surgical team confirmed the neuroma's inability to conduct via intra-operative electrical stimulation. The appearance of her neuroma-in-continuity was classic: the neuroma was fusiform in shape and felt thickened and hard, unlike the proximal and distal, soft and pliable uninjured nerve (Fig. 4a).

The upper extremity surgeons treated the neuroma-in-continuity with microsurgical resection, followed by reconstruction. After the damaged, scarred nerve was removed, there was a 3 cm gap between healthy sections of the ulnar nerve (Fig. 4b). The patient retained three uninjured nerve fascicles which made up less than 20% of the normal diameter of the nerve. The healthy fascicles were dissected free and preserved (Fig. 5b). To bridge the nerve gap, the patient's sural nerve was harvested from her lower leg, cut into 3 cm long segments and bundled together to recreate the caliber and fascicles of the resected ulnar nerve (Fig. 5). This cabled sural nerve autograft was sutured into place using a surgical microscope and 9–0 Nylon sutures.

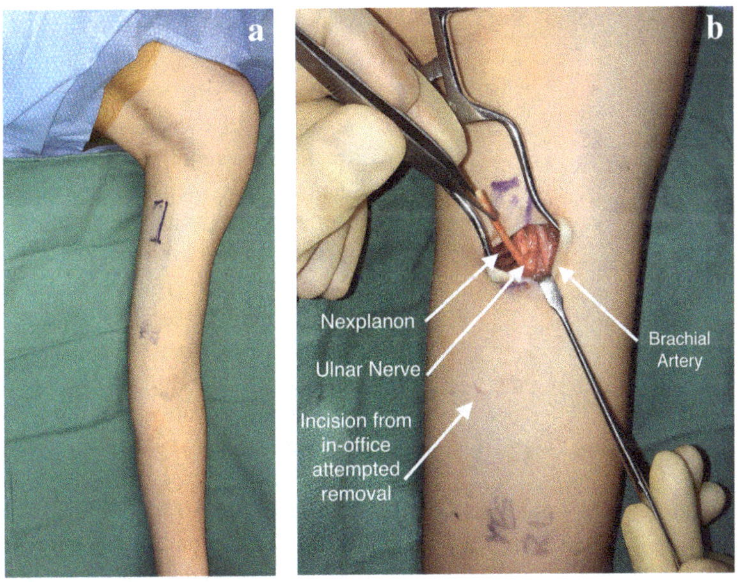

Fig. 3 Nexplanon removal. The location of the Nexplanon was marked using intra-operative fluoroscopy before incision (**a**). Surgical removal of the Nexplanon was then undertaken at this location (**b**). The ulnar nerve was just deep to the Nexplanon and the brachial artery was in close proximity. Note the location of the Nexplanon in relation to the incision used for the attempted in-office removal

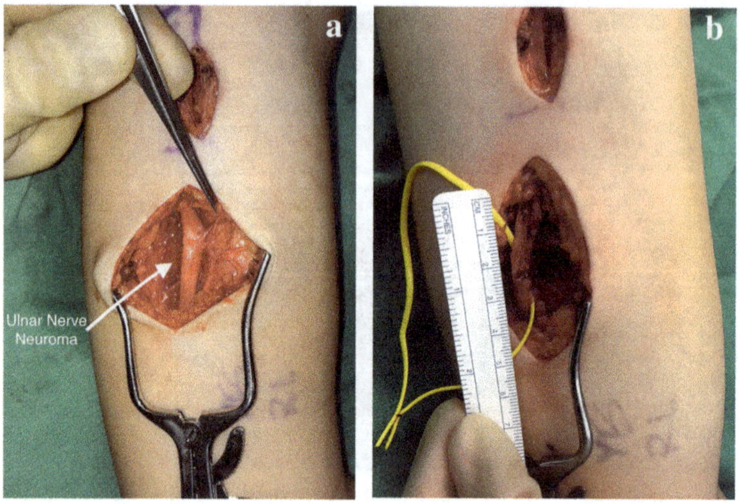

Fig. 4 Identification and resection of ulnar nerve neuroma. An ulnar nerve neuroma in continuity was identified by fusiform swelling and fibrotic nerve (**a**). After resection of the traumatic neuroma, 3 undamaged deep ulnar nerve fascicles were left intact, but a 3 cm gap was left in the majority of the nerve (**b**)

At 7 months after nerve reconstruction, the patient had weak grade 2/5 function of ulnar innervated muscles. She still had dense numbness in an ulnar nerve distribution. She did have an advancing Tinel's sign on physical exam and reported intermittent paresthesias in an ulnar nerve distribution in her hand.

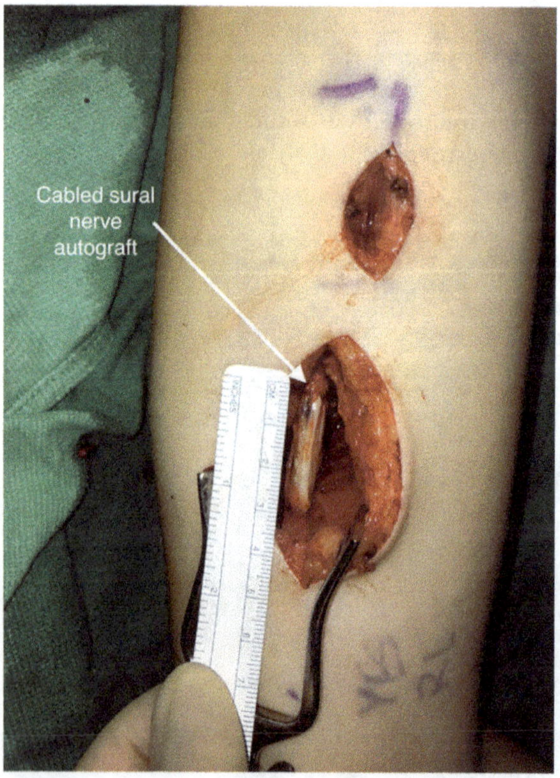

Fig. 5 Ulnar nerve reconstruction using cabled autologous sural nerve graft. Sural nerve autograft was harvested from the patient's leg and used to create a reversed, cabled nerve graft of matching length and diameter. It was placed into the ulnar nerve defect using a surgical microscope, 9–0 Nylon sutures, and fibrin glue

Discussion and conclusions

The presented case is an example of an uncommon, but serious complication from implantable contraception. Peripheral nerve injury from any cause often carries a poor prognosis and causes significant disability for patients. For this patient, both deep implantation and in-office removal of a non-palpable device contributed to the iatrogenic nerve injury. The medial arm is a dense anatomic area where precise device implantation and extraction are required to maximize patient safety. Our patient's limited recover 7 months after nerve reconstruction is unfortunately not uncommon: the prognosis for recovery after repair or reconstruction is particularly poor for the ulnar nerve [16, 17]. Prompt diagnosis and treatment is crucial to preserve treatment options and maximize a patient's outcome. It is also important to keep in mind that delayed or incomplete treatment of nerve injuries, particularly of iatrogenic nerve injuries, can result in significant liability [18, 19].

Peripheral nerves of the arm can be at risk with either insertion or extraction of a contraceptive implant into the arm. The majority of cases have been described with older implantable devices. Specifically, Norplant has been reported to cause transient paresthesias that resolve with removal [20, 21]. Norplant removal has be associated with ulnar nerve injury and with significant scar tissue around the ulnar nerve causing nerve compression with motor and sensory symptoms [22]. Implanon® (Organon International INC, Roseland, NJ) insertion and removal has been linked to sensory-only medial antebrachial cutaneous nerve injury, medial cutaneous nerve of the forearm injury, and transient ulnar nerve sensory deficit after device removal [6, 8, 23]. And, as in our case, the currently available Nexplanon® with it's updated delivery system and specific insertion and removal technique has been associated with median nerve injury in two cases [3]. Other recently reported cases do not mention the specific device used, but describe injury to the median nerve, medial antebrachial cutaneous, and ulnar nerves in a single patient and structural injury to the ulnar nerve in another patient [4, 5].

We emphatically agree with the current manufacturer recommendations: insertion should avoid the sulcus between the biceps and triceps where the median nerve, ulnar nerve, brachial artery and vein are located [10]. Furthermore, our case strongly supports the manufacturer's recommendation that extraction should not be attempted without knowing the exact location of the device [10]. It is the senior author's opinion that in-office placement and removal should be performed or directly supervised by an experienced physician who has undergone the appropriate implant-based training.

Since deep implantation and migration are possible, imaging studies should be used to precisely localize migrated or non-palpable devices before removal. In one paper describing operative removal of 28 implantable contraceptive devices, 30% of implants had migrated from the insertion site with 37% lying intramuscular and 11% lying in the neurovascular sheath [8]. Imaging studies should also be done for any patient who develops neurologic symptoms. X-ray, CT, MRI, and ultrasound can all be used to precisely identify an implant's location. X-ray and ultrasound are both inexpensive, accessible, and non-invasive imaging modalities. While ultrasound offers a zero-radiation technique for localization, X-ray machines and radiologist interpretation are widely available and relatively inexpensive. Although X-ray does involve ionizing radiation, two standard views of the humerus only exposes a patient to 0.001 mSv of radiation [24]. This is the same amount of radiation an average US habitant sees by simply being exposed to our environment for 3 h [24].

Multidisciplinary care involving family planning practitioners and peripheral nerve surgeons for complex removal improves patient care and optimizes safety [25]. Nerve surgeons can have a hand surgery, orthopaedic surgery, plastic surgery, or neurosurgery background. Symptoms that can indicate an iatrogenic nerve injury at the time of placement or removal include electric or shock-like pain, numbness, or weakness in the distribution of a peripheral nerve. Physical exam findings can include decreased sensation to touch and hand or forearm weakness. Late signs of untreated nerve injury include visible muscle wasting or abnormal posturing such as our patient's ulnar claw hand.

Prompt referral to a peripheral nerve surgeon is crucial because the motor end plates and end target muscles irreversibly degenerate without nerve input [26]. After nerve repair or grafting, nerves regenerate at a rate of approximately 1 mm per day [26]. As a rule of thumb, if the newly advancing axons do not reach the muscle by 12 months after injury, the damage is permanent and no meaningful functional recovery is made [26].

Even though there are surgical options for timely nerve repair and reconstruction, normal sensation and strength almost never return. Loss of ulnar nerve function is devastating for patients as the ulnar nerve is responsible for extrinsic and intrinsic hand muscles, as well as crucial hand sensation [27]. Sural nerve autograft is the current gold standard in major peripheral nerve reconstruction. Taking the sensory sural nerve from the leg universally results in lateral foot numbness [26]. In addition, a small percentage of patients have lasting neuropathic pain from this iatrogenic sural nerve injury [26].

In conclusion, Nexplanon® related major peripheral nerve injuries are an uncommon but possible complication. We recommend documenting the precise location of the implant with careful physical exam after insertion and before extraction. If a patient develops nerve symptoms in the setting of a non-palpable implant or migrated device, imaging and prompt referral to a peripheral nerve and upper extremity surgeon is strongly recommended. Experienced referral centers can be located by contacting the manufacturer.

Author's contributions

RL assisted in operative and perioperative care of the patient. RL was a major contributor in writing the manuscript, reviewing the literature, and creating figs. MH was a major contributor in writing the manuscript and reviewing the literature. HL assisted in operative care of the patient. He provided clinical images and contributed to writing and editing the manuscript. MS was the attending physician for the patient for the patient's perioperative and operative care. He contributed to manuscript outline and editing. All authors read, edited, and approved the final manuscript.

Author details

[1]Department of Orthopaedic Surgery, Division of Hand Surgery, University of Southern California, 1200 N State Street A7-CT, Los Angeles, CA 90033, USA. [2]Department of Obstetrics and Gynecology, University of Southern California, 2020 Zonal Ave., IRD Room 512, Los Angeles, CA 90033, USA. [3]Department of Plastic and Reconstructive Surgery, University of Southern California, 1510 San Pablo St., Suite 415, Los Angeles, CA 90033, USA.

References

1. Belyea C, Ernat J, Gumboc R. Removal of a contraceptive implant from the brachial neurovascular sheath. J Hand Surg [Am]. 2017;42:e115–7.

2. Christensen JM, Caggiano NM, Giladi AM, Iorio ML. Median nerve injury after removal of subdermal implantable contraceptive. Hand (N Y). 2017; https://doi.org/10.1177/1558944717744335.
3. Gillies R, Scougall P, Nicklin S. Etonogestrel implants - case studies of median nerve injury following removal. Aust Fam Physician. 2011;40:799–800.
4. O'Grady EE, Power DM. Ulnar nerve injury on removal of a contraceptive implant. Practitioner. 2016;260:21–4.
5. Restrepo CE, Spinner RJ. Major nerve injury after contraceptive implant removal: case illustration. J Neurosurg. 2016;124:188–9.
6. Wechselberger G, Wolfram D, Pulzl P, Soelder E, Schoeller T. Nerve injury caused by removal of an implantable hormonal contraceptive. Am J Obstet Gynecol. 2006;195:323–6.
7. Creinin MD, Kaunitz AM, Darney PD, Schwartz L, Hampton T, Gordon K, Rakers H. The US estrogestrel implant mandatory clinical training and active monitoring programs: 6-year experience. Contraception. 2017;95:205–10.
8. Vidin E, Garbin O, Rodriguez B, Favre R, Bettahar-Lebugle K. Removal of estogestrel contraceptive implants in the operating theater: report on 28 cases. Contraception. 2007;76:35–9.
9. Kang S, Niak A, Gada N, Brinker A, Jones SC. Etonogestrel implant migration to the vasculature, chest wall, and distant body sites: cases from a pharmacovigilance database. Contraception. 2017;96:439–45.
10. Merck. Nexplanon prescribing information. New Jersey: Whitehouse Station; 2017. p. 1–23.
11. Mommers E, Blum GF, Gent TG, Peters KP, Sordal TS, Marintcheva-Petrova M. Nexplanon, a radiopaque etonogestrel implant in combination with a next-generation applicator: 3 year results of a noncomparative multicenter trial. Am J Obstet Gynecol. 2012;207(388):e381–6.
12. Bragg TW, Jose RM, Bland JW, Matthews RN, Srivastava S. Implantable contraceptive devices: primum non nocere. J Fam Plann Reprod Health Care. 2006;32:190–2.
13. Mansour D. Nexplanon: what Implanon did next. J Fam Plann Reprod Health Care. 2010;36:187–9.
14. Park SY, Kang JW, Yang DH, Lim TH. Intracardiac migration of a Kirschner wire: case report and literature review. Int J Card Imaging. 2011;27:85–8.
15. Pillai M, Gazet AC, Griffiths M. Continuing need for and provision of a service for non-standard implant removal. J Fam Plann Reprod Health Care. 2014;40:126–32.
16. He B, Zhu Z, Zhu Q, Zhou X, Zheng C, Li P, Zhu S, Zhu J. Factors predicting sensory and motor recovery in the repair of upper limb peripheral nerve injuries. Neural Regen Res. 2014;2014(6)
17. Ruijs AC, Jaquet JB, Kalmijn S, Giele H, Sovius SE. Median and ulnar nerve injuries: a meta-analysis of predictors of motor and sensory recovery after modern microsurgical nerve repair. Plast Reconstr Surg. 2005;116:484–94.
18. Rowlands S. Legal aspects of contraceptive implants. J Fam Plann Reprod Health Care. 2010;36:243–8.
19. Rowlands S. Nerve injuries related to etonogestrel implant. Contraception. 2013;88:431.
20. Chang A, Edlich RF, Himel NH. Local reactions at the insertion site of the Norplant contraceptive system. J Long-Term Eff Med Implants. 1993;3:305–12.
21. Hueston WJ, Locke KT. Norplant neuropathy: peripheral neurologic symptoms associated with subdermal contraceptive implants. J Fam Pract. 1995;40:184–6.
22. Marin R, McMillian D. Ulnar neuropathy associated with subdermal contraceptive implant. South Med J. 1998;91:875–8.
23. Brown M, Britton J. Neuropathy associated with etonogestrel implant insertion. Contraception. 2012;86:591–3.
24. Radiological Society of North America Inc. Radiology Info for Patients. 2018 2/20/18]; Available from: https://www.radiologyinfo.org/en/pdf/safety-xray.pdf.
25. Odom EB, Eisenberg DL, Fox IK. Difficult removal of subdermal contraceptive implants: a multidisciplinary approach involving a peripheral nerve expert. Contraception. 2017;96:89–95.
26. Birch R, Quick T, Nerve injury and repair in Green's Operative Hand Surgery 2017: Philadelphia.
27. Kim S, Moran SL. Ulnar Nerve Repair. In: Slutsky D, editor. Upper extremity nerve repair - tips and techniques: a master skills publication. Rosemont: ASSH; 2008. p. 113–24.

6

Perception, pattern of use, partner support and determinants of uptake of family planning methods among women in rural communities in Southeast Nigeria

Ifeyinwa Chizoba Akamike[1*], Ugochukwu Chinyem Madubueze[1], Ijeoma Nkem Okedo-Alex[1], Chika Julius Anyigor[1], Benedict Ndubueze Azuogu[1,2], Chukwuma David Umeokonkwo[1] and Chinyere Ojiugo Mbachu[3]

Abstract

Background: Family planning is a cost-effective strategy for achieving population development. Family planning uptake is low in sub-Saharan Africa, including Nigeria. We assessed the perception, pattern of use, partner support and determinants of uptake of family planning methods among married women of reproductive age in rural communities of Ebonyi state.

Methods: This is part of a baseline report of a quasi-experimental study. A total of 484 married women of reproductive age were recruited using multistage sampling method. Four focus group discussions (men and women) and pre-tested semi-structured interviewer-administered questionnaires were used to collect information from the participants. Data were analysed using Statistical Package for Social Sciences (SPSS) version 20 software and thematic analysis. Chi-square test and logistic regression were carried out at 5% significance level.

Results: Only 26.2% of respondents were currently using any method of family planning. The most commonly used method was the natural method (57%). Amongst those who reported using artificial methods, 32.7% used condoms, 27.3% used implant while 23.64 and 16.4% used injectables and pills respectively. Predictors of current use of any family planning method were: older age (AOR = 1.7, 95%CI = 1.01–3.00), having more than five children (AOR = 1.7, 95%CI = 1.05–2.83), minimum of secondary level of education for respondent (AOR = 3.3, CI = 1.60–6.96) and their husband/partner (AOR = 2.0, 95%CI = 1.05–3.92). Qualitative findings showed that only few families were using a method of family planning and those who did not practice family planning perceived it to interfere with God's plan for fruitfulness and to be counter-productive to household income due to decreased manpower for agricultural activities. Poor partner involvement and support for family planning was also cited as a deterrent by both male and female participants.

(Continued on next page)

* Correspondence: ifeyakamike@gmail.com
[1]Department of Community Medicine, Alex Ekwueme Federal University Teaching Hospital, Abakaliki, Ebonyi State, Nigeria

(Continued from previous page)

Conclusions: Perception and use of family planning methods is poor in rural communities of Ebonyi state. Improving uptake of family planning methods in these rural communities will require proper demographic targeting as well as debunking fatalistic views, and cultural and religious myths around family planning.

Keywords: Perception, Pattern of use, Partner support, Determinants, Family planning

Background

Family planning allows people to attain their desired number of children and determine the spacing of pregnancies. This is achieved through the use of family planning methods and treatment of infertility [1, 2]. Family planning is voluntary, and available methods of contraception (previously referred to as birth control) can be customized to individual needs with a range of methods that are acceptable to all and effective if used correctly [2]. The choice and use of a particular family planning method and their sources vary globally. Family planning can be categorized into two: natural and artificial methods. The natural methods include abstinence, coitus interruptus, safe period, and lactational amenorrhoea. Common artificial methods used are; condoms, injectables, pills and Intra Uterine Contraceptive Devices (IUCD) [1]. Over200 million women of reproductive age in developing countries who want to avoid pregnancy are not using a modern contraceptive method [1–3]. This is due to limited choice of methods; limited access to contraception, particularly among young people, poorer segments of populations, or unmarried people; fear or experience of side-effects; cultural or religious opposition; poor quality of available services; user and provider bias and, gender-based barriers [1].

Globally, among the 1.9 billion women of reproductive age (15–49 years) living in the world in 2019, 1.1 billion have a need for family planning. Of the number who need family planning, 842 million (44%) use artificial methods of contraception, 80 million use traditional methods of family planning, while 190 million (10%) women have an unmet need for contraception [4]. In 2018, the prevalence rate for any contraceptive use among Nigerian women was 17% and this was more among sexually active single women (28%) than currently married women (12%) [5]. Although currently married women may have more sexual exposure, overall contraceptive use has only marginally increased from 15% in 2013 to 17% in 2018 while use of any modern method of contraception also increased, from 10 to 12%. In addition, there has been a slight rise in the use of implants since 2008, from 0 to 3% [5].

Some studies have reported variations in preference and pattern of use of family planning methods. In south-eastern Asia, the most common contraceptive method used was Intra-uterine device, 18.6% of women rely on this method [4]. In Europe and Northern America, the pill and female condom are the most commonly used methods (17.8 and 14.6% of women, respectively), while in Latin America and the Caribbean it is female sterilization and the pill (16.0 and 14.9%, respectively) [4]. Sub-Saharan Africa is the only region in which injectables are the dominant method with a prevalence of 9.6% among women of reproductive age [4]. A three year review of pattern of contraceptive use among women aged 15 to 52 years in southwest Nigeria revealed that majority (46.3%) preferred Jadelle implant while the least used implant was Norplant (0.5%) [6]. In that study married women were more likely to seek family planning methods and the motivating factor was based on the increasing challenge in raising children and the need to reduce family size [6].

Although there has been slight improvement in contraceptive use in Nigeria, the uptake is still very low. The Nigerian demographic health survey of 2018 reported a contraceptive uptake ranging from 2 to 7% for Ebonyi State with lower values in rural areas compared to urban areas [5]. Therefore, this study seeks to understand the perception, pattern of use, partner support and determinants of uptake of family planning methods among married women in rural areas of Ebonyi state, Nigeria. Findings from this study will be useful in informing the design of family planning interventions for married women in similar rural contexts.

Materials and methods

Study area

The study was conducted in Igbeagu in Izzi local government area (LGA) and Ezzamgbo in Ohaukwu LGA, both in Ebonyi State in South Eastern Nigeria. The State has a land mass of about 5935 km^2. Majority of the people of Ebonyi State live in the rural area and are predominantly of Roman Catholic faith. About 75% of the population is involved in some form of agriculture, and this constitutes the key occupation of people in the study communities where there is a preference for crops such as rice, yam, cassava, maize and some other economic crops. The staple foods include locally prepared cassava, rice, and yam. Family planning services are provided at all levels of healthcare in the State.

Study design

This is part of a baseline report of a quasi-experimental study. Detailed description of the study design has been published elsewhere [7].

Study population

The study population included women of reproductive age (15–49 years) who were either married or in a union. Pregnant women were excluded from the study. Women within the reproductive age, who had achieved menopause, were also excluded.

Sample size and sampling technique

A total of 484 women of reproductive age were approached to participate in this survey. Respondents were selected from the two rural LGAs in Ebonyi north senatorial zone using a multistage sampling technique. Detailed description of the sample size determination and sampling technique have been presented in another paper [7].

Data collection

A pre-tested, semi structured interviewer administered questionnaire was used to collect information from respondents. Information collected include socio-demographic characteristics of the respondents such as age, level of education and spouse's level of education; use of family planning; pattern of use including method used, frequency of use and duration of use. The focus group discussion (FGD) was used to better understand community perceptions and practices (including sources) of family planning and to explore in-depth the factors that influence acceptability and use of modern methods of family planning. A total of four FGDs were conducted, two for the men and two for the women. Participants for the FGD were married and within the reproductive age group. Men and women who are outspoken and willing to participate were identified and purposively selected with the help of community health workers. Outspoken people were selected for the FGD because of the need to explore in-depth and so required people who can articulate and voice out their opinions so as to better understand the phenomenon under study. A total of seven questions with probes were discussed. There were about 10–12 discussants per FGD. Permission was obtained from the discussants to audio record the sessions to assist the researcher obtain details of the discussion. The researcher was the moderator and a research assistant was the note-taker who recorded key issues raised in the sessions. Each FGD lasted about 35 min.

Measurement of variables

The independent variables were: socio-demographic and household characteristics of women such as age, level of education, religion, husband's education, number of living children, family type, household head and main decision maker on health issues. These variables were measured using the structured questionnaire. Age was measured using age as at last birthday. Mean and standard deviation were calculated for age. All the other independent variables were measured either on the nominal or ordinal scale and were later recoded into two categories. Frequencies and proportions were calculated for categorical variables. Religion was coded into two categories: Roman Catholic denomination and other denominations since only Christians participated in the survey.

The dependent variables include: pattern of use and uptake of family planning. Pattern of use was measured using self-reports of commonly used method of family planning (that is type of method used); frequency of use; and duration of use.

Uptake of modern methods of family planning refers to the use of modern methods of family planning. This was measured by: proportion currently using a method. Questions with "Yes" or "No" was used to determine respondents' uptake of family planning.

Data analysis

Quantitative data analysis was carried out using the Statistical Package for Social Sciences (SPSS) for the Microsoft Window version 20 software. Frequencies and proportions were calculated for categorical variables while means and standard deviations were calculated for numeric/quantitative variables. Chi square test was carried out to determine relationships between categorical variables and statistical significance was said to be present at *P* value of less than 0.05. The independent variables were socio-demographic characteristics of women (age category, level of education, partner's/husband's education, number of living children, and religion). The dependent variables were uptake of any family planning method and pattern of use of family planning methods.

Qualitative data analysis commenced with verbatim transcription of audio recordings and review of transcripts with hand-written notes to ensure completeness of information and inclusion of non-verbal responses. Pre-conceived themes were then generated from the interview guide to develop a coding framework. The four transcripts were then read to achieve familiarization and identify any themes that were not in the coding framework. The final coding framework was then applied to all 4 transcripts. The themes in the final coding framework are: i) Perceptions of family planning and artificial methods of contraception, ii) Attitude towards artificial methods of family planning and methods commonly used, iii) Partner involvement in family planning.

Table 1 Socio-demographic and household characteristics of respondents

Variable	*n* = 484	(%)
Age (Mean ± SD)	29.2 ± 6.1	
Religious denomination		
Roman Catholic	278	57.4
Other denominations	206	42.6
Educational level		
Primary and less	99	20.5
Secondary and more	385	79.5
Spouse's Educational level		
Primary and less	104	21.5
Secondary and more	380	78.5
Number of living children		
< 5 children	348	71.9
≥ 5 children	136	28.1
Type of household		
Monogamous	443	91.5
Polygamous	41	8.5
Household head		
Husband/partner	458	94.6
Others*	26	5.4
Decision maker on health matters		
Husband/partner	449	92.80
Others*	35	7.20

*father in-law, mother in-law, Self, Parents

Result

Table 1 shows the socio-demographic characteristics of the respondents. Mean age of the respondents was 29.2 ± 6.1. Over half (57.4%) of the respondents were of the Roman Catholic denomination. Majority of the respondents and their spouses had at least secondary education. Greater proportion (71.9%) of the respondents had less than five children. Almost all the respondents (91.5%) were in a monogamous family setting. The husband/partner was the household head and decision maker on health matters for most of the respondents (94.6 and 92.8% respectively). Figure 1 shows that only 26.2% of the respondents were using a method of family planning. In Table 2, among those using a method of family planning, majority were using the natural method and amongst the 43% who reported using artificial methods, 32.7% used condoms, 27.3% used implant while 23.64 and 16.4% used injectables and pills respectively. Most of those using any method of family planning did so consistently (79.53%) and had used a method for at least 6 months (77.17%). Older age (AOR = 1.7, 95%CI = 1.01–3.00), having more than five children (AOR = 1.7, 95%CI = 1.05–2.83), and attaining secondary education by husband (AOR = 2.0, 95%CI = 1.05–3.92), and respondent (AOR = 3.3, CI = 1.60–6.96) were predictors of use of family planning methods (Table 3).

FGD result

Perceptions of family planning and artificial methods of contraception

Majority of the respondents demonstrated a good knowledge of family planning and its benefits. They reported that family planning is used for child spacing and is beneficial for child health and family size. Some supporting quotes are: "*Family planning is a way of delaying pregnancy so that the child grows before another comes*" (Female).

> "*It* (family planning) *helps women take care of the children and also helps them decide the number of children to have*" (Female).

However, contraception is not practiced by families in the community due to fatalistic reasons and

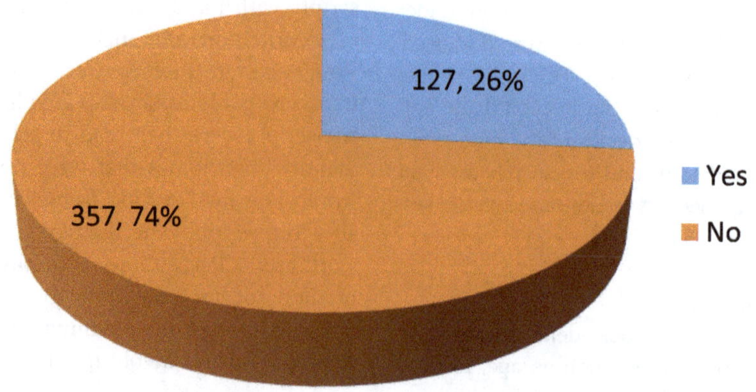

Fig. 1 Proportion of respondents using a method of family planning

Table 2 Pattern of use of family planning methods

Variable	*n* = 127	%
Method used		
Natural method	72	56.60
Artificial method	55	43.40
Type of artificial method used		
Pills	9	16.36
Barrier	18	32.72
Injectable	13	23.64
Implant	15	27.27
Frequency of use of any family planning method		
Consistent	101	79.53
When affordable	3	2.36
If I remember	11	8.66
If partner permits	12	9.45
Duration of use of any method of family planning		
< 6 months	29	22.83
6- < 12 months	17	13.39
1–5 years	61	48.03
> 5 years	20	15.75

misconceptions about side effects of modern methods of contraception. One respondent said:

> *"Some families in this community do not accept family planning because they believe it causes bleeding and barrenness"* (Female).

Some respondents stated that people may not practice family planning because they believe that limiting family size has negative implications for economic and food productivity of the household. Also, family planning goes against God's plan of fruitfulness and the church does not support modern methods of contraception.

> *"Villagers say it is not good, people should deliver all the children in their womb, be it 10 or 20. Children should fill the home so that farming would be more productive and there will be food everywhere. If family planning is done, there will be no productivity and thus hunger"*(Female).

The respondents also reported the position of their religious denominations about family planning. Some affirmed that the church supports only the natural method of family planning. *"Church says if you stop it will make church members to be small. The bible says go and fill the earth so give birth to all in your womb. Church says go natural but modern methods are not natural"* (Female).

The men also appeared to share similar views as the women with respect to family planning and contraception. For instance, they perceived limiting family size as interfering with God's plan for procreation. They were also of the opinion that having more children is a form of assurance in the event of death. In the words of one of the men,

> *"Family planning is not good. If God has said you'll have many children and you do family planning and have only two, if one dies, you'll be left with only one. We should allow God so that we can have the number of children he wants us to have"*(Male).

Participants also highlighted that women who practiced family planning were perceived as being selfish and denying men their rights and reported as follows:

> *"The men do not accept it, they feel they're being denied their right"* (Female).

Others stated that it is believed that women who make use of family planning do not have feelings for their spouses. One of the respondents quoted as follows: *"Some people do not accept family planning. They believe that women who have done family planning do not have feelings for their husbands"* (Male).

Table 3 Predictors of uptake of any family planning method

Independent variable	AOR	CI
Age in years		
≥ 35 years	1.7	1.01–3.00
< 35 years	1	
Respondent's education		
≥ Secondary	3.3	1.60–6.96
≤ primary	1	
Spouse's education		
≥ Secondary	2.0	1.05–3.92
≤ primary	1	
Number of living children		
≥ 5 children	1.7	1.05–2.83
< 5 children	1	
Religion		
Other denominations	1.1	0.73–1.70
Roman catholic denomination	1	

Attitude towards artificial methods of family planning and methods commonly used

Attitude towards artificial methods of family planning was reported to be generally poor. The attitudes of the respondents towards family planning arise from perceptions about side effects which appeared to vary depending on the type of contraceptive. One of the male respondents commented as follows:

> *"Men feel negative impact, for example, Condom they say it can burst and if it bursts can lead to disease; if injectable is used it leads to difficulty in getting pregnant; and IUD leads to bleeding"* (Male).

However, the women had genuine concerns about the side effects of modern methods of contraception that influence their attitude. One of the women said:

> *"It is good but has much side effects, fat, ceases menses and if it comes there's heavy flow, enlargement of breast"* (Female)

The respondents also revealed the fact that community support for family planning is lacking. Some men in the community could go to the extent of sending their wives away because of family planning. One of the supporting quotes is shown below:

> *"Villagers say husbands won't agree when wife does it, and when some wives do it their husbands chase them away"* (Male).

Although a few of the participants stated that they use artificial methods of family planning, majority of them preferred and used natural methods. Some of the reasons for the preference of natural method were perception of safety, effectiveness and absence of side effects. Additionally, some women stated that their partners did not oppose natural methods.

> *" ... Natural method is safer and has no side effect"*(Male)

> *" ... Natural method is what I will use, it is the best"*(Male)

Women who used modern methods did so for various reasons. Some had no ugly experiences or adverse effects from the methods they used and therefore continued using these methods. Some of their quotes are shown below:

> *" ... I use Condom, it has no side effects and my husband does not complain"*(Female);

> *" ... I use implants and no much side effects, once removed, I take in"* (Female)

Partner involvement in family planning

The respondents reported that family planning is not discussed except among literate men. Most of the men do not want to discuss about family planning especially when they have not completed their family size. Many men do not support nor give approval for their wives to practice family planning. Some supporting quotes are:

> *"I have a friend that has six children but as soon as she mentioned family planning to her husband, he shouted at her and bluntly refused"*. (Female)

> *"The men see having as many children as they want as their right and so any one talking about family planning is like an enemy"*(Male)

Although discussions around family planning in the home are raised by women, a few of the participants affirmed that when they discuss family planning with their husbands they are supportive of their choices, even if it takes a while to happen. *"My husband and I talk about it and decide on which method to use .... Females are always the ones that bring it up"*(Female)

> *"My husband told me it is good to wait for 2-3 years so he will save enough and I agreed. My husband pays for it"*.(Female)

Discussion

This study assessed the perception, pattern of use, and partner support for family planning and equally identified predictors of uptake of family planning.

This study revealed that only few of the respondents were using any method of family planning at the time of the survey and majority of these were using the natural method. Previous studies have also reported low family planning use [8–16]. Uptake of family planning is still low in developing countries including Nigeria [5]. The low uptake reported in the quantitative survey was also affirmed by the FGD participants. Although all of the women who participated in the FGDs perceived family planning as beneficial, they reported that most families did not practice it. FGD respondents expressed various reasons for not using contraceptives. Some of the reasons given for non-use of family planning methods include: desire for more children, fear of side effects, religious beliefs and the fact that reduction in family size has a negative effect on economic and food productivity. This shows the need to identify and intensify interventions which are multi-sectoral to increase uptake of family planning.

Use of natural method by majority of the respondents is a pointer to the fact that these women are probably having fears about side effects of modern methods. The

FGD respondents also concurred with the fact that natural method of family planning is mostly encouraged in the community with majority having a generally poor attitude towards the artificial methods. Consequently, it is necessary that information on various methods of family planning including their mechanisms of action be included in the content of the health education usually delivered to women both during antenatal, post natal clinics, and during community outreaches. It may also be of benefit to pay attention to teaching women about the natural family planning method so that those who choose this method can use it correctly and effectively. Additionally, unavailability and cost of artificial methods could also play a role in the preference for natural methods. Among those using a method of family planning, majority were consistent in using a method. This finding disagrees with a study carried out in Rivers State which showed that only 22.6% of respondents used a method consistently [17]. This disparity may be due to the fact that the study in Rivers State assessed only use of modern methods of contraceptives. It's been shown that women's use-related behaviors, especially the consistency with which they take pills is associated with effectiveness of contraceptives [18].

The independent variables found to predict the use of family planning methods in this study were age, respondents' education, husband's education, and number of living children. Those that were ≥ 35 years were 1.7 times more likely to use a method of family planning than those who were less than 35 years. This may be because older women might have completed their family size considering the fact that women marry early in the African culture, particularly those who live in the rural areas [5, 19, 20].

Husband's education was positively correlated with current use of family planning for those with at least secondary-level of education compared to those with a primary-level of education or less. This is similar to the finding in a study carried out in Pakistan which reported that husband's education positively correlated with current contraceptive use among women [21]. The FGD further supports the fact that education has an influence on family planning use as some women reported that family planning discussions come up mainly among literate men. This study further revealed that men were the main decision makers on health matters. This was further buttressed by the FGD respondents. Therefore, the importance of men's education cannot be overemphasized because it has a huge role to play in improving uptake of family planning and other health services. Partner support for family planning including spousal communication is a crucial factor that can influence use [15, 21, 22]. Evidence shows that men's awareness of, and support for, use of contraceptives are associated with their spouses' desire to use contraception [23]. It is therefore essential to address the problem of literacy among men while also emphasizing female education. Some FGD respondents however stated that they get their husband's support even if it takes some time to convince them. This shows the need for persistence in the efforts to improve male involvement in family planning.

Those that had five or more children were more likely to be family planning users. This finding was also supported by the FGD respondents who believed that women should have as many children as they want, it is therefore unlikely for women who have few children or who have not achieved their desired family size to use a method of family planning. A Ghanaian study found a positive predictive correlation between number of living children and uptake in a study on correlates of contraceptive use among women of reproductive age [24].

Although religion has been reported as a factor that affects uptake of family planning [9, 12, 25] and our FGD also reported religion as a reason for non-use, paradoxically, religion was not found to be a predictor of family planning use in this study. This could be because individuals are beginning to take decisions that are beneficial to their health without being clouded by the decision of third parties.

One strength of this study is that it employed a mixed method design which makes it possible to understand better the topic under study. This study was however carried out in rural communities and therefore limits the extent to which the findings can be generalized.

Conclusion

The study has shown that natural family planning methods were most used with age, parity, self and partner education as predictors of current use of any method. Religion on the contrary was not found to be a predictor of family planning. Desire for more children, fear of side effects, religious beliefs and the perceived negative effect of small family size on economic and food productivity are some reasons why uptake of family planning is low in rural communities. Improving uptake of family planning methods in these rural communities will require proper demographic targeting as well as debunking fatalistic views, and cultural and religious myths around family planning. Family planning interventions should therefore target older and grand-multiparous women. It is also necessary to explore ways of improving the educational status of men and women in the community.

Abbreviations

SPSS: Statistical Package for Social Sciences (IBM-SPSS); IUCD: Intrauterine Contraceptive Device; LGA: Local Government Area; FGD: Focus Group Discussion

Acknowledgements
Not applicable.

Authors' contributions
ICA, BNA and COM worked on study conception and design. ICA, COM and INO led efforts for data collection activities. ICA, COM, CDU conducted data analysis and interpretation. The first draft of the manuscript was written and prepared by ICA, UCM, INO and CA. All authors significantly contributed to, and approved of, the final version.

Author details
[1]Department of Community Medicine, Alex Ekwueme Federal University Teaching Hospital, Abakaliki, Ebonyi State, Nigeria. [2]Department of Community Medicine, Ebonyi State University, Abakaliki, Nigeria. [3]Department of Community Medicine, College of Medicine, University of Nigeria, Nsukka, Nigeria.

References

1. World Health Organisation. Family planning / contraception factsheet. http://www.who.int/mediacentre/factsheets/fs351/en/ Accessed July 2016.
2. WHO | The ABC's of family planning. WHO. World Health Organization; 2013.
3. Pack AP, McCarraher DR, Chen M, Okigbo CC, Albert LM, Wambugu S. Factors associated with unmet need for modern contraception in post-conflict Liberia. Afr J Reprod Health. 2014;18(2):58–67.
4. United Nations, Department of Economic and Social Affairs. Contraceptive Use by Method 2019 Data Booklet. 2019. www.un.org › sites › files › documents › Jan › u...Accessed March 5 2020.
5. National Population Commission. Nigeria Demographic And Health Survey 2018. 2018.
6. Okunade K, Daramola E, Ajepe A, Sekumade A. A 3-year review of the pattern of contraceptive use among women attending the family planning clinic of a university teaching hospital in Lagos, Nigeria African. J Med Heal Sci. 2016;15(2):69.
7. Akamike IC, Mbachu C, Onwasigwe C, Okedo-Alex I, Eze I, Eze N. Role of community resource persons in improving use of modern family planning methods among women of reproductive age in a rural area in Ebonyi state, Nigeria. Int J Health Plann Manage. 2019:1–10.
8. Nwachukwu I, Obasi OO. Use of modern birth control methods among rural communities in Imo state, Nigeria. Afr J Reprod Health. 2008;12(1):101–8.
9. Oye-Adeniran BA, Adewole IF, Umoh A, Oladokun A, Gbadegesin A, Ekanem EE, et al. Community-based study of contraceptive behaviour in Nigeria. Afr J Reprod Health. 2006;10(2):90–104.
10. Sanusi A, Akinyemi O, Onoviran O. Do knowledge and cultural perceptions of modern female contraceptives predict male involvement in Ayete, Nigeria? Afr J Reprod Health Women's Health Act Res Center. 2015;18:105–14.
11. Avidime S, Aku-Akai L, Mohammed A, Adaji S, Shittu O, Ejembi C. Fertility intentions, contraceptive awareness and contraceptive use among women in three communities in northern Nigeria. Afr J Reprod Health Women's Health Act Res Center. 2014;14:65–70.
12. Egede JO, Onoh RC, Umeora OUJ, Iyoke CA, Dimejesi IBO, Lawani LO. Contraceptive prevalence and preference in a cohort of south-east Nigerian women. Patient Prefer Adherence. 2015;9:707–14.
13. Doctor H, Findley SE, Afenyadu GY, Uzondu C, Ashir GM. Awareness, use, and unmet need for family planning in rural northern Nigeria. Afr J Reprod Health. 2013;17(4):107–17.
14. Wendo BM. Barriers to uptake of long term and permanent family planning methods among HIV infected postpartum mothers in Kenyatta national hospital. Department of Obstetrics and Gynaecology, University of Nairobi; 2013. http://erepository.uonbi.ac.ke/handle/11295/71463?show=full. Accessed Jan 2017.
15. Choge MC. Contraceptive uptake among women of reproductive age in Kakuma refugee camp in Turkana county, Kenya. Kenyatta University; 2012. http://ir-library.ku.ac.ke/handle/123456789/7680. Accessed April 2020.
16. Namazzi G. Missed Opportunities for Modern Family Planning Services among women attending Child health clinics in Iganga/ Mayuge Demographic Surveillance site. 2013. www.musphcdc.ac.ug › files › pdf ›. Accessed April 2020.
17. Osaro BO, Tobin-West CI, Mezie-Okoye MM. Knowledge of modern contraceptives and their use among rural women of childbearing age in Rivers state Nigeria. Ann Trop Med Public Heal. 2017;10(4):1043–8.
18. Benagiano G. Introduction: enhancing oral contraceptive compliance and efficacy. Adv Contracept. 1992;8(1):1–3.
19. National Bureau of Statistics and UNICEF. Multiple Indicator Cluster Survey 2016–17, Survey Findings Report. 2017.
20. UNFPA & UNICEF. Child Marriage in West and Central Africa: At a Glance. September 2018.
21. Azmat SK, Ali M, Ishaque M, Mustafa G, Hameed W, Khan OF, et al. Assessing predictors of contraceptive use and demand for family planning services in underserved areas of Punjab province in Pakistan: results of a cross-sectional baseline survey. Reprod Health. 2015;12(1):25.
22. Sileo KM. Determinants of family planning service uptake and use of contraceptives among postpartum women in rural Uganda. Int J Public Health. 2015;60(8):987–97.
23. Ezeanolue EE, Iwelunmor J, Asaolu I, Obiefune MC, Ezeanolue CO, Osuji A, et al. Impact of male partner's awareness and support for contraceptives on female intent to use contraceptives in Southeast Nigeria. BMC Public Health. 2015;15(1):879.
24. Nketiah-Amponsah E, Arthur E, Abuosi A. Correlates of contraceptive use among Ghanaian women of reproductive age (15-49 yrs). Afr J Reprod Health. 2012;16(3):154–69.
25. Ankomah A, Anyanti J, Adebayo S, Giwa A. Barriers to contraceptive use among married young adults in Nigeria : a qualitative study. Int J Trop Dis Health. 2013;3(3):267–82.

7

Prevalence and determinants of post-abortion family planning utilization in a tertiary Hospital of Northwest Ethiopia

Enyew Abate[1*], Yolanda R. Smith[2], Walelign Kindie[1], Addisu Girma[3] and Yonas Girma[4]

Abstract

Background: Provision of post abortion contraception following an abortion is an excellent opportunity to address unmet family planning needs of women. In Ethiopia, post abortion family planning is minimal and underutilized. The objective of this study is to assess determinant factors for utilization of contraception following any abortion process (induced and/or spontaneous) among reproductive age women (15–49 years) in a tertiary hospital of North West Ethiopia.

Methods: A cross-sectional study was conducted on 423 clients who presented for either spontaneous or induced abortion care from September 2016 to August 2017 in Felege Hiwot referral hospital, North West Ethiopia. Respondents were identified using a consecutive sampling method. Data was collected in clinic using an interviewer administered pre-tested questionnaire administered after services were completed. Factors associated with use of post-abortion family planning were explored using multivariable logistic regression analysis.

Results: 64.8% of clients who presented for abortion care received family planning services before discharge from the hospital. Family planning counseling during service provision [AOR: 25.47, 95% CI: (9.11, 71.58)], having previous information about family planning [AOR: 2.16, 95% CI: (1.09, 4.23)], gestational age of index pregnancy less than 3 months [AOR: 1.78, 95% CI:(1.13, 3.05)], being a housewife [AOR: 0.32, 95% CI: (0.16, 0.65)] and monthly income > 5000 ETB [AOR: 0.38, 95% CI:(0.16,0.98)] are significantly associated with post abortion family planning utilization.

Conclusions: The proportion of post abortion family planning utilization is good but could be improved. Education before and especially at the time of abortion services strongly influenced the usage of family planning services. The government and regional health bureau at large as well as health care providers at each health system level have an opportunity to provide information and counsel women on family planning methods to increase utilization of post abortion contraception.

Keywords: Post abortion family planning, Abortion services, Bahir Dar, Ethiopia

* Correspondence: enyewabate@gmail.com
[1]College of Medicine and Health Sciences, Department of Obstetrics and Gynecology, Bahir Dar University, Bahir Dar, Ethiopia

Background

The World Health Organization (WHO) estimates that abortion related complications are responsible for the deaths of approximately 800,000 women each year worldwide, which accounts for 19.6% of all maternal deaths [1, 2].

Ethiopia has one of the world's highest maternal mortality ratios, 412 per 100,000 live births [3]. In Ethiopia, 38% of pregnancies are unintended, with an estimated 620,300 induced abortions performed each year. Among these pregnancy terminations, 53% occur in health facilities and 47% are performed outside of health facilities [4].

Family planning is a successful strategy to address this issue, and overall prevents 32% of maternal deaths from all causes [5]. Post abortion family planning is family planning that is provided to clients or individuals after a spontaneous or an induced abortion [6]. This post abortion period is a time when women are highly motivated to avoid or delay another pregnancy [7, 8]. This provides an opportunity to offer services immediately after the provision of abortion care.

Most unwanted pregnancies in developing countries occur as a result of restricted access to family planning services [9, 10]. In Ethiopia, 22% of women have an unmet need for family planning [3]. Providing voluntary post abortion family planning options generally reduces subsequent unintended pregnancies and further decreases maternal mortality [1, 6]. A consensus statement developed by Post Abortion Care Consortium and International Conference on Population and Development (ICPD) stated that the pregnancy-abortion-pregnancy cycle must be broken by providing post-abortion contraception to those who are in need of it [11].

Multiple studies done in Asia, South America and Africa on post-abortion family planning utilization showed wide variations in use, ranging from 61 to 97% [10, 12, 13]. A cross-sectional study performed in three health facility based settings in Ethiopia demonstrated that 48–59% of clients left their institution with post-abortion family planning services which showed wide variations in the percentage of women who received post-abortion contraception [14–16]. In addition, comparative studies from countries outside Ethiopia reveal a greater acceptance and use of modern contraceptives in women who received post abortion family planning counseling and services relative to the no-program group [17–19].

Several factors are associated with women's decisions regarding starting post-abortion family planning. Studies done in Ethiopia indicate that urban residence, higher maternal education level, occupation, undergoing spontaneous abortion, receiving post abortion family planning counseling, good knowledge of family planning, and availability of family planning are significantly associated with uptake of family planning in the post-abortion period [16, 20–24].

Research performed around the world shows variation in the utilization of post-abortion family planning and type of methods offered and identified determinant factors. The majority of the research done in Ethiopia is community based and or health facility based studies.

No identified Ethiopian studies have sampled patients only from a tertiary teaching hospital to assess family planning utilization following abortion, where more complicated cases of abortion and women with advanced gestational age will come and where medical training occurs which may reflect what happens to the community after trainees leave.

Therefore, this study was done to provide information on the proportion and determinant factors for utilization of post abortion contraception in a tertiary teaching hospital in Ethiopia.

Methods and materials

Study setting, design and population

The study was an institutional cross-sectional study using quantitative data collection methods. It was conducted at Felege Hiwot referral hospital (FHRH), Bahir Dar, northwest Ethiopia from September 1, 2016 to August 31, 2017. FHRH is comprehensive specialized referral and teaching hospital found in Bahir Dar city, the capital of Amhara regional state which is located 563 Km away from the capital city Addis Ababa. It serves as referral hospital for South Gondar, East and West Gojjam, Awi zone and Benshangul Gumuz region providing service for about nine million populations.

We included all women who came for abortion care to get abortion services from FHRH. The sample size was calculated with the single population proportion formula: using 95% CL, 5% marginal error [25]. Using data on proportion of post-abortion family planning utilization done in Dessie, North East Ethiopia, which was 47.5% [15] and adding a 10% non-response rate, the planned sample size was 423.

Data collection

Women were approached sequentially by trained bachelor degree holder nurses after their clinical visit was completed and while preparing to leave the hospital, until the desired sample size was achieved. Women who consented to participate completed a semi-structured interviewer administered questionnaire with 24 questions. The questionnaire was initially prepared in English and translated to Amharic language on a printout paper. The questions covered socio demographic characteristics, reproductive performance, previous abortion history, previous knowledge and utilization of any contraceptive methods, interest in future fertility, current pregnancy and abortion related circumstances which were obtained from the clients and health care provider information which was obtained from the abortion registration logbook.

Data analysis

Data was entered and cleaned using Epi-data version 3.1, independently verified, exported and analysis was done using SPSS Version 22.0.

Descriptive statistics were used to assess the percentage of individual client characteristics and percentage of utilization of post-abortion family planning.

Bivariable analyses were performed, examining the association of selected independent variables with the outcome of post-abortion family planning utilization. Predictors with p values less than 0.25 were entered into subsequent multivariable models employing forward selection approach. The final multivariable logistic regression modelling was built by including predictors with p value less than 0.05 was undertaken to evaluate the net effects of set of predictor variables over the utilization of post abortion family planning.

Results

Sociodemographic characteristics

A total of 423 post abortion women participated in the study. Among the study participants, the majority of women were in the age group between 25 and 29 years (33.3%), resided in urban areas (58.9%), married (74%) and had access to at least one communication media (86.1%) (Table 1).

Table 1 Sociodemographic characteristics of study participants in Felege Hiwot referral hospital from Sep 2016- Aug 2017

Characteristics	Total	
	Number	Percent %)
Age in years		
Less than 19	62	14.7
20–24	111	26.2
25–29	141	33.3
30–34	63	14.9
> 35	46	10.9
Place of residence		
Urban	249	58.9
Rural	174	41.1
Current marital status		
Married	313	74
Not married	110	26
Religion		
Orthodox	361	85.3
Islam	57	13.5
Others	5	1.2
Educational status		
illiterate	162	38.3
Primary school	83	19.6
Secondary school	95	22.5
Higher education	83	19.6
Occupation		
Employed	117	27.7
Student	71	16.8
House wife	132	31.2
Daily laborer	27	6.4
Farmer	76	17.9
Monthly income in birr[a]		
< 5000	372	87.9
≥ 5000	51	12.1
Availability of communication media		
Yes	364	86.1
No	59	13.9

[a]One Ethiopian Birr is 0.027 United states Dollar as of September 22, 2020

Obstetric and contraceptive history

Among the women participants, most of them had no child, had no previous abortion and wanted to be pregnant with in the next 6 months following the abortion process. Two thirds of women had spontaneous abortion and for majority abortion was done and/or completed by male nurses or midwives by using surgical methods. Most of the study participants had received counseling on family planning (Table 2).

Utilization of post abortion contraception

Of all the study participants, nearly two third (274, 64.8%) had left the hospital after they have received family planning service. A little more than one third of women (35.2%) didn't receive any type of family planning and among them,30% of women said nobody discussed the issue of contraception and another one third (30%) said they wanted to be pregnant in the near future.

Among women who received post abortion family planning services, majority (82.5%) had received upon discharge to their home and only 17.5% received services immediately after treatment. From the different contraceptives given to those women, Depo Provera injectable contraception was the most chosen method (138, 50%) and the least chosen method was traditional method (6, 2%).

Factors associated with post abortion contraceptive utilization

The result of the Bivariate and Multivariable logistic regression analysis is displayed in Table 3. The Adjusted

Table 2 Description of obstetrics, contraceptive and abortion related factors of study participants in Felege Hiwot referral hospital from Sep 2016- Aug 2017

Characteristics	Total	
	Number	Percent (%)
Number of alive children		
None	217	51.3
One to four	170	40.2
≥ five	36	8.5
Need for near future pregnancy		
Yes	200	47.3
No	223	52.7
Previous history of abortion		
Yes	86	20.3
No	337	79.7
Previous history of abortion care service		
Yes	60	14.2
No	363	85.8
Previous information about FP		
Yes	345	81.6
No	78	18.4
Currently counseled on FP		
Yes	380	89.8
No	43	10.2
Pregnancy planned		
Yes (Planned)	225	53.2
No (Unplanned)	198	46.8
Pregnancy wanted and supported		
Yes (Wanted and supported)	290	68.6
No (Unwanted and unsupported)	133	31.4
Gestational age of current pregnancy		
Less than three months	185	43.7
Three to seven months	238	56.3
Type of current abortion		
Spontaneous	292	69
Induced	131	31
Type of abortion procedure		
Medication abortion	115	27.2
MVA	242	57.2
Both	66	15.6
Sex of service provider		
Male	349	82.5
Female	74	17.5
Profession of service provider		
Nurse or midwifery	279	66
General practitioner and above	144	34.1

Odds Ratio (AOR) revealed that receiving family planning counseling during service provision (25.47[95% CI: 9.11, 71.58]), occupation of the patient (0.32[95% CI: 0.16,0.65]), having previous information about family planning (2.16 [95% CI: 1.09, 4.23]), gestational age of current pregnancy (1.78[95% CI: 1.13, 3.05]) and monthly income of the family (0.38[95% CI: 0.16,0.98]) have a significant impact on the utilization of post abortion family planning. Particularly, among Sociodemographic characteristics, women who are house wife were twenty times less likely to utilize PAFP. Similarly, the odds of using of PAFP in women whose monthly income was 5000 Ethiopian birr (ETB) and above were thirty-eight times less likely than their counter parts.

The odds of utilization of post abortion family planning by women who received family planning counseling during service provision was 25.47 times than those women who didn't. Likewise, the odds of using PAFP in women who have previous information about family planning was 2.16 times to those women who didn't have previous information. Similarly, the odds of using PAFP in women whose current gestational age of pregnancy was less than 3 months was 1.78 times those whose gestational age was 3 to 7 months.

Discussion

This cross-sectional study was conducted to assess the utilization of post-abortion family planning and associated factors in women who receive abortion care service. Accordingly, the proportion of use of post abortion family planning in this study was 64.8%. When compared with the studies done in Dessie (47.5%), Debre Markos (59.2%) and Gurage (56.5%), it is higher [14–16]. The possible explanations for these could be differences in study set up and time difference. In Dessie and Debre Markos studies, the study was performed in public, private and Non-Government Organization (NGO) clinics and in Gurage; they studied utilization in facilities at all levels of health system, whereas the current study was done in tertiary hospital. However, the studies done in Mexico (82%) and Brazil (97%), both had utilization above our study [10, 12]. This might be as result of different study design and set up. In Brazilian study they used a cohort study [10]. Another explanation might be excellent quality of service and health service coverage. On the other hand, our results are comparable with other studies done in Ghana (65%) and Burkina Faso (65.7%) [19, 26].

Client occupation is one factor which was identified to be associated with PAFP. On the contrary, in prior studies in Dessie [15] and Debre Markos [16] occupation had no statistically significant association with utilization of post abortion family planning. Our study found that women who are housewives were less likely to utilize

Table 3 Factors associated with utilization of post abortion contraception, logistic regression analysis, Felege Hiwot referral hospital, Ethiopia, from Sep 2016- Aug 2017

Variables	COR (95%)	AOR (95%)	AOR *P*-value
Occupation			
Employed	1	1	.
House wife	1.10 (0.78, 1.54)	0.32 (0.16,0.65)	002
Monthly income in birr			
< 5000	1	1	
≥ 5000	1.41 (0.51,2.31)	0.38 (0.16,0.98)	.037
Previous information about FP			
Yes	2.05 (1.64,2.57)	2.16 (1.09,4.23)	.028
No	1	1	
Currently counseled on FP			
Yes	2.59 (2.07,3.24)	25.47 (9.11,71.58)	<.001
No	1	1	
Gestational age of current pregnancy			
Less than three months	2.36 (1.72, 3.24)	1.78 (1.13, 3.05)	.038
Three to seven months	1	1	

PAFP. The possible reason could be that housewives have more time and support at home to raise a child, while women who are employed may intend to delay pregnancy.

Women whose monthly income was 5000 ETB and above were less likely to use PAFP than those women whose monthly income was less than 5000 ETB. This is contrary to another Ethiopian study from Addis Ababa, which found no significant association between use of post-abortion contraception and monthly income of the client [23].

Respondents who have previous information about family planning and those who were provided with post abortion family planning counseling were more likely to use PAFP than those who did not have previous information and were not counseled. These results are similar to those from other studies done in Debre Markos, Kenya and Turkey [1, 16]. This emphasizes the impact that post-abortion family planning counseling has on utilization of post abortion family planning.

Clients whose gestational age is less than 3 months in the current pregnancy were more likely to use post abortion family planning than those whose gestational age is 3 to 7 months. However, the studies from Dessie and Addis Ababa did not find a similar association [15, 20]. One possible explanation may be that our second trimester abortions have included women who had an induced abortion for medical reason following planned pregnancy. Therefore, these women may not wish to delay another pregnancy following the abortion process.

This was a single site study done in a referral hospital where generalization could be compromised as single hospital will not represent the community. The study also may not give the real utilization of post abortion family planning service because perhaps clients might show courtesy bias during the exit interview even if they were assured that all their words will be kept confidential.

Conclusions and recommendations

In this study post-abortion contraceptive prevalence in a tertiary hospital was low as compared with studies done outside the country, even if it is higher than studies done in our country. Still there is more to be done to increase post-abortion contraception utilization. Family planning counseling during service provision, being a housewife, having previous information about family planning, monthly income and gestational age of index pregnancy are significantly associated with post-abortion family planning utilization. The type of abortion, miscarriage or induced, did not impact the interest and acceptance of contraception. We strongly recommend the government and regional health bureau at large and health care providers at each health system level in particular to provide family planning counseling for those women who come for any type of abortion related service.

Abbreviations

AIDS: Acquired Immune Deficiency Syndrome; ARHB: Amhara Regional Health Bureau; CIRHT: Centers for International Reproductive Health Training; EDHS: Ethiopian Demographic Health Survey; ETB: Ethiopian birr; FHRH: Felege Hiwot Referral Hospital; HIV: Human Immune Virus; ICPD: International Conference on Population and Development; IUCD: Intra Uterine Contraceptive Device; MVA: Manual Vacuum Aspiration; PAFP: Post Abortion Family Planning; WHO: World Health Organization

Acknowledgments
We would like to express our gratitude to Pre-Publication Support Service (PREPSS) for pre-publication peer review and copy editing of the manuscript. Authors are very grateful for the funding provided by CIRHT and training of the authors at each step of the study. We would like to thank the study participants too.

Authors' contributions
EA contributed in the proposal write up, data analysis and manuscript writing. WK and AG involved in proposal development and write up. YRS and YG involved in commenting data analysis and manuscript writing. All authors read and approved the final manuscript for submission.

Author details
[1]College of Medicine and Health Sciences, Department of Obstetrics and Gynecology, Bahir Dar University, Bahir Dar, Ethiopia. [2]Department of Obstetrics and Gynecology, University of Michigan and Centers for International Reproductive Health Training (CIRHT), Ann Arbor, Michigan, USA. [3]Debre Birhan Referral Hospital, Debre Birhan, Ethiopia. [4]Centers for International Reproductive Health Training (CIRHT), Addis Ababa, Ethiopia.

References

1. Ceylan A, Ertem M, Saka G, Akdeniz N. Post abortion family planning counseling as a tool to increase contraception use. BMC Public Health. 2009;9(20). https://doi.org/10.1186/1471-2458-9-20.
2. Tessema G, Laurence C, Melaku Y, Misganaw A, Woldie SA, Hiruye A, et al. Trends and causes of maternal mortality in Ethiopia during 1990–2013: findings from the global burden of diseases study 2013. BMC Public Health. 2017. https://doi.org/10.1186/s12889-017-4071-8.
3. Ethiopian stastical agency, Ethiopian democratic health survey. 2016. Available at < https://datacatalog.worldbank.org/dataset/ethiopia-demographic-and-health-survey-2016-0>.
4. Moore A, Gebrehiwot Y, Fetters T, Bado Y, Bankole A, Singh S, et al. The estimated incidence of induced abortion in ethiopia,2014: changes in the provision of services since 2008. Int Perspect Sex Reprod Health. 2016;42(3): 111–20.
5. Minstry Of Health of Ethiopia, National Guideline for Family Planning Services in Ethiopia. 2011: Available at https://www.scirp.org/reference/ReferencesPapers.aspx? ReferenceID=1317212>.
6. Guttmacher Institute. Facts on Induced Abortion Worldwide. Geneva, Switzerland. 2007. Available at < https://www.guttmacher.org/fact-sheet/induced-abortion-worldwide>.
7. FIGO, Post abortion family planning:a key component of post abortion care. 2013. Available at <https://www.figo.org/news/post-abortion-family-planning-key-component-post-abortion-care-0014665>.
8. Gizaw A, Regassa N. Family planning service utilization in mojo town, Ethiopia: a population based study. J Geography Regional Planning. 2011; 4(6):355–63.
9. Sedgh G, Singh S, Hussain R. Intended and unintended pregnancies worldwide in 2012 and recent trends. Stud Fam Plan. 2014;45(3):301–14.
10. Ferreira A, Souza A, Lima R, Braga C. Choices on contraceptive methods in post-abortion family planning clinic in the northeast Brazill. Reprod Health J. 2010;7(5) http://www.reproductive-health-journal.com/content/7/1/5.
11. International Conference on Population and Development. Post abortion Care Consortium. Cairo; 1994. Available at < https://www.ncbi.nlm.nih.gov/books/NBK138200/ >.
12. Becker D, Olavarrieta C, Garcia S, Harper C. Women's reports on postabortion family-planning services provided by the public-sector legal abortion program in Mexico City. Int J Gynaecol Obstet. 2013;121(2):149–53.
13. Azmat S, Hameed S, Ishaque M, Mustafa G. Post-abortion care family planning use in Pakistan. Pakistan J Public Health. 2012;2(2):4–9.
14. Tesfaye G, Oljira L: Post abortion care quality status in health facilities of Guraghe zone, Ethiopia. Bio med central reproductive health, 2013. http://www.reproductive-health-journal.com/content/10/1/35.
15. Seid A, Gebremariam A, Abera M. Integration of family planning services within post abortion Care at Health Facilities in Dessie –north East Ethiopia. Sci Technol Arts Res J. 2012;1(1):38–46.
16. Kokeb L, Admassu E, Kassa H, Seyoum T. Utilization of Post Abortion Contraceptive and Associated Factors among Women who Came for Abortion Service: a Hospital Based Cross Sectional Study. J Fam Med Disease Prev. 2015;1:022.
17. Tripney J, Kwan I, Schucan Bird K. Postabortion family planning counseling and services for women in low-income countries: a systematic review. Contraception. 2013;87(1):17–25. https://doi.org/10.1016/j.contraception.2012.07.014.
18. Khanal V, Joshi C, Neupane D, Karkee R. Practices and percepions on contraception acceptance among clients availing safe abortion services in Nepal. Kathmandu Univ Med J. 2011;35(3):179–84. https://doi.org/10.3126/kumj.v9i3.6301.
19. Kiemtoré S, Zamane H, Sawadogo YA, Ouédraogo CM, Kaïn DP, Diallo A, et al. Integration of post abortion care package in the activity of 56 health facilities by the Burkina Faso Society of Obstetricians and Gynecologists. Open J Obstetr Gynecol. 2016;6:457–62.
20. Prata N, Bell S, Holston M, Gerdts C, Melkamu Y. Factors associated with choice of post-abortion contraception in Addis Ababa, Ethiopia. Afr J Reprod Health. 2011;15(3):51.
21. Amentie M, Abera M, Abdulahi M. Utilization of family planning services and influencing factors among women of child bearing age in assosa district, benishangul gumuz regional state, West Ethiopia. Sci J Clin Med. 2015;4(3): 52–9.
22. Assefa H, Fikrewold H. Factors affecting unmet need for family planning in southern nations, nationalities and peoples region, Ethiopia. Ethiop J Health Sci. 2011;21(2):77–89.
23. Zemene A, Feleke A, Alemu A, Yitayih G, Fantahun A. Factors Influencing Utilization of Post Abortion Care in Selected Governmental Health Institutions, Addis Ababa, Ethiopia. Fam Med Med Sci Res. 2014;3(115). https://doi.org/10.4172/2327-72.1000115.
24. Abamecha A, Shiferaw A, Kassaye A. Assessment of post abortion contraceptive intention and associated factors among abortion clients in gambella health facilities, gambella town, south West Ethiopia. Int J Med Sci Clin Inventions. 2016;3(8):2061–70.
25. DH., S. Statistics: A first course, ed. t. edition. New York: McGraw Hill; 1995.
26. Maxwell L, Voetagbe G, Paul M, Mark A. Does the type of abortion provider influence contraceptive uptake after abortion? An analysis of longitudinal data from 64 health facilities in Ghana. BMC Public Health. 2015;15:586. https://doi.org/10.1186/s12889-015-1875-2.

8

Intrauterine lidocaine and naproxen for analgesia during intrauterine device insertion

Shana M. Miles[1*], Katerina Shvartsman[2] and Susan Dunlow[3]

Abstract

Background: This study evaluates oral naproxen and intrauterine instillation of lidocaine for analgesia with intrauterine device (IUD) placement as compared to placebo.

Methods: This was a randomized, double-blind, placebo-controlled trial. Patients desiring levonorgestrel 52 mg IUD or Copper T380A IUD were randomized into treatment groups. Patients received either oral naproxen 375 mg or placebo approximately 1 h prior to procedure in conjunction with 5 mL of 2% lidocaine or 5 mL of intrauterine saline. The primary outcome was pain with IUD insertion measured on a visual analog scale immediately following the procedure. Prespecified secondary outcomes included physician pain assessment, post procedure analgesia, satisfaction with procedure, satisfaction with IUD, and pain assessment related to IUD type.

Results: From June 4, 2014 to October 28, 2016 a total of 160 women desiring Copper T380A or levonorgestrel 52 mg intrauterine device insertion and meeting study criteria were enrolled and randomized in the study. Of these, 157 (78 in the Copper T380A arm, 79 in the levonorgestrel 52 mg) received study treatment medication. There were 39 in naproxen/lidocaine arm, 39 in placebo/lidocaine arm, 40 in naproxen/placebo arm, and 39 in placebo/placebo arm. There were no differences in the mean pain scores for IUD placement between treatment groups (naproxen/lidocaine 3.38 ± 2.49; lidocaine only 2.87 ± 2.13; naproxen only 3.09 ± 2.18; placebo 3.62 ± 2.45). There was no difference in self-medication post procedure or in satisfaction with the procedure and IUD among women in the treatment arms or by type of IUD.

Conclusion: Naproxen with or without intrauterine lidocaine does not reduce pain with IUD placement.

Keywords: Intrauterine device, IUD, Pain, Lidocaine, NSAID

Background

Approximately 50% of pregnancies in the United States are unintended [1, 2] with over 4 million women at risk of unintended pregnancy not utilizing contraception [3]. Intrauterine devices (IUDs) are among the most effective long-acting reversible contraceptives [4]. Currently, five IUDs are available in the United States: the Copper T380A (Paragard), levonorgestrel 52 mg (Mirena), levonorgestrel 52 mg (Liletta), levonorgestrel 19.5 mg (Kyleena) and levonorgestrel 13.5 mg (Skyla). The safety, efficacy, convenience, and cost of long acting reversible contraception, including IUDs, has led the Institute of Medicine to include contraception as part of women's preventive care in the Affordable Care Act in an effort to decrease barriers to care [5].

While IUD and contraceptive implant use has grown over the past decade, the current usage is only 14% in the United States [6]. One of the barriers to IUD insertion is discomfort, or anticipation of pain, during device insertion [7–9]. While most patients tolerate pain to complete the procedure, studies show that pain scales on IUD insertion range from 2 to 7 on a 10 point visual analog score [10–15]. Surprisingly, adequate pain control during gynecologic outpatient office procedures including hysterosalpingography, endometrial biopsy, and IUD

* Correspondence: shana.m.miles2.mil@mail.mil
[1]Second Medical Group, 243 Curtiss Rd, Barksdale AFB, Louisiana 71110, USA

insertion and removal have been addressed in only a limited way in the literature. Moreover, despite the discomfort associated with IUD insertion, endometrial biopsy, and other office gynecology procedures, there is no standard of care for pre/intra/post procedure analgesia. In our institution, depending on provider preference and previous patient counseling, many patients receive no pain medication for their IUD insertion procedure.

Autonomic innervation to the uterus and cervix is provided via S2-S4, and the T10-L1 afferent visceral pain fibers [16]. Intrauterine instilled anesthetic is thought to act on nerve endings within the endometrium [17]. As such, analgesia for common office outpatient gynecologic procedures that have been investigated include: intracervical or paracervical injections, nonsteroidal anti-inflammatory drugs (NSAIDs), intrauterine instillation. Despite efficacy with intracervical/paracervical injections [18], the injection is painful and is a deterrent to use [19–21]. NSAIDs block prostaglandin synthesis and have been shown to be effective in relief of mild-moderate pain associated with gynecologic procedures [20]. A 2015 Cochrane review examining analgesia with IUD insertion found that naproxen may have an effect at reducing pain during IUD insertion [22] however, subsequently, Ngo et al. found that while naproxen did not reduce pain with IUD insertion it did reduce pain post-insertion [13].

Intrauterine instillation of lidocaine has been shown to be efficacious in endometrial biopsy [23–25], saline sonogram [26], and retrieval of "lost" IUD [27]. Another study showed that intrauterine lidocaine in conjunction with naproxen significantly decreased the pain associated with endometrial biopsy [25]. If the administration of oral and/or intrauterine analgesia was efficacious for intrauterine device insertion, this would be a low cost and a low risk intervention. The aim of this study was to determine efficacy of NSAID and intrauterine analgesia, either singly or doubly, during intrauterine device insertion on patients' pain perception.

Materials and methods

This study was approved by the Walter Reed National Military Medical Center Institutional Review Board (#384645–3) prior to enrollment of the first patient and the study was posted on Clinicaltrials.gov (NCT 02769247) on May 11, 2016. This was a factorial design, randomized, double blind, placebo-controlled study with women who were recruited from our outpatient obstetrics and gynecology clinics. Prior to their enrollment in the study for the intrauterine device of their choice (Copper T380A or Mirena levonorgestrel 52 mg), subjects signed procedure consent. After subjects completed a study consent form with a study physician in accordance with the Declaration of Helsinki, they completed a demographics form to ensure that they met inclusion criteria and had no exclusion criteria. Inclusion criteria included Defense Enrollment Eligibility Reporting System (DEERS)-eligible women aged 18 years and older desiring Copper T380A or levonorgestrel 52 mg intrauterine device insertion. DEERS eligibility would allow them to receive care at a Military Treatment Facility. Exclusion criteria were current pregnancy, history of cervical stenosis, severe medical illness, known allergy or sensitivity to lidocaine or naproxen, peptic ulcer disease, current pelvic inflammatory disease, patients with known renal insufficiency, and patients using chronic NSAIDs or on chronic pain medication. Due to the infrequency of Skyla IUD use in our clinic and the non-availability of Liletta and Kyleena at the time of the study, women desiring these devices were also excluded.

Each subject was then assigned a study number and was randomized to a treatment within the Copper T380A or Levonorgestrel 52 mg arms by the investigational pharmacy on the day of enrollment. The patient chose which IUD they desired prior to enrollment and was not randomized to IUD type. The investigational pharmacist, who was otherwise not involved in the study, used computer generated block randomization. The pharmacy provided study packets that included an unlabeled syringe and oral medication so that physicians and patients were blinded to the assigned treatment group. The subject took the oral medication (naproxen 375 mg prepared in a capsule or similarly prepared placebo capsule) 1 h prior to the procedure. After performing a bimanual exam, placing a speculum and cleansing the cervix with betadine, the study physician then instilled 5 ml of the intrauterine solution (2% lidocaine or similarly prepared normal saline) through the endocervix using an 18-gauge angiocatheter advanced to the hub. The angiocatheter was left in place for 3 min before it was removed. Single tooth tenaculum was then placed and the uterus was measured with a metal sound. The intrauterine device was then inserted according to manufacturer's instruction. To maintain consistency, three study physicians (KS, SD, SM) used the same technique to place the IUDs.

Immediately after the procedure, each patient completed a post procedure survey rating their pain during the procedure, satisfaction with the insertion, and whether they would have an IUD placed again. The survey included a visual analog scale (VAS) where 0 represented no pain and 10 being the worst pain they could imagine. The satisfaction ratings were scored on a scale from 1 to 5 with 5 being extremely satisfied with the procedure. The patients completed another survey at day 30 post insertion. The physician also recorded and scored visible signs of the women's discomfort during the procedure (gripping table, lifting off table) using a 3-point observer scale for each of the parameters [24]. On this scale 0 was no response, 1 was patient admits to some discomfort but procedure is not interrupted, 2 was patient in discomfort but after briefly halting the procedure, the IUD is inserted while 3 the patient is visibly uncomfortable, gripping the table or squeezing the attendant's hand. The difficulty of insertion was also noted. Lidocaine and saline were packaged in identical syringes and oral placebo tablets were encased in same capsule as the naproxen. Patients and physicians were blinded to treatment groups but not IUD type.

Power calculation was based on other studies assessing pain with IUD placement and endometrial biopsy [11, 21, 25]. Power calculation was done for treatment groups of 34 patients, assuming pain rating in placebo group of 4, standard deviation of VAS scores is 2.9 points, with a two-sample t test with 5% two-sided significance level will have 80% power to detect a difference of 2 points between the groups. Clinically significant difference in VAS pain score has been defined as 2 on a 0–10 VAS scale [28, 29]. To allow room for missing data, non-completion of procedure and loss to follow up, we planned to recruit 80 women in each IUD type (levonorgestrel 52 mg vs Copper T380A) and 40 women in each treatment arm (placebo/normal saline; naproxen/normal saline, placebo/lidocaine; naproxen/lidocaine), for a total of 160 patients.

Demographics and survey data were compared using the t test or Wilcoxon two-sample test for continuous variables. X^2 or Fisher exact test was used for categorical variables. Additional statistical analysis was performed using Kruskal-Wallis test to evaluate the differences of the mean pain scores between the groups. $P < 0.05$ was considered statistically significant.

Results

There were 160 women enrolled in the study between June 2014 and October 2016, with 80 desiring the levonorgestrel 52 mg IUD and 80 desiring Copper T380A IUD with 40 randomized in each treatment arm. Patients chose their desired IUD prior to enrollment. Enrollment was closed for either levonorgestrel 52 mg IUD or Copper T380A IUD after 80 women were enrolled in each respective arm. Two patients decided against study participation after enrollment, another took non-study medication prior to her IUD insertion excluding her from the analysis, and another was unable to have her IUD placed due to difficulty with IUD insertion (Fig. 1). All other patients analyzed received the assigned study medication and completed IUD insertion. A total of 157 patients were analyzed (79 patients desiring levonorgestrel 52 mg IUD, 78 patients desiring Copper T380A IUD). Within treatment groups there were 39 in the combined treatment arm, 39 in the intrauterine lidocaine only arm, 40 in the naproxen only arm, and 39 in the placebo arm. There were no statistically significant differences among treatment groups in age, body mass index (BMI), parity, history of cervical procedures, vaginal parity, ease of insertion, use of pain medication post-procedure as shown in Tables 1 and 2. There was a significant difference of distribution of patients with history of c-section ($p = 0.031$) between treatment groups.

Pain perceived by patients in the treatment groups was not statistically significant between the groups with mean VAS in the placebo arm of 3.62 ± 2.45 (Fig. 2) as compared to the naproxen only (3.09 ± 2.18), lidocaine only (2.87 ± 2.13), naproxen and lidocaine (3.38 ± 2.49) arms. Pain assessment during the procedure rated by the

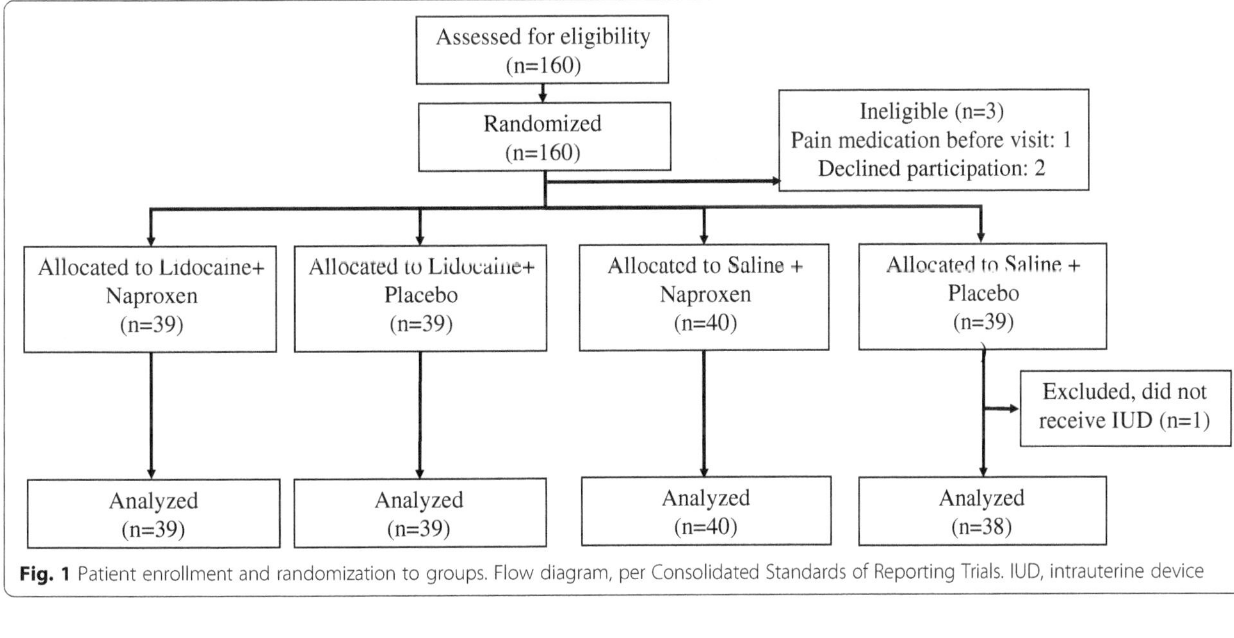

Fig. 1 Patient enrollment and randomization to groups. Flow diagram, per Consolidated Standards of Reporting Trials. IUD, intrauterine device

Table 1 Patient demographics

Characteristic	Lidocaine/Naproxen (*n* = 39)	Lidocaine/Placebo (*n* = 39)	Saline/Naproxen (*n* = 40)	Saline/Placebo (*n* = 39)	P
Age (y)	31.1 ± 8.5	31.1 ± 7.4	31.2 ± 6.5	29.7 ± 6.9	0.788
BMI (kg/m^2)	27.6 ± 6.4	26.0 ± 4.1	27.1 ± 5.1	25.9 ± 4.4	0.340
Parity					0.510
Nulliparous	13 (33.3)	17 (43.6)	11 (27.5)	14 (35.9)	
Parous	26 (66.7)	22 (56.4)	29 (72.5)	25 (64.1)	
Vaginal parity	18 (46.1)	15 (38.4)	12 (30.0)	14 (35.9)	0.408
Prior c-section	10 (25.6)	9 (23.1)	20 (50.0)	14 (35.9)	0.031
Prior IUD insertion					0.605
Yes	6 (15.4)	9 (23.0)	12 (30.0)	8 (20.5)	
No	33 (84.6)	30 (76.9)	28 (70.0)	31 (79.5)	
Prior Cervical procedures					0.298
Yes	5 (12.5)	12 (30)	6 (15)	6 (15.4)	
No	34 (85)	27 (67.5)	34 (85)	33 (84.6)	
Ease of insertion					0.99
Easy	38 (97.4)	38 (97.4)	38 (95)	36 (94.7)	
Difficult	1 (2.6)	1 (2.6)	2 (0.5)	2 (5.2)	

Data are n%, unless otherwise specified
BMI body mass index, *IUD* intrauterine device

Table 2 Analgesic outcomes

Characteristic	Lidocaine/Naproxen	Lidocaine/Placebo	Saline/Naproxen	Saline/Placebo	P
Physician pain assessment	0.77 ± 0.11	0.56 ± 0.09	0.48 ± 0.11	0.59 ± 0.8	0.238
Visual analog pain score	3.38 ± 2.49	2.87 ± 2.13	3.09 ± 2.18	3.62 ± 2.45	0.456
Post procedure analgesia					0.568
Yes	10 (25)	8 (20)	9 (22.5)	12 (30.8)	
No	28 (70)	28 (70)	31 (77.5)	22 (56.4)	
Satisfaction with procedure	4.36 ± 0.84	4.26 ± 0.94	4.3 ± 0.94	4.4 ± 0.9	0.910
Satisfaction with IUD (Day 30)					0.701
Levonorgestrel 52 mg	4.40 ± 0.75	4.36 ± 0.97	4.35 ± 1.1	4.38 ± 0.89	
Copper T380A	4.31 ± 0.95	4.16 ± 0.92	4.3 ± 0.81	4.47 ± 0.94	
Physician pain assessment					0.31
Levonorgestrel 52 mg	0.90 ± 0.72	0.50 ± 0.11	0.55 ± 0.18	0.53 ± 0.12	
Copper T380A	0.63 ± 0.13	0.63 ± 0.14	0.40 ± 0.11	0.63 ± 0.11	
Visual analog pain score					
Levonorgestrel 52 mg	3.55 ± 0.55	2.45 ± 0.44	2.85 ± 0.45	3.26 ± 0.54	0.09
Copper T380A	3.26 ± 0.59	3.32 ± 0.52	3.35 ± 0.52	4.00 ± 0.58	
Post procedure analgesia					
Levonorgestrel 52 mg					0.65
Yes	3 (16) [0.33]	3 (17) [0.23]	5 (25) [0.09]	5 (31) [0.64]	
No	16 (84) [0.09]	15 (83) [0.06]	15 (75) [0.02]	11 (69) [0.18]	
Copper T380A					0.43
Yes	7 (41) [0.45]	5 (28) [0.10]	4 (20) [0.89]	7 (41) [0.45]	
No	10 (59) [0.21]	13 (72) [0.05]	16 (80) [0.42]	10 (59) [0.21]	

Data are mean ± standard deviation, n%, [X^2] unless otherwise specified

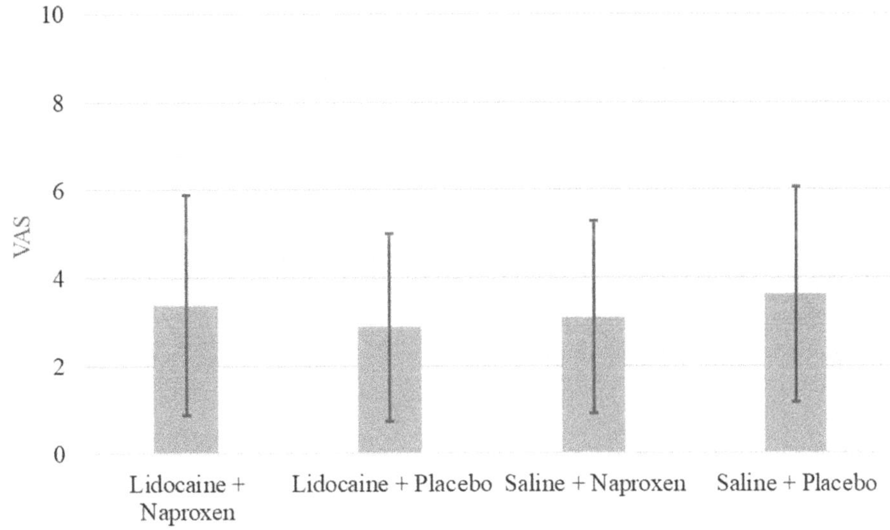

Fig. 2 Mean visual analog scores within 30 min of IUD insertion. Bars denote treatment groups with standard deviation. Treatment groups are lidocaine instillation and naproxen, lidocaine instillation and placebo capsule, placebo instillation and naproxen, placebo instillation and placebo capsule

physician inserting the device was not significantly different between treatment groups or type of IUD (Table 2) . There was no statistically significant difference in patients' use of post procedure analgesia regardless of IUD type ($p = 0.19$) or treatment groups ($p = 0.568$) when surveyed approximately 30 days post-insertion. This study was not powered to detect differences between treatment groups between types of IUDs nor were patients randomized to type of IUD.

Overall satisfaction for the IUD procedure was high with 98% of the patients scoring they were satisfied to extremely satisfied with their procedure and 97% would have an IUD placed again. Satisfaction scores were not different between treatment groups or IUD type. There was one patient that was diagnosed with pelvic inflammatory disease approximately 1 week after her IUD insertion and her IUD was inadvertently removed during her requested clipping of strings. Patient's IUD was not replaced at that visit. Another patient returned with vasovagal symptoms approximately 1 h following placement of her IUD however this did not affect her retention of the device. This study was not powered to detect differences in the low rates of adverse events or measures of patient satisfaction.

Discussion

Consistent with other studies, the data suggests that there is no significant difference in pain control during IUD insertion using NSAIDs like naproxen [11, 13, 30–32]. The average VAS of 3.6 in our placebo group is consistent with other studies [30, 31]. The wait time of 1 h after administration of naproxen and three minutes with intrauterine instillation should have been appropriate to achieve peak levels of analgesia at time of IUD insertion [33]. To our knowledge, this is the first randomized, double-blind, placebo-controlled study comparing the use of NSAIDs and intrauterine instillation of anesthetic for IUD insertion. There was no observed multiplicative effect as had been previously shown with the same regimen for endometrial biopsy [25].

There was no difference in post-procedure analgesia usage in our treatment groups or between IUD type (Table 2). However, only 26% of our patients used any analgesia post procedure ($X^2 = 0.568$) and there were no differences between patients who received naproxen versus placebo. This suggests that naproxen did not have an effect on post procedure analgesia despite its up to 12 h duration of analgesia [33]. However, recall bias may have contributed to this finding since the patients were asked if they took anything additional for pain after their IUD insertion during their 30-day post-procedural survey. There were also no differences in pain ratings or post procedure analgesia in patients receiving the intrauterine lidocaine as compared to saline. This suggests that the lidocaine also does not have a significant effect on analgesia for IUD insertion either during or post-procedure. Interestingly, there was a trend towards decreased usage of post-procedure analgesics in the lidocaine instillation arms within the levonorgestrel IUD treatment groups, however this study was not adequately powered for this outcome measure (Table 2).

Limitations of this study include the fact the placebo group still received instillation of saline which itself may have been a treatment modality. Given the pain ratings of our patients at the lower end of the reported range, this may suggest that the instillation and distension of the uterus may affect the nerve endings within the endometrium and, consequently, patients' perceived pain rating. The hydro-distention accomplished by the intrauterine instillation may have affected the dilation of the insertion path, thereby making the insertion of the IUD devices easier. This distension may also contribute to the finding of no differences in pain perception between devices. Usage of the 18-gauge angiocatheter was a separate procedure and possible treatment modality. While not specifically tracked there was a small proportion of patients that noted cramping during the instillation though none required the procedure to be paused or halted during this step. Including a separate arm with no intervention other than IUD insertion would have improved this study and addressed this potential confounding factor of intrauterine instillation.

While we had no differences in distribution of parous women throughout our treatment groups, it is also possible that if subjects had been limited to nulliparous women, differences in pain perception may have been noted between the treatment groups in a similarly powered study. This study was not randomized to type of IUD or powered to detect differences between the two devices but we did observe a trend of increased pain ($p = 0.09$) in the Copper T380A patients as compared to the levonorgestrel recipients in conjunction with decreased pain in our naproxen and lidocaine treatment groups. Our findings were similar to Dogan et al. [25], in that the combined treatment group was not superior to single agent. However, unlike the findings from Dogan et al., our naproxen/lidocaine arm was not superior to the placebo/saline arm which maybe secondary to our overall lower pain scores during IUD insertion compared to endometrial biopsy in their study. This study was also similar to the 2015 Cochrane review that found no benefit to pre-treatment with naproxen (NSAID) for analgesia for IUD insertions though patients in the Cochrane review were less likely to note the insertion experience as unpleasant [22].

In conclusion, our study showed that naproxen alone or in combination with intrauterine lidocaine does not reduce pain during IUD insertion. Intrauterine instillation of lidocaine is not superior to saline. A future study examining the difference of intrauterine instillation of saline and no instillation may help elucidate these differences.

Abbreviations

BMI: Body mass index; DEERS: Defense Enrollment Eligibility Reporting System; IUD: Intrauterine device; NSAID: Nonsteroidal anti-inflammatory drug; VAS: Visual analog scale

Acknowledgements

Statistical support was provided by Robin Howard, Uniformed Services University.

Authors' contributions

SMM, SD, and KS all contributed to study design, clinical implementation, data analysis, and authorship of this paper. All authors read and approved the final manuscript.

Author details

[1]Second Medical Group, 243 Curtiss Rd, Barksdale AFB, Louisiana 71110, USA. [2]Department of Obstetrics and Gynecology, Uniformed Services University, 4301 Jones Bridge Rd, Bethesda, MD 20814, USA. [3]Department of Obstetrics and Gynecology, Walter Reed National Military Medical Center, 8901 Wisconsin Ave, Bethesda, MD 20889, USA.

References

1. Finer LB, Henshaw SK. Disparities in rates of unintended pregnancy in the United States, 1994 and 2001. Perspect Sex Reprod Health. 2006. p. 90–6.
2. Trussell J. Contraceptive failure in the United States. Contraception. 2011. p. 397–404.
3. Mosher WD, Jones J. Use of contraception in the United States : 1982 – 2008 Library of Congress cataloging-in-publication data. Vital Health Stat 23. 2010. p. 1–44.
4. Trussell J, Wynn LL. Reducing unintended pregnancy in the United States. Contraception. 2008. p. 1–5.
5. Kuehn BM. Institute of medicine outlines priorities for comparative effectiveness research. JAMA. 2009. p. 936–7.
6. Kavanaugh ML, Jerman J. Contraceptive method use in the United States: trends and characteristics between 2008, 2012 and 2014. Contraception. 2018. p. 14–21.
7. Bracken J, Graham CA. Young women's attitudes towards, and experiences of, long-acting reversible contraceptives. Eur J Contracept Reprod Health Care. 2014. p. 276–84.
8. MLCSGAWKL J. Myths and misconceptions about intrauterine contraception among women seeking termination of pregnancy. TT. J Fam Plan Reprod Health Care. 2013. p. 36–40.
9. Asker C, Stokes-Lampard H, Beavan J, Wilson S. What is it about intrauterine devices that women find unacceptable? Factors that make women non-users: a qualitative study. J Fam Plan Reprod Health Care. 2006. p. 89–94.
10. Ngo LL, Ward KK, Mody SK. Ketorolac for pain control with intrauterine device placement: a randomized controlled trial. Obstet Gynecol. 2015. p. 29–36.
11. Hubacher D, Reyes V, Lillo S, Zepeda A, Chen PL, Croxatto H. Pain from copper intrauterine device insertion: randomized trial of prophylactic ibuprofen. Am J Obstet Gynecol. 2006. p. 1272–7.
12. Dijkhuizen K, Dekkers OM, Holleboom CAG, De Groot CJM, Hellebrekers BWJ, Van Roosmalen GJJ, et al. Vaginal misoprostol prior to insertion of an intrauterine device: an RCT. Hum Reprod. 2011. p. 323–9.
13. Ngo LL, Braaten KP, Eichen E, Fortin J, Maurer R, Goldberg AB. Naproxen sodium for pain control with intrauterine device insertion: a randomized controlled trial. Obstet Gynecol. 2016. p. 1306–13.
14. Sääv I, Aronsson A, Marions L, Stephansson O, Gemzell-Danielsson K. Cervical priming with sublingual misoprostol prior to insertion of an intrauterine device in nulliparous women: a randomized controlled trial. Hum Reprod. 2007. p. 81–4.
15. Edelman AB, Schaefer E, Olson A, Van Houten L, Bednarek P, Leclair C, et al. Effects of prophylactic misoprostol administration prior to intrauterine device insertion in nulliparous women. Contraception. 2011. p. 234–9.
16. Origoni M, Leone Roberti Maggiore U, Salvatore S, Candiani M. Neurobiological mechanisms of pelvic pain. Biomed Res Int. 2014. p. 1–9.
17. Tokushige N, Markham R, Russell P, Fraser IS. High density of small nerve fibres in the functional layer of the endometrium in women with endometriosis. Hum Reprod. 2006. p. 782–7.
18. Mody SK, Farala JP, Jimenez B, Nishikawa M, Ngo LL. Paracervical block for intrauterine device placement among nulliparous women: a randomized controlled trial. Obstet Gynecol. 2018.p p. 575–82.
19. Costello MF, Horrowitz S, Steigrad S, Saif N, Bennett M, Ekangaki A. Transcervical intrauterine topical local anesthetic at hysterosalpingography: a prospective, randomized, double-blind, placebo-controlled trial. Fertil Steril. 2002. p. 1116–22.
20. Davies A, Baskett TF, Richardson RE, Nagele F, O'Connor H, Magos AL. Lignocaine aerosol spray in outpatient hysteroscopy: a randomized double-blind placebo-controlled trial. Fertil Steril. 1997. p. 1019–23.

21. Mody SK, Kiley J, Rademaker A, Gawron L, Stika C, Hammond C. Pain control for intrauterine device insertion: a randomized trial of 1% lidocaine paracervical block. Contraception. 2012. p. 704–9.
22. Lopez LM, Bernholc A, Zeng Y, Allen RH, Bartz D, O'Brien PA, et al. Interventions for pain with intrauterine device insertion. Cochrane Database Syst Rev. 2015.
23. Mercier RJ, Zerden ML. Intrauterine anesthesia for gynecologic procedures: a systematic review. Obstet Gynecol. 2012. p. 669–77.
24. Güney M, Oral B, Mungan T. Intrauterine lidocaine plus buccal misoprostol in the endometrial biopsy. Int J Gynecol Obstet. 2007. p. 593–8.
25. Dogan E, Celiloglu M, Sarihan E, Demir A. Anesthetic effect of intrauterine lidocaine plus naproxen sodium in endometrial biopsy. Obstet Gynecol. 2004. p. 347–51.
26. Guney M, Oral B, Bayhan G, Mungan T. Intrauterine lidocaine infusion for pain relief during saline solution infusion sonohysterography: a randomized, controlled trial. J Minim Invasive Gynecol. 2007. p. 304–10.
27. Güney M, Oral B, Mungan T. Efficacy of intrauterine lidocaine for removal of a "lost" intrauterine device: a randomized, controlled trial. Obstet Gynecol. 2006. p. 119–23.
28. Rowbotham MC. What is a "clinically meaningful" reduction in pain? Pain. 2001. p. 131–2.
29. Todd KH, Funk KG, Funk JP, Bonacci R. Clinical significance of reported changes in pain severity. Ann Emerg Med. 1996. p. 485–9.
30. Chor J, Bregand-White J, Golobof A, Harwood B, Cowett A. Ibuprofen prophylaxis for levonorgestrel-releasing intrauterine system insertion: a randomized controlled trial. Contraception. 2012. p. 558–62.
31. Bednarek PH, Creinin MD, Reeves MF, Cwiak C, Espey E, Jensen JT. Prophylactic ibuprofen does not improve pain with IUD insertion: a randomized trial. Contraception. 2015. p. 193–7.
32. Jensen HH, Blaabjerg J, Lyndrup J. Prophylactic use of prostaglandin synthesis inhibitors in connection with IUD insertion. Ugeskr Laeger. 1998; 160(48):6958–61.
33. Davies NM, Anderson KE. Clinical pharmacokinetics of naproxen. Clin Pharmacokinet. 1997. p. 268–93.

9

Removal of a missing intrauterine contraceptive device after location through an ultrasound

Mesele Damte Argaw[1]*, Hailemariam Segni Abawollo[1], Binyam Fekadu Desta[1], Zergu Taffesse Tsegaye[1], Dejene Mengistu Belete[2] and Melkamu Getu Abebe[1]

Abstract

Background: In the last decade, (2000–2019), the modern contraceptive prevalence among married women of reproductive age (14–49 years), has increased by only 2.1%. The slow progress was due to limited access to services and myths surrounding methods held by both users and providers. This case report was identified, diagnosed and managed by a midwife working in rural health center in low resource setting. However, literature is scare on the management of missing Intra-Uterine Contraceptive Device (IUCD) thread removal services of confirmed diagnosis using Vscan or limited ultrasound services in rural health centers. The aim of reporting this case report was developed to enhance easy access to intra-uterine contraceptive method removals, which may address myths associated with difficulties of undergoing the services in rural set-up.

A 26 year-old married woman, Gravida 1 and Para 1, attended Mekoy Health Center for IUCD removal service after 7 years of protection and internally referred to limited obstetric ultrasound service room due to non- visualization of IUCD thread with Vaginal Speculum examination. An ultrasonography scan however, showed a centrally located copper-T 380A IUCD in the endometrial cavity. As a result, after dilatation of the cervix, a successful removal of the Copper-T 308A was conducted. The client received followed up care for 2 hours post-procedure and was then discharged.

Conclusions: This case highlights the importance of availing diagnostic and removal services in rural set ups to mitigate myths in the community. The availability of limited obstetric ultrasound scanning services can improve the diagnoses and management of conditions in clients. The reported case shows that although, the basic infrastructure was limited, ultrasound scanning and Long Acting Reversible Contraception (LARC) trained midwives can ensure the provision of safe IUCD removal services in rural areas.

Keywords: Missing threads, Intra uterine contraceptive device, Ultrasonography, Ethiopia

* Correspondence: mdamte5@gmail.com; mesele_damte@et.jsi.com
[1]USAID Transform: Primary Health Care, JSI Research & Training Institute, Inc., Addis Ababa, Ethiopia

Introduction

The global trend of modern contraceptive prevalence among married women of reproductive age has increased slowly from 55.0% (95% CI 53.7–56.3%) in 2000 to 57.1% (95% CI 54.6–59.5%) in 2019. The limited progress was explained by poor quality of available services, limited access to services, and myths against methods held by users and providers [1].

Ethiopia is the second most populous country in Africa, with an estimated population of 114 million. In the year 2017, with a total fertility rate of 4.99, the country assumed the 15th rank among twenty countries with the highest fertility rates in the world [2]. According to the Health Sector Transformation Plan (2015–2020), the country aims to achieve modern contraceptive method coverage of 80%, where, 40% of mothers will use long-acting reversible contraceptives through informed choices [3]. However, among currently married women, the modern contraceptive acceptance rate is 41.0% and only 2.0% of them use IUCDs [4]. Quality of care affected not only the uptake of IUCD services but its removal too. A misplaced IUCD usually presents as missing threads and remains asymptomatic in most cases [5]. This report is of a case of missing IUCD threads that was diagnosed and managed with the help of portable ultrasound services following a short training in a rural set up in Ethiopia.

Case

A 26-year-old married woman, Gravida I and Para 1, was evaluated at Mekoye Health Center's limited obstetric ultrasound service room on May 03, 2020. The client was internally referred from the family planning service unit for non-visualization of an IUCD thread upon undergoing a vaginal speculum examination. The client attended the clinic to get an IUCD removal service and was showing no signs and symptoms of abnormal health conditions. Seven years ago, she had experienced a normal vaginal delivery and an IUCD was inserted 42 days after delivery. The client had no history of known medical or surgical health abnormalities and had no history of reported expulsion of IUCD. After providing a brief explanation of the speculum vaginal examination procedure and its purpose, the provider obtained verbal consent. The speculum examination revealed a normal looking vaginal wall and cervix. To complete the gynecological workup, a bimanual examination was performed revealing that her uterus was anteverted and was a normal non-pregnant uterus size. An ultrasonography scan however, (Fig. 1), showed a centrally located copper-T 380A IUCD in the endometrial cavity. As a result, after dilatation of the cervix, a successful removal of the IUCD was conducted. The client received followed up care for 2 hours post-procedure and was then discharged.

Discussion

Intrauterine contraceptive device is one of the types of long-acting reversible contraceptive (LARC) methods. IUCD is a safe and effective contraceptive method and fertility of women returns promptly after removal [6]. Ethiopia - like many low-income countries - strives to address its unmet family planning need and control its population growth through promoting modern contraceptive methods [3].

According to the mini-Ethiopian Demographic and Health Survey (2019), the overall modern contraceptive prevalence rate (CPR) among married women is 41.0%, while IUCD use remains low at 2.0% [4]. The Ministry

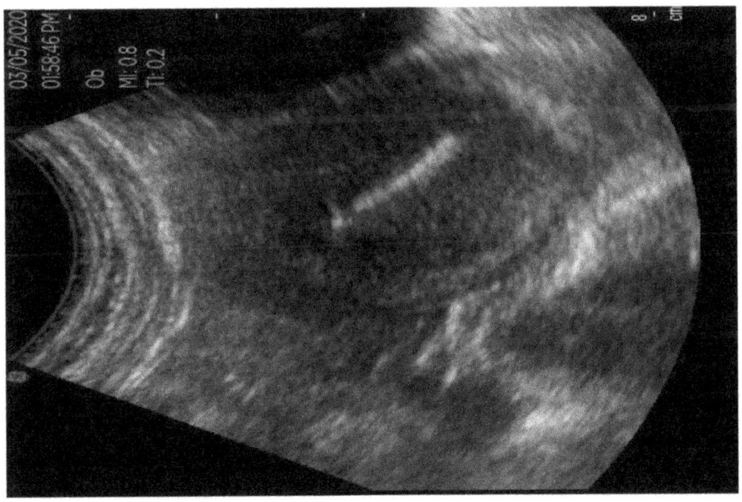

Fig. 1 Transabdominal ultrasonic image of the intrauterine contraceptive device (copper-T 380A IUCD). Ultrasound image showed a centrally located copper-T 380A IUCD in the endometrial cavity

of Health and its development partners work to strategically improve quality and equity for, and access to LARC services. Some of the interventions applied to achieve this are promoting task shifting/sharing between health extension workers and facilitating community back-up services by trained clinical staff of health centers and primary hospitals [3, 4]. However, the proportion of IUCD use among LARCs is about 7.3%. One of the factors influencing uptake of IUCD services includes misconception on delays to returning to normal fertility [7]. Among the many reasons for low uptake, the delay in getting access to removal services and more specifically, patients with missing threads may create myths in the community.

The client in the reported case who was asymptomatic was attending the health center to receive an IUCD removal service. The string, which can be used to remove the IUCD, was not visible to the family planning unit's service providers. This finding was in line with an estimation of up to 30 to 85% of patients with displaced or migrated IUCDs being asymptomatic cases [5, 8]. Mishra (2017), confer the causes of lost strings as expulsion curling and indrawing into the uterine cavity [6]. The incidence of complications of IUCD strings can be affected by several factors which includes the timing of IUCD insertion, uterine position, past history of abortion, and the operator's experience [5]. Similarly, Mishra (2017) explored that missing strings after post-placental intrauterine contraceptive device and low segment caesarian section insertion is a common problem. They pointed out that it is important to follow up on infrequently occurring complications on a regular basis with the increasing use of IUCDs [6]. Sowmya, et al., (2016) confer the importance of performing post-insertion close follow up care after a month, subsequent 3 months and on a yearly basis for the exclusion of infection, abnormal bleeding, and the proper positioning of copper-T. In addition, IUCD users should receive proper counseling services to make them aware of the need to contact health care providers in cases where IUCD threads cannot be felt, for persistent abdominal pain and missed periods [9].

The United States Agency for International Development funded Transform: Primary Health Care Activity has enhanced access to limited obstetric ultrasound services at the primary health care, (health center level) in rural Ethiopia [10]. Cognizant of the low number of available specialized senior health professionals in the country and their maldistribution, i.e. concentration in large cities, the Activity trained midwives and other mid-level health professionals recruited from 100 health centers and supplied portable ultrasound machines [10]. This is in line with the Sikolia et al., (2017) recommendation that enhanced point of care through the provision of portable ultrasound services help healthcare providers to make evidence-based decisions for mothers [11]. A midwife working in Mekoy Health Center identified and removed the IUCD in the reported case using narrow-type forceps (Spencer Wells or alligator forceps). This procedure was in line with the Moro et al., (2015) novel ultrasound-guided procedure for successful retrieval of lost IUCDs and is well tolerated by women [12]. The use of narrow-type forceps for removal of missing threads is also referenced by Dalby et al., (2017) [13]. In addition, the availability of limited obstetric ultrasound services helps the health system to avert unnecessary referrals and reduces costs associated with referral services for clients [14].

Conclusion

Long-acting reversible contraceptive methods are promoted to address the high unmet family planning needs among reproductive aged married women and control the population growth of low-income countries. This case highlights the importance of availing diagnostic and removal services in rural set ups to mitigate myths in the community. The availability of limited obstetric ultrasound scanning services can improve the diagnoses and management of conditions in clients. The reported case shows that although, the basic infrastructure was limited, ultrasound scanning and LARC trained midwives can ensure the provision of safe IUCD removal services in rural areas. In addition, close follow up to alleviate pain and observation of any resulting complications were carried out. After the safe removal of the IUCD, family planning counseling services were also provided.

Abbreviations

CPR: Contraceptive Prevalence Rate; FMOH: Federal Ministry of Health IUCD Intra-Uterine Contraceptive Device; LARC: Long-Acting Reversible Contraceptive; USAID: United States Agency for International Development

Acknowledgements

The authors are very grateful for the case to voluntary participated in this study. The authors thank Heran Demissie for English language editing.

Authors' contributions

The authors of this manuscript are MDA, HSA, BFD, ZTT, DMB and MGA. All authors substantial contribution to conceiving and designing the study, and MDA, DMB and MGA was responsible for overseeing the field work, cleaning the data, analysing the data, interpreting the analysis and drafting the manuscript. All authors read the final document and approved it. MDA, the corresponding author, submitted the manuscript for publication.

Authors' information

MDA: Ph.D.; Senior Health Systems Strengthening Advisor at USAID Transform: Primary Health Care, JSI Research & Training Institutes, Inc., Addis Ababa, Ethiopia.

HAS: MD, Gyn/Obs, MPH: Senior Maternal and Newborn Advisor at USAID Transform: Primary Health Care, JSI Research & Training Institutes, Inc., Addis Ababa, Ethiopia.

BDF: Ph.D.; Deputy Chief of Party at USAID Transform: Primary Health Care, JSI Research & Training Institutes, Inc., Addis Ababa, Ethiopia.
ZTT: MPH; Programs Director at USAID Transform: Primary Health Care, JSI Research & Training Institutes, Inc., Addis Ababa, Ethiopia.
DMB: BSc Midwife, Delivery Case team process owner at Mekoy Health Center, North Eastern Amhara, Ethiopia.
MGA: MPH; Health Systems Strengthening Program Officer at USAID Transform: Primary Health Care, JSI Research & Training Institutes, Inc., Bahir Dar, Ethiopia.

Author details
[1]USAID Transform: Primary Health Care, JSI Research & Training Institute, Inc., Addis Ababa, Ethiopia. [2]Mekoy Health Center, Mekoy, Antsokiya Gemza District, Ethiopia.

References

1. Kantorová V, Wheldon MC, Ueffing P, Dasgupta ANZ. Estimating progress towards meeting women's contraceptive needs in 185 countries: a Bayesian hierarchical modelling study. PLoS Med. 2020;17(2):e1003026 https://journals.plos.org/plosmedicine/article?id=10.1371/journal.pmed.1003026.
2. The World Fact Book. County Comparison: total fertility rate. Accessed From: https://www.cia.gov/library/publications/the-world-factbook/rankorder/2127rank.html (29 Jun 2020).
3. Ethiopian Federal Ministry of Health. Health sector transformation plan. Addis Ababa: EFMoH; 2015.
4. Ethiopian Public Health Institute (EPHI) [Ethiopia] and ICF. Ethiopia mini demographic and health survey 2019: key indicators. Rockville: EPHI and ICF; 2019.
5. Varun N, Nigam A, Gupta N. Misplaced IUCD: a case report. Int J Reprod Contracept Obstet Gynecol. 2017;6(11):5155–7.
6. Mishra S. Tale of the tails, the missing postpartum IUCD strings. J Obstetrics Gynecol India. 2017;67(3):202–7.
7. Alemayehu M, Belachew T, Tilahun T. Factors associated with utilization of long acting and permanent contraceptive methods among married women of reproductive age in Mekelle town, Tigray region, North Ethiopia. BMC Pregnancy Childbirth. 2012;12(1):6.
8. Cheung ML, Rezai S, Jackman JM, Patel ND, Bernaba BZ, Hakimian O, Nuritdinova D, Turley CL, Mercado R, Takeshige T, Reddy SM, Fuller PN, Henderson CE. Retained Intrauterine Device (IUD): triple case report and review of the literature. Case Rep Obstet Gynecol. 2018;2018:9362962.
9. Sowmya Shruthi D, Manoli N. A case report of successful retrieval of missing copper T by laparoscopic approach. J Med Sci Health. 2016;2(1):37–9.
10. USAID Transform: Primary Health Care Activity. Theory of change in practice 2017. Addis Ababa: USAID Transform: Primary Health Care; 2017.
11. Wanyonyi SZ, Mariara CM, Vinayak S, Stones W. Opportunities and challenges in realizing universal access to obstetric ultrasound in sub-Saharan Africa. Ultrasound Int Open. 2017;3:E52–9.
12. Moro F, Knez J, Pateman K, Derdelis G, Foo X, Jurkovic D. Ultrasound-guided retrieval of lost intrauterine devices using very fine grasping forceps: a case series. J Fam Plann Reprod Health Care. 2015;41(3):205–9.
13. Dalby J, Dihlmann-Malzer E. What methods are most effective in the office setting for removing IUDs with missing strings? Evidence-Based Pract. 2017;20(3):5.
14. Adewale FB, Ashimi A. Missing intrauterine contraceptive device string: diagnosis and management at federal medical center Bida, Northcentral, Nigeria. Trop J Obstet Gynaecol. 2018;35(3):298–303.

10

Infertility knowledge and treatment beliefs among African American women in an urban community

Ashley Wiltshire[1*], Lynae M Brayboy[2], Kiwita Phillips[1], Roland Matthews[1], Fengxia Yan[3] and Desiree McCarthy-Keith[1]

Abstract

Background: To assess infertility knowledge and treatment beliefs among African American women in an urban community in Atlanta, Georgia.

Methods: This was a cross sectional study at a safety net hospital. A convenience sample of a total of 158 women receiving outpatient obstetrical or gynecologic care from March–April 2017 were recruited. Infertility knowledge and treatment beliefs were assessed using a previously applied and field-tested survey from the International Fertility Decision Making Study.

Results: The mean infertility knowledge score was 38.15% for total subjects. Those with a higher level of education ($p < 0.0001$) and those with paid employment ($p = 0.01$) had a significantly higher level of infertility knowledge. Those who had a history of infertility therapy were significantly more likely to agree with negative treatment beliefs ($p = 0.01$). There was no significant difference in infertility knowledge or treatment beliefs based on age, sexuality, parity or being pregnant at the time of survey completion.

Conclusions: African American women in our urban clinic setting seem to have a limited level of knowledge pertaining to infertility. Further research is needed to understand how differences in knowledge and beliefs translate into infertility care decision-making and future childbearing.

Keywords: Infertility, African American, Women, Reproduction

Introduction

Infertility is a disease of numerous etiologies, which can affect both men and women of every ethnic group and race around the world [1]. Though it is rarely considered a health issue of serious concern, infertility can lead to distress and depression, as well as discrimination and ostracism in certain cultures [2]. An estimated 48.5 million couples worldwide were infertile in 2010 [1]. According to the Centers for Disease Control and Prevention (CDC), approximately 6% of married women of reproductive age are infertile and approximately 12% of reproductive age women, regardless of marital status, have impaired fecundity in the United States (US) [3].

Similar to many other health conditions in the US, infertility is intertwined with multifactorial racial disparities [4]. Studies show that African American (AA) women are disproportionately affected by infertility in terms of prevalence, utilization of treatment, and access to care [4–7]. Even after adjusting for socioeconomic status, risk factors, and pregnancy intent, a US population-based study showed that AA women ages 33–44 years are still two-fold more likely to experience infertility in comparison to Caucasian American (CA) women [4, 6]. This issue has been of even greater concern, as statistical trends have shown that infertility rates were increasing among AA women while simultaneously decreasing among CA women (5).

This racial disparity persists, in regard to pursuit of infertility care and success rates of Assisted Reproductive Technology (ART). It is well documented in the literature that AA women usually have a longer duration of infertility

* Correspondence: ashleyfimrc@gmail.com
[1]Morehouse School of Medicine, Department of Obstetrics and Gynecology, 720 Westview Drive, Atlanta, GA 30310, USA

before seeking care and they also pursue medical care for infertility significantly less often than CA women [4–7]. Currently, there are 15 states in the US with varying degrees of ART insurance coverage, as mandated by law [8]. Even in insurance mandated states, AA women seek infertility care less often than CA women [4]. Of the AA women who do seek care, live birth rates after IVF are disproportionately lower [4, 5, 7]. The trend of poor outcomes in AA women is particularly illustrated by the Society for Assisted Reproductive Technology (SART) database [5, 7]. Trend analysis has shown that live births after fresh embryo transfer occurs significantly less often in AA than CA women. The difference was calculated to be as high as 31% between 2000 and 2004 [5]. In an analysis of SART data from 2004 to 2013, AA women had higher rates of SAB and significantly lower rates of live birth after autogolous and third party ART [7].

Numerous studies have confirmed that there is a racial disparity regarding infertility, which prevails through access, pursuit, utilization and success rates of treatment [4–7]. Nevertheless, the answer as to why these disparities exist and persist remains unclear. Just as unclear, is our understanding of what AA women know of the disease. Likewise, when it comes to patient perspectives of infertility and infertility care, there is a dearth of research on this topic with adequate representation of AA women. Therefore, characterizing this subpopulations' understanding of infertility and infertility management would likely yield a valuable first step in tackling these issues.

Our objectives in this study were to assess infertility knowledge and treatment beliefs specifically among AA women in an urban setting in Atlanta, Georgia. The ultimate goal was to establish a generalized knowledge level and to uncover unique belief patterns within this subpopulation to use as a foundation for educational intervention, as well as a tool to help shape optimum patient care.

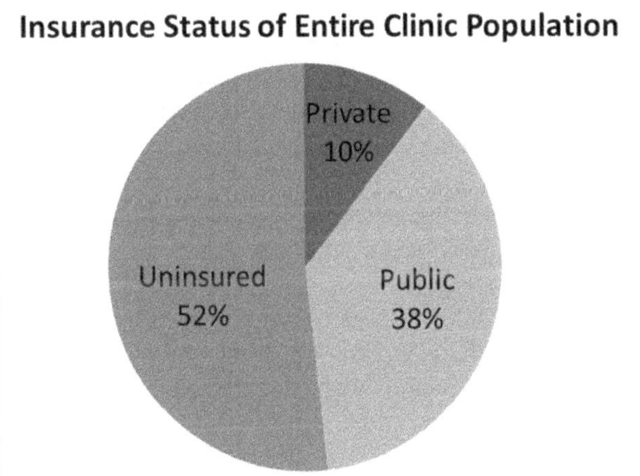

Fig. 1 Insurance status of entire clinic population

Material and methods

Study population

This study was conducted at a Historically Black College/University (HBCU) affiliated safety-net hospital in an urban community in Atlanta, Georgia. The study participants were recruited from the Obstetrics and Gynecology clinics, staffed by resident physicians, attending physicians, nurse midwives and physician assistants. The insurance status of our patient population at this location is 52% uninsured, 38% public, and 10% private (Fig. 1). From March to April 2017, women presenting for either obstetrical or gynecologic evaluation were recruited to participate in the study. Recruitment was performed by the provider or clinic nurse after the clinic visit was completed to avoid the perception of coercion. Patients were provided with a cover letter describing the study. The cover letter also explained that participation was completely voluntary and would have no impact on their medical care. If the patient decided to participate, a paper copy of the survey was provided for them to complete privately in a separate room before discharge. Inclusion criteria consisted of female gender, age ≥ 18 years, English literacy, and self-identification as Black or African American. Participants were not compensated.

Survey instrument

The survey instrument consisted of 13 items on infertility knowledge statements answered with True/False/Don't Know and 6 items of infertility treatment belief statements answered with a Likert scale (Additional file 1). For infertility treatment beliefs, the first two items were considered positive beliefs (ex. "treatment is safe") and last four items were considered negative beliefs (ex. "treatment is a scary experience"). These 19 questions were taken directly from the published survey administered in the FKBF-IFDM study, with the author's permission (Fertility Knowledge and Beliefs about Fertility Treatment: Findings from the International Fertility Decision-Making Study). We decided to incorporate these particular infertility knowledge and belief questions because this survey has been previously applied and field tested in 79 different countries, including the US [9]. In addition to those 19 questions, we added an additional 12 questions pertaining to patient demographics and personal obstetrical history. Our final survey was considered to be at the 7th grade reading level per the Flesche-Kincaid scale. It was self-administered and self-paced, requiring approximately 10 min to complete.

Statistical analyses

The data was coded, logged into a Microsoft Excel and then analyzed using Statistical Analysis Software (SAS 9.4). For infertility knowledge, the patient was given a score of 1 if answered correctly and 0 if the answer was incorrect or if they chose "don't know", as done in the original study. The final knowledge score was calculated using summation of the number of correctly answered questions divided by total number of questions and multiplied by 100. The score range was 0–100%. For infertility treatment beliefs, the answer range for both the positive and negative statements were based on a Likert score of 1–5. A selection of "1" signified strongly disagree and "5" signified strongly agree. The mean Likert score was calculated and used for comparisons.

Descriptive statistics was performed to summarize the demographic characteristics and other related measurements. The frequency with percentage was used for categorical variables and the mean with standard deviation was used for numerical variables. Two independent sample t-tests were used to compare the knowledge and belief difference between two level categorical variables (i.e., age, race, education, employment status, pregnant status and parity). An analysis of variance test was used to examine the knowledge and belief differences among three types of sexual orientation. A multiple linear regression analysis was performed to examine the individual effect of different factors by controlling other factors for positive beliefs, negative beliefs and knowledge. All the data analyses were performed using SAS 9.4 and $p < 0.05$ was considered to be statistically significant.

Results

A total of 158 completed questionnaires were collected meeting our inclusion criteria. The mean age of the subjects was 35 years, with an age range from 18 to 72 years. Fifty-three and a half percent (53.5%) of the total participants were younger than 35 years. Twenty-nine percent (29%) had a higher-level education (university or post-graduate). Fifty-nine percent (59%) had paid employment. Sexual orientation was as follows: heterosexual (90%), homosexual (6%), bisexual (4%). Eleven percent (11%) of subjects reported a history of difficulty conceiving and 3% of total participants required infertility therapy for conception in the past. Forty-seven percent (47%) of participants were pregnant at the time of questionnaire completion. The average age of first pregnancy/delivery was 20 years, and the average parity was 2. Socio-demographic details are displayed in Table 1.

The mean infertility knowledge score was 38.15% for total participants in our study (Tables 2 and 3). Those with a higher level of education ($p = < 0.0001$) and those with paid employment ($p = 0.01$) had a significantly higher level of infertility knowledge (Table 4). The mean positive belief score was 3.31 and the mean negative belief score was 2.96 in our study (Table 2). Those who had a history of infertility treatment had significantly stronger agreement with negative treatment beliefs ($p = 0.01$) (Table 4). There was no significant difference in infertility knowledge or treatment beliefs based on age, sexuality, parity or being pregnant at the time of survey completion. There was no correlation between the fertility knowledge score and having a stronger agreement with negative or positive treatment beliefs. Fertility knowledge and treatment beliefs in relation to socio-demographic factors are displayed in Table 4. The frequency and percentage of participants who correctly answered each item in the knowledge section of the survey is displayed in Table 3.

Table 1 Results of infertility survey ($N = 158$)

Baseline Characteristics	Frequency (%) or mean ± SD
Age < 35 years	84 (53.5)
Age	35.03 ± (12.24)
University or Post Graduate Education	46 (29)
Have paid employment	92 (59)
Sexuality	
Heterosexual	142 (90)
Homosexual	9 (6)
Bisexual	7 (4)
Pregnant currently	65 (47)
History of difficulty becoming pregnant	16 (11)
History of fertility therapy	4 (3)
Gravidity	3.04 ± 2.39
Parity	2.04 ± 1.62
Number of miscarriage/abortions	1 ± 1.26
Age at first delivery	20.33 ± 5.46

A multiple linear regression analysis was performed to examine the individual effect of different factors by controlling other factors for positive beliefs, negative beliefs and knowledge (Table 5). Based on the multiple linear regression analysis, for negative infertility treatment beliefs, having a history of infertility treatment remained a significant factor. For positive infertility treatment beliefs, age remained a significant factor. Lastly, for infertility knowledge, education remained a significant factor. Results of the multiple linear regression are displayed in Table 5.

Discussion

Infertility knowledge

Despite being disproportionately affected by infertility, African American women seem to have a limited level of infertility knowledge. In a comparison to the original study by Bunting et al., our participants had a lower level

Table 2 Fertility knowledge and treatment beliefs total results

Survey Section	Mean ± SD
Fertility Knowledge	38.15 ± 20.36
Positive beliefs	3.31 ± 0.90
Negative beliefs	2.96 ± 0.88

Table 3 Frequency and percentage of participants who correctly answered each knowledge item

Question	Total	Frequency	Percentage (95% CI)
1. A woman is less fertile after the age of 36 years. (True)	157	38	24.2 (17.7–31.7)
2. A couple would be classified as infertile if they did not achieve a pregnancy after 1 year of regular sexual intercourse (without using contraception). (True)	156	59	37.8 (30.2–46.0)
3. Smoking decreases female fertility. (True)	157	55	35.0 (27.6–43.0)
4. Smoking decreases male fertility. (True)	158	39	24.7 (18.2–32.2)
5. About 1 in 10 couples are infertile. (True)	157	89	56.7 (48.6–64.6)
6. If a man produces sperm he is fertile. (False)	157	70	44.6 (36.7–52.7)
7. These days a woman in her 40s has a similar chance of getting pregnant as a woman in her 30s. (False)	157	18	11.5 (6.9–17.5)
8. Having a healthy lifestyle makes you fertile. (False)	157	31	20.0 (13.8–26.8)
9. If a man has had mumps after puberty he is more likely to later have a fertility problem. (True)	157	67	42.7 (34.8–50.8)
10. A woman who never menstruates is still fertile. (False)	158	70	44.3 (36.4–52.4)
11. If a woman is overweight by more than 28 pounds then she may not be able to get pregnant. (True)	158	90	57.0 (48.9–64.8)
12. If a man can achieve an erection then it is an indication that he is fertile. (False)	158	83	52.5 (44.5–60.5)
13. People who have had a sexually transmitted disease are likely to have reduced fertility. (True)	158	72	45.6 (37.6–53.7)

of infertility knowledge (score 38%) when compared to their total number of women ($n = 8355$, average score 59.1%, 79 countries). Our participants also had a lower knowledge score in comparison to their female participants specifically representing the USA ($N = 427$, average score approximately 65%) [9].

While infertility is a disease of many etiologies, a commonly cited cause of infertility among AA women is tubal factor, which is often secondary to a history of sexually transmitted infection or pelvic inflammatory disease [5]. Interestingly, only 45.6% of total participants in our study knew that sexually transmitted diseases could adversely affect fertility. This reflects a concerning lack of sexual health awareness among the women in our study. Our results are consistent with those found by Deatsman et al., who found that AA women were less aware, in comparison to other racial groups, that a history of STI can be risk factor for infertility [10].

As delayed childbearing has become the norm in our society, patient awareness of how age affects infertility is becoming increasingly more important [11]. In our study, 24% percent of participants knew that a woman's fertility decreases after the age of 36 years. Furthermore, only 11.5%of subjects knew that the probability of conceiving is different between a woman age 30 vs. 40 years. This was also consistent with Deatsman et al's study, showing AA women were significantly less aware of the impact age has on infertility [10].

Obesity (defined as BMI > 30) is another health condition disproportionately affecting African Americans in the US. In the US approximately 56.5% of African American women are obese compared to 35.3% of Caucasian American women. When including those who are overweight (defined as BMI 25–30), the percentage surges to 82% of AA women and 63.5% of CA women [12]. The survey instrument included the threshold of "greater than 28 pounds overweight", as this was previously determined in a preliminary study by Bunting et al., to be the point at which there is a significant association with infertility [13]. In our study, 57% of participants correctly associated increased difficulty with fertility and being overweight by > 28 lbs. This is of clear concern as obesity is a modifiable risk factor and the vast majority of AA women have a BMI > 25 [12].

Infertility treatment beliefs

Overall, our subjects had a relatively neutral response to both negative and positive treatment beliefs. There was no significant difference in treatment beliefs based on age, education level, and parity. Interestingly, those with a history of infertility therapy were significantly more likely to agree with negative treatment beliefs. Detailed questions to characterize the experiences of those who reported a history of infertility treatment were not included in the survey. Therefore, this finding may be due to a personal history of poor success with treatment. However, this finding also raises questions of how their infertility care experiences may differ from other racial groups. It is important to consider the commonly found mistrust of the

Table 4 Two sample T Test/ANOVA to test mean scores for fertility knowledge and treatment belief ($N = 158$)

	Fertility knowledge mean score (SD)	*p*-value	Negative treatment belief mean score (SD)	*p*-value	Positive treatment belief mean score (SD)	*p*-value
Age		0.56		0.05		0.07
< 35 years	37.41 (18.36)		2.81 (0.89)		3.44 (0.77)	
≥35 years	39.32 (22.50)		3.10 (0.82)		3.16 (1.02)	
Education		< 0.0001*		0.08		0.26
University or post graduate	47.55 (23.25)		3.15 (0.88)		3.44 (0.73)	
High school graduate or less	33.98 (17.53)		2.87 (0.88)		3.25 (0.97)	
Paid employment		0.01*		0.9		0.58
Yes	41.58 (20.84)		2.97 (0.97)		3.34 (0.82)	
No	33.06 (18.78)		2.95 (0.75)		3.26 (1.01)	
Have sexual relationship with				0.94		0.05
Males	38.88 (20.83)	0.35	2.95 (0.85)		3.25 (0.89)	
Females	29.06 (13.75)		2.97 (1.37)		3.56 (0.82)	
Both	35.16 (15.92)		3.07 (0.92)		4.07 (0.93)	
Pregnant now		0.76		0.22		0.98
Yes	37.20 (20.25)		2.83 (0.77)		3.25 (0.84)	
No	38.25 (20.88)		3.01 (0.93)		3.25 (0.93)	
Deliver baby before		0.66		0.41		0.79
Yes	38.22 (20.12)		2.93 (0.89)		3.26 (0.91)	
No	36.12 (23.01)		2.81 (0.56)		3.20 (0.80)	
Have difficulty becoming pregnant		0.75		0.84		0.2
Yes	36.54 (22.21)		2.98 (0.90)		3.54 (0.66)	
No	38.30 (20.44)		2.93 (0.86)		3.22 (0.90)	
Require fertility therapy		0.17		< 0.0001*		0.25
Yes	51.92 (26.18)		4 (0.20)		3.75 (1.26)	
No	37.70 (20.37)		2.9 (0.85)		3.24 (0.87)	

***Significant statistical difference was detected**

Table 5 Multiple regression model outcomes for infertility beliefs and knowledge

	Negative belief		Positive belief		Knowledge	
Source	*F* Value	*P* value	*F* Value	*P* value	*F* Value	*P* value
Age	2.74	0.1009	8.82	0.0036*	0.74	0.3908
Education	0.8	0.4956	1.33	0.269	3.85	0.0112*
Work	0.09	0.7655	0.41	0.521	2.94	0.0889
Sexuality	1.92	0.1506	2.64	0.076	0.22	0.8004
Currently Pregnant	0.23	0.6304	0.63	0.4275	0.48	0.4911
Infertility History	2.57	0.1115	0.18	0.6717	1.81	0.1807
Infertility Treatment History	4.78	0.0308*	0.82	0.3675	1.44	0.2319
Parity	0.13	0.7179	0.55	0.4616	0.16	0.6925

The outcome of the multiple regression model was performed on negative beliefs positive beliefs and knowledge separately. The input variables include age, education level, employment, gender, current pregnancy status, Infertility History, Infertility Treatment history and parity. *Significant statistical difference was detected

US healthcare system held among many AAs. This general mistrust is often attributed to the AA response to institutionalized racism and the history of medical maltreatment in the US [14]. It is possible that these negative beliefs result from underlying mistrust rooted in AA history.

Strengths and limitations

Our study is unique because it includes solely women who self-identify as African-American or black, which is currently the third largest racial ethnic group in the US [15]. This group is often underrepresented in the literature, especially in qualitative studies focused on infertility. Further strengths include the diversity of our subjects, with respect to age, parity and education levels.

There were limitations to this study, which may affect the generalizability of our results. Our survey was administered to a convenience sample at a single location in a safety net hospital. The results of our study may not reflect the infertility knowledge and beliefs of privately insured AA women, those with a higher socioeconomic status or those living in the suburbs, rural or other urban areas. We did not include insurance type as a part of the survey instrument. Therefore, a sampling bias may have been created as the majority of the patients at our clinic are insured by Medicaid or are uninsured. Though we are unable to incorporate specific insurance types per participant, we were able to calculate the proportion of insurance types used across our entire clinic patient population (Fig. 1). Also not included in the survey instrument, were detailed questions to characterize experiences of those who reported a history of infertility treatment.

Unfortunately, the participation rate was not tracked and therefore cannot be calculated or analyzed. However, most patients who were invited to participate in this study completed the survey. Additionally, a sample selection bias may have been created on exceptionally busy clinic days when recruitment occurred less often. Lastly, the sociodemographic composition of our patient population differed greatly from the original study and the proportion of African American representation in the original study was not published. Due to this, we were unable to make a stronger/statistical comparison. Though this is a limitation, it also underscores our disposition to further characterize this subpopulation's perspective of infertility.

Conclusion

Our study contributes a unique perspective of a significant yet underrepresented population of American women. Numerous studies have confirmed that there is a racial disparity for infertility, which prevails through access, pursuit, utilization and success rates of treatment [4–7]. Our study shows that African American women within our healthcare setting have a limited level of infertility knowledge. The consistent finding of poor infertility knowledge is of particular importance because being able to understand the basics of fertility and reproduction can shape a woman's fertility decision-making and planned childbearing.

One of the biggest modifiable factors for the disparities associated with infertility is likely knowledge. Regardless of socioeconomic status, women's health providers should routinely include culturally sensitive fertility awareness and education for all of their patients. Both the American College of Obstetricians and Gynecologists and the Centers for Disease Control and Prevention recommend inclusion of "Reproductive Life Planning" as part of the annual well woman visit [16]. Additional educational outreach modalities include infertility workshops, brochures, online modules and smartphone mobile applications. A worthwhile future investigation would be to incorporate a wider sociodemographic patient population, provide the aforementioned educational modalities and compare pre and post-test knowledge and beliefs.

Though increased awareness and education is likely a promising preventative strategy, the disparity in infertility care should not be ignored. The full spectrum of infertility care is not commonly provided in low-income communities. These services are also not readily available at our hospital. Hence, clear patient inequities are easily appreciated in the attempt to counsel those who require ART for their infertility but are unable to afford subspecialty fertility care elsewhere. One strategy to correct this issue would be through the implementation of more low-cost IVF programs. With the creation of low-cost yet high quality ovarian stimulation protocols and IVF techniques, the prospect of providing full spectrum infertility care to those living in low resource settings has become feasible [17]. As the outcomes of these new techniques and programs materialize in the literature, hopefully additional programs with similar goals will begin to disseminate throughout the US and worldwide.

In conclusion, African American women in our urban clinic setting seem to have a limited level of knowledge pertaining to infertility. This finding is likely generalizable to other minority groups within similar settings and warrants a great need for further research, as well as effective, culturally relevant educational interventions. It is our responsibility, as women's health providers, to work in unison not only to improve patient awareness but to also strive for changes that will ensure equal quality infertility care for all.

Acknowledgements
The authors would like to thank the Grady Memorial Hospital Obstetrics and Gynecology Clinic staff for their support.

Authors' contributions
AW: Study Development and Execution, Writing. LMB: Study Development, Editing. KP: Editing. RM: Statistical Support. FY: Statistical Analysis. DM-K: Study Development, Editing. All authors read and approved the final manuscript.

Author details
[1]Morehouse School of Medicine, Department of Obstetrics and Gynecology, 720 Westview Drive, Atlanta, GA 30310, USA. [2]Department of Obstetrics and Gynecology Division of Reproductive Endocrinology and Infertility Women & Infants Hospital, Alpert Medical School of Brown University, 101 Dudley Fl 1, Providence, RI 02905, USA. [3]Morehouse School of Medicine Department of Community Health & Preventive Medicine, 720 Westview Drive, Atlanta, GA 30310, USA.

References
1. Mascarenhas MN, Flaxman SR, Boerma T, Vanderpoel S, Stevens GA. National, regional, and global trends in infertility prevalence since 1990: a systematic analysis of 277 health surveys. PLoS Med. 2012. https://doi.org/10.1371/journal.pmed.1001356.
2. Inhorn MC, Patrizio P. Infertility around the globe: new thinking on gender, reproductive technologies and global movements in the 21st century. Hum Reprod Update. 2015. https://doi.org/10.1093/humupd/dmv016.
3. Chandra A, Copen CE, Stephen EH. Infertility and impaired fecundity in the United States, 1982–2010: data from the National Survey of family growth. Natl Health Stat Report. 2013;67:1–18.
4. Eichelberger KY, Doll K, Ekpo GE, Zerden ML. Black lives matter: claiming a space for evidence-based outrage in obstetrics and gynecology. Am J Public Health. 2016. https://doi.org/10.2105/AJPH.2016.303313.
5. Seifer DB, et al. Trends of racial disparities in assisted reproductive technology outcomes in black women compared with white women: Society for Assisted Reproductive Technology 1999 and 2000 vs. 2004–2006. Fertil Steril. 2010. https://doi.org/10.1016/j.fertnstert.2009.02.084.
6. Wellons MF, Lewis CE, Schwartz SM, et al. Racial differences in self-reported infertility and risk factors for infertility in a cohort of black and white women: the CARDIA Women's study. Fertil Steril. 2008. https://doi.org/10.1016/j.fertnstert.2007.09.056.
7. Shapiro AJ, Darmon SK, Barad DH, Albertini DF, Gleicher N, Kushnir VA. Effect of race and ethnicity on utilization and outcomes of assisted reproductive technology in the USA. Reprod Biol Endocrinol. 2017. https://doi.org/10.1186/s12958-017-0262-5.
8. Hornstein M. Is insurance coverage forin vitro fertilization a good thing? Fertil Steril. 2018. https://doi.org/10.1016/j.fertnstert.2018.02.012.
9. Bunting L, Tsibulsky I, Boivin J. Fertility knowledge and beliefs about fertility treatment: findings from the international fertility decision-making study. Hum Reprod. 2013. https://doi.org/10.1093/humrep/des402.
10. Deatsman S, Vasilopoulos T, Rhoton-Vlasak A. Age and fertility: a study on patient awareness. JBRA Assist Reprod. 2016. https://doi.org/10.5935/1518-0557.20160024.
11. American College of Obstetricians and Gynecologists. Female age-related fertility decline. Committee Opinion No. 589. Obstet Gynecol. 2014;123:719–21.
12. U.S Department of Health and Human Services Office of Minority Health. Obesity and African Americans. 2017. https://minorityhealth.hhs.gov/omh/browse.aspx?lvl=4&lvlid=25. Accessed 19 July 2019.
13. Bunting L, Boivin J. Development and preliminary validation of the fertility status awareness tool: FertiSTAT. Hum Reprod. 2010. https://doi.org/10.1093/humrep/deq087.
14. Sule E, Sutton RM, Jones D, et al. The Past Does Matter: a Nursing Perspective on Post Traumatic Slave Syndrome (PTSS). J Racial Ethn Health Disparities. 2017. https://doi.org/10.1007/s40615-016-0328-7.
15. United States Quick Facts. Race and Hispanic Origin. https://www.census.gov/quickfacts/fact/table/US/RHI825218#viewtop. Accessed 20 July 2019.
16. American College of Obstetricians and Gynecologists. Well-woman visit. ACOG Committee Opinion No. 755. Obstet Gynecol. 2018;132:e181–6.
17. Herndon CN, Anaya Y, Noel M, Cakmak H, Cedars M. Outcomes from a university-based low-cost in vitro fertilization program providing access to care for a low-resource socioculturally diverse urban community. Fertil Steril. 2017. https://doi.org/10.1016/j.fertnstert.2017.06.035.

11

Determinants of intrauterine contraceptive device utilization at primary health care facilities in Mekelle City, northern Ethiopia

Gebremaryam Temesgen Birgoda[1], Haftom Gebrehiwot[2], Sultan Hussen Hebo[3*], Birhane Hagos[4], Genet Assefa[5], Negussie Boti Sidamo[3] and Mulugeta Shegaze Shembri[3]

Abstract

Background: Each year, the current level of modern contraceptive use averts 188 million unintended pregnancies, which in turn results in 112 million fewer abortions. Of the 867 million women in the developing world who are sexually active and want to avoid becoming pregnant, approximately 222 million of them have an unmet need for modern contraception. In spite of several advantages and potential effectiveness of Intra Uterine Contraceptive Device, its utilization still too low in Sub Saharan African countries including Ethiopia.

Objectives: To identify the determinant factors for utilization of intra uterine contraceptive device among women visiting primary health care facilities in Mekelle city.

Method: Facility based unmatched case-control study design was conducted among 234 women (78 cases and 156 controls). Data was collected by structured questionnaire. Data entry and cleaning was done using EPI- Info version 5.3.1 and analysis done using SPSS version 20.0 statistical software. During analysis the variables were defined, categorized and the difference in variables was determined. Odds ratio used to show degree of association between independent variables with Intra Uterine Contraceptive Device.

Result: Marital status ([AOR (95%CI) =8.59(2.60–28.43)], number of pregnancies (AOR (95%) CI = 5.69(1.020–31.802), number of alive children [AOR (95%CI) =3.5 (1.03–11.9) are variables continued to have statistically significant association with use of Intra Uterine Contraceptive Device. Other determinants found to have significant association includes awareness about Intra Uterine Contraceptive Device, visual exposure to Intra Uterine Contraceptive Device, and participants told about availability of health care provider able to insert Intra Uterine Contraceptive Device.

Conclusion: This study has identified marital status, Gravidity, number of alive children and awareness to Intra Uterine Contraceptive Device as major determinants for use of Intra Uterine Contraceptive Device. Thus, it is vital at addressing the aforementioned determinants will be vital to improve utilization of Intra Uterine Contraceptive Device.

(Continued on next page)

* Correspondence: Sultanhussn@gmail.com
[3]Department of Public Health, College of Medicine & Health Sciences, Arba Minch University, Arba Minch, Ethiopia

(Continued from previous page)

Plain English summary: Among long acting reversible modern contraceptive methods, Intra Uterine Contraceptive Devices (IUCDs) are the most reliable and effective as well as with fewer side effects. Despite these advantages and cost effective potential of Intra Uterine Contraceptive Device its utilization is still too low in Sub Saharan countries like Ethiopia. Thus, this study intended to identify the factors that limit the utilization of Intra Uterine Contraceptive Device among women of Ethiopia in Mekele City. The study identify that the utilization of Intra Uterine Contraceptive Device was determined by the marital status of the women, the number of previous pregnancy and recent alive children and the level of awareness about Intra Uterine Contraceptive Device of the women. Therefore, providers training that focus on promoting Intra Uterine Contraceptive Device, centering on increasing awareness and practice about Intra Uterine Contraceptive Device is very important.

Keywords: Intra uterine contraceptive device, Case control, Determinant factors

Introduction

Family planning is defined as the use of contraceptive methods enables couples to have desired number of children, to control the timing and spacing of pregnancy [1]. Modern contraceptives methods are categorized into three: Long acting reversible contraceptive methods which consists of development and introduction of modern intrauterine devices (IUCDs) and Implants, permanent contraceptive methods which includes tubal ligation and vasectomy and short term contraceptives methods constitutes predominant method in developing countries (inject-able), oral pill, male and female condoms, foam tablet and cervical cap [2].

The development and introduction of modern intrauterine devices (IUDs) in 1960, shortly after the advent of oral contraceptives, makes the beginning of the modern era of long-acting reversible contraception. Then rapidly became the method of choice in pioneering programs in Taiwan, Korea, and other countries like United States [3].

It is estimated about 500 million women in the developing world are using some form of family planning. From 113 million married women of reproductive age in sub-Saharan Africa, 21 million (one in five) married women use family planning. 14.7 million less than one of seven) women currently use modern contraception only 2.7 million women use long-acting or permanent contraception [4].

Copper IUCD are the most reliable and effective form of LARC have several advantages over other forms including implanone (it serves us both long and short acting as fertility return immediately after removal, fewer side effect than hormonal methods, fewer discontinuation rate (13%) than other forms oral contraceptives (43.5%),injectable (40.6%) and condom 50.4% over 12 months. It can be inserted immediately after delivery and abortion, has no adverse effect with other medications like anti-retroviral therapy and can be inserted by trained health providers at all level. In spite of these advantages and cost effective potential of IUCD its utilization is still too low only 8% in Sub Saharan countries and 9% in South Central Asia, even as high as 22% in South east Asia [5].

Fertility rate is 2.5 children per woman World fertility pattern (WFP 2015). According to WHO estimate about global MMR is 216 and 800 maternal death every day occur with preventable causes related with pregnancy and child birth. Ninety Nine Percent of this death is in developing countries, Sub-Saharan Africa contributes 66% followed by south Asia [5]. Each year, the current level of modern contraceptive use averts 188 million unintended pregnancies, which in turn results in 112 million fewer abortions, 1.1 million few newborn deaths and 150,000 fewer maternal deaths [6].

Africa remains the region with the highest fertility at 4.7 children per woman, which is the fastest growth from any other region and projected to account 21% of the global population by 2050 [7]. The Federal Democratic Republic of Ethiopia is the second most populous country in sub Saharan Africa with an estimated population of approximately 92.08 million people1 and total fertility rate (TFR) of 4.6 children per woman (2.3 in urban areas and 5.2 in rural areas) and the tenth largest by area with its 1.1 million square kilometers [8].

Globally, 163 million (15% of reproductive aged women use IUCD [9]. Countries with the higher number of IUCD user includes Cuba (43.5%), Vietnam (37.7%), Egypt (36.5%) and China (44.9%) (World Bank Africa Region,), the lowest use of the IUCD is observed in Africa, where few countries show more than one or 2 % use of the method [10].

By now the progress of CPR in Ethiopia is increased from 6% in 2000 to 35% by 2016. However, The CPR is highly dependent on short-term family planning methods (e.g. Nearly 23% for inject able followed by implant 8% and IUCD constitute 2%),and unmet need for family planning is still high for spacing births (13%) and limiting (9%) [11]. The CPR in Tigray is similar with the national Average (35%) in EDHS 2016,and dependent on injectable (19%) followed by implant (11%) and pills

(4%),but the prevalence of IUCD (1%),which is below the national level [12].

Recent evidence related to intrauterine contraception provides various assumptions as to the reasons for low and declining use of the IUCD. Among various reasons, incorrect perceptions and knowledge of IUCDs, skills of providers and facility readiness for IUCD service have been considered as a major limitation [13].

Although the IUCD is available free of charge in the public sector services, it is not being utilized adequately. Various studies suggest that lack of clients knowledge and/or misunderstanding about IUCD method, reluctance of service providers in providing information about IUCD, in adequately trained health care providers, and absence of continuing education and awareness of clients have been suggested to be major limiting factors to improve acceptability of this safe and effective contraceptive method of IUCD [14].

Recognizing this situation, the Federal Ministry of Health (FMOH), under Health service development program IV, has set a target CPR of 66% by 2015, besides, the FMOH has considered the important role of long-acting nonpermanent and permanent methods and aims to provide 20% of all family planning clients with these long-acting methods [12]. But it remained un attainable as CPR in the country is 35% which relies on injectable [13].

In general, it is possible to conclude from the above discussions that modern contraceptive use in Ethiopia is dependent on short acting contraceptive methods and IUCD methods share of use remains below or else underutilized in most women in Ethiopia (19, 20). Thus, understanding the factors that limits the use of IUCD in women in Mekelle city, therefore, can help to inform interventions that can strengthen women's empowerment in ways to plan their pregnancies to achieve desired family size.

Methods and materials

Study setting, design and population

Study was done in Mekelle town, which is the capital of Tigray region from October 25–November 25, 2017 where the overall prevalence IUCD in the city is 1.5% (27). Facility based unmatched case-control study design was used. Participant number is determined by using formula for comparison of two population proportions with unequal proportion and EPINFO Version 3.5.3 statistical software. Based on the assumption of level of significance, $\alpha = 0.05$, Power $1\text{-}^{\beta} = 90\%$, Control to case ratio, = 2:1 and the study done in Debremarkos town partner discussion about modern contraceptive is determinant factor for utilization of IUCD, in that study women who have discussion are 2.5 times more likely to use CI (0.143,0.833)(62.5% of users and 40% of non-users have partner discussion about contraceptives [2]. Using this reference the calculated sample size become 234(78 IUCD users and 156 non users). It is taken since it increases my sample size.

Sampling procedures

In the town there are 9 health centers, 2 facilities that are providing reproductive health services (marry stops international and family guidance association) and 2 primary hospitals that facilities are selected randomly and cases are allocated based on their last 2 months provision (August and September, 2017). In each facility, all women who are IUCD users during the study were selected as cases for this study, if the selected case was not fulfill the inclusion criteria, she would be dropped before controls selected. For each case, two controls that used OCPs or injectable during the study were selected after the new IUCD user and if the selected control did not fulfill the inclusion criteria, the next woman who uses OCPs or Injectable during the study were included in the study as a control.

Data collection procedures and tools

A structured questionnaire containing four parts (Socio-demographic and socio-economic variables, Reproductive variables, Knowledge, practice and, decision making variables and Health system variables) was used to interview study participants. It was prepared in English and translated to Tigrigna language. Questionnaires were pre-test and edited. One day training was given for data collectors. Pretest was done in the next day after training of data collectors at Mekele general hospital which is not the actual study settings. Seven trained female clinical nurses and Midwives collected the data immediately after the client obtained the service (exit interview). Before starting the interview, the data collectors took informed verbal consent from the client to participate in the study and registered the chart number of the client for checking any missed or incomplete data.

During the supervision, quality and completeness of gathered information by the data collectors was checked periodically by the principal investigator and timely corrections made which could help a lot in improving the quality, consistency and completeness of data of subsequent interviews. The collected data cleaned manually by the investigator.

Data analysis

After manual cleaning, data entry were done using EPI-Info version 3.5.3. and analysis was done using SPSS version 20.0 statistical software. During analysis the variables defined, categorized and recoded then frequencies of the different variables and cross- tabulations determined. Odds ratio used to show statistical significant level of association between independent variables with

IUCD utilization at p-value < 0.25 and < 0.05 for Binary and Multivariate Logistic Regression respectively.

Ethical considerations

Ethical clearance was obtained from the Health Research Ethics Review Committee at the college of health sciences. Formal recommendation letter was written from department of Midwifery for Tigray Regional Health bureau (TRHB) in turn TRHB wrote similar letter to each selected PPHC and permission obtained from the main office of selected health facility. The issue of consent, privacy and confidentiality were given due emphasis during the training of data collectors. Informed written consent was sought from all study participants at all levels.

Result

Socio-demographic characteristics

A total of 234 women of reproductive age attending the selected Primary health care facilities were interviewed giving response rate of 100%. The age of respondents showing that it is normally distributed at mean (±SD) is 32 ± 6.22 (range 20–43) and 26.28 ± 5.83 (range 17–40) for case and control respectively. Less than 10% of cases and controls can read and write but more than half 52.6% of respondents in each group had secondary education. The following table summarizes the socio-demographic characteristics of the respondents (Table 1).

Table 1 Socio-demographic characteristics of clients visiting family planning clinic at Primary Health Care Facilities in Mekelle city. Northern Ethiopia, Tigray region, 2017

Variables	Cases (78)	Controls (156)	Total (234)
Age (years)			
15–24	9 (11.5)	69 (44.3)	78 (33)
25–29	23 (29.5)	42 (26.8)	65 (27)
30–34	17 (21.8)	26 (16.7)	43 (18)
35–39	16 (20.5)	13 (8.3)	29 (12)
40–44	13 (16.7)	6 (3.8)	19 (8)
Religion			
Christian	69 (88.5)	134 (85.9)	171 (73.1)
Muslim	9 (11.5)	22 (14.1)	31 (13.5)
Ethnicity			
Tigray	64 (82.2)	130 (83.3)	194 (82.9)
Amhara	10 (10.6)	19 (12.2)	29 (12.4)
Others	6 (7.7)	12 (7.7)	18 (7.7)
Educational status			
Primary school	10 (12.8)	37 (23.7)	47 (19.3)
Secondary school	41 (52.6)	82 (52.6)	123 (52.6)
Above secondary	27 (34.6)	37 (23.7)	64 (27.4)
Marital status			
Married	73 (93.6)	101 (64.7)	174 (74.4)
Single	5 (6.4)	55 (35.3)	60 (25.6)

Reproductive health characteristics of the women

Ninety Seven Point Four percent of cases and Seventy Five Point Six Percent of controls experienced pregnancy. More than half 56.6% of cases experienced pregnancy 3 to 4 times and less than 10% of controls were pregnant for 5 and more times. Among those who had history of pregnancy, the majority of cases 72(98.6%) and controls 105(93.8%) had history of normal birth. Majority 58(80.6%) of cases and 82(78.1%) of controls were planned to space birth. All of the case have no history of STI, but 15(9.6%) of controls had STIs history having treated for all of them (Table 2).

Awareness and practice to IUCD

The most majority 76(97.4%) of cases and three-quarter (66%) of controls have heard about IUD. Seventy Nine point Seven Percent of cases and Thirty Four point Six Percent of controls has seen IUCD. Regarding partner discussion about modern contraception 79.2% of cases and 69% of controls have husband discussion.

The above graph shows that health workers are source of information for 29(37.2%) of cases and 63(40.4%) of controls followed by mass media for around quarter of (24.4%) of cases and friends for 40(25.6%) of controls (Fig. 1).

Among 234 respondents the majority of controls 110(70.5%) and less than one third use Injectable and OCP respectively.

Health system factors

76.9% of cases and less than half (42.6%) of controls were told about the effectiveness of IUCD up to 12 years. Majority 85% of cases and around half (53.8%) of controls were told about the availability of health care providers able to insert IUCD.

Factors associated with IUCD utilization

Variables considered for multiple logistic regressions were those with a p-value < 0.05 at bivariate logistic regression analysis and those variables included were age, occupation, marital status, ever heard about IUCD, Visual experience of IUCD, information given about (availability of IUCD, availability health care providers able to insert IUCD, protect pregnancy to 12 years and IUCD require minimal follow up after insertion.

Multiple logistic regression analyses identified that, marital status, number of pregnancy, number of alive children, Awareness about IUCD, visual exposure of IUCD and information given about the availability of Health Care provider able to insert IUCD were

Table 2 Reproductive health characteristics of clients visiting family planning clinic at Primary Health Care Facilities in Mekelle city. Northern Ethiopia, Tigray region, 2017

Variables	Cases(78)	Controls(156)	Total (234)
History of pregnancy (234)			
Have experienced pregnancy	76 (97.4)	118 (75.6)	194 (82.9)
No Experience of Pregnancy	2 (2.6)	38 (24.4)	40 (17.1)
Number of pregnancy (*N* = 194)			
1 to 2 times	19 (25)	67 (57.35)	86 (44.6)
3 to 4 times	43 (56.6)	40 (34.2)	83 (43)
≥5 times	14 (18.4)	10 (8.5)	24 (12.4)
History of abortion (*N* = 194)			
Experienced abortion	37 (48.7)	56 (47.9)	93 (48.2)
No experience of abortion	39 (51.3)	61 (52.1)	100 (51.8)
Number of Abortion (*N* = 93)			
Experienced Abortion Once	32 (86.5)	51 (91.2)	83 (89.4)
Experienced Abortion Twice	5 (13.5)	5 (8.8)	10 (10.6)
History of birth (*N* = 194)			
experienced birth	72 (98.6)	105 (93.8)	177 (95.7)
No experience of birth	1 (1.45)	7 (6.2)	8 (4.3)
Number of Birth (*N* = 177)			
Once	6 (8.2)	33 (31.4)	38 (21.9)
Twice	22 (30.1)	30 (28.6)	52 (29.2)
>Twice	45 (61.6)	42 (40)	87 (48.9)
Number of alive children (*N* = 177)			
1 child	6 (8.2)	33 (31.4)	39 (21.9)
2 children	25 (34.2)	30 (28.6)	55 (30.9)
> 2 children	42 (57.5)	42 (40)	4 (47.2)
Future plan of fertility (234)			
Spacing Birth	58 (80.6)	82 (78.1)	140 (79.1)
Limiting Birth	14 (19.4)	23 (21.9)	37 (20.9)
History of STI			
No history of STI	78 (100)	141 (90.4)	219 (93.6)
History of STI	–	15 (9.6)	15 (6.4)
Screening for HIV			
screened for HIV	76 (33.5)	151 (66.55)	227 (97)
Not screened for HIV	2 (2.6)	5 (3.2)	7 (3)
Test result to HIV			
Reactive	2 (2.6)	5 (3.2)	7 (3)
Non-reactive	76 (97.4)	149 (96.8)	225 (97)

independent predictors that had statistically significant association with the current use of IUCD after adjusted for other covariates (Table 3).

Discussion

The percent distribution of IUCD among ever-married and currently married women is difficult to estimate since there is continuous shift from one method to the other. However, the type of selection of contraceptive method is related to the couple relationship status. By this study marital status is significant determinant of IUCD utilization, those women who are married are 8.6 times more likely to use IUCD than those single and divorced ([AOR (95%CI) =8.59(2.598–28.42)]. This finding is higher than studies conducted in Addis Ababa; Women who had married were 1.89 times more likely to

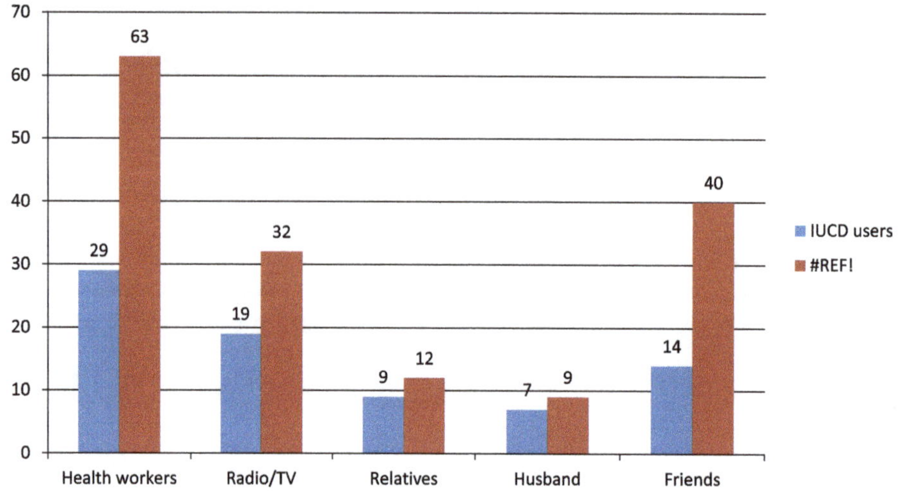

Fig. 1 Source of information to modern contraception for women visiting family planning clinic at primary health care facilities in Mekelle city, Northern Ethiopia, Tigray region, 2017

use IUCD than women who are not married. It could be because of women who are married and in long term relation are more likely to choose IUCD for its ability to act as long term contraceptive methods, on the other hand those who are unmarried not think IUCD is necessary for their infrequent sexual activity or they may perceive their short term relation do not need the effect of IUCD. It also may be due to joined decision with their husband to prefer IUCD. But this finding is contrasted by study done based on Evidence from EDHS 2011, women who were temporarily live with their partners are about Two times more likely to use LARC([AOR (95%CI) =1.9(1.2,3.0) [15]. This may be a result of social and cultural in acceptability of giving birth before formal marriage at most part of Ethiopia.

Another strong predictor of IUCD utilization is awareness about IUCD 97% of users and 66% of non-users have ever heard about IUCD which implies those have awareness are about 14 times more likely to utilize the method than their counter parts ([AOR (95%CI) =14.2 (2.814–71.184). this is higher compared with the result of the 2 studies done in Mekelle town before 5 years that shows 55.3% of the respondents heard about IUCD and another evidence based study done Ethiopia which shows 48.5% of cases and 19.4% of controls have heard about IUCD [9, 15, 16]. The might be a result of continuous promotion and advertisement through media increases through time and the difference in the educational background of clients as the most of the clients are with secondary and tertiary education.

Number of alive children is the strong predictor for IUCD utilization, as this study implies those having > 2 children are more than three times more likely to use IUCD compared with women having a unit child [AOR (95%CI) =3.5 (1.03–11.9). This finding oppose with study done in India which states woman acceptance of IUCD are highest after first child (73.70%), 22.3% after two children and declined thereafter and 84% of users were in the peak child bearing age of 20–29 years this can be the resulted from women with increased parity may achieve desired family size and choose the most effective and permanent method (female sterilization) [17].

This finding is supported by studies done in Nepal and Hosanna towns. Comparative cross sectional study done in urban area of Nepal shows that women having more than 2 children are about 2 times more likely to utilize IUD compared with those having ≤2 children [AOR (95%CI) = 2.20 (1.12–4.32)] and other higher finding reported from case control study done on LACs utilization those who have 1–2 and 3–4 children are around six times to use IUCD compared with those hiving no child [AOR (95%CI) =5.5 (2.7, 11.0) and 6(3.0–12.0) [11, 15]. This positive association can be a result of logical governance of reproductive intentions by the total number of children and the discrepancy in Odds might be the difference in the sample size of the studies.

Information told about the availability of health care provider able to insert IUCD stay strong predictor in multivariate logistic regression. Those respondents who are told about this information are about four times more likely to use IUCD [AOR (95%CI) =3.89 (1.55, 9.74)].This finding is relatively lower compared with case control study conducted in Addis Ababa city, which states that those who provided with this information are five and half times more likely to utilize the method [AOR (95%CI) =5.765(1.646, 51.486) [18]. This can the problem with health care providers in counsel each aspects of IUCD and/or could be relatively higher awareness and sociodemographic difference between the Two Cities. It also might be a result of providers simply do

Table 3 Determinants of IUCD utilization in Primary health care facilities in Mekelle city, Northern Ethiopia, Tigray region, 2017

Variables	Cases (78)(%)	Controls 156(%)	COR (95% CI)	AOR (95% CI)
Age (years)				
40–44	13 (16.7)	6 (3.8)	16.61 (5.05,54.65)*	7.23(.74, 70.79)
35–39	16 (20.5)	13 (8.3)	9.43 (3.44, 25.88)*	2.75(.46, 16.35)
30–34	17 (21.8)	26 (16.7)	5.01 (1.99,12.65)*	1.34(.26, 6.81)
25–29	23 (29.5)	42 (26.8)	4.19 (1.78, 9.93)*	1.14(.28, 4.65)
15–24	9 (11.5)	69 (44.3)	1	-
Occupation				
House wife	10 (12.8)	47 (30.1)	1.97 (0.57–6.78) *	0.1 (0.01–1.26)
Merchant	26 (33.3)	24 (15.4)	10.02 (3.11–32.33)*	0.62 (0.05–7.29)
Govt. Employee	23 (29.5)	29 (18.6)	7.34 (2.28–23.58)*	0.43 (0.04–4.89)
Private Employee	15 (19.2)	19 (12.2)	7.30 (2.13–25.08)*	0.65 (0.06–7.76)
Student	4 (5.1)	37 (23.7)	1	1
Marital status				
Married	73 (93.6)	101 (64.7)	7.95 (3.03–20.84)	8.59 (2.6–28.4) **
Single	5 (6.4)	55 (35.3)	1	1
Number of pregnancy ($N = 194$)				
≥5 times	14 (18.4)	10 (8.5)	4.94 (1.89–12.87)	5.7 (1.02–31.80) **
3-4 times	43 (56.6)	40 (34.2)	3.79 (1.95–7.39) *	2.04 (0.67–6.23)
1–2 times	19 (25)	67 (57.35)	1	1
Number of alive children ($N = 177$)				
> 2 children	42 (57.5)	42 (40)	5.50 (2.08–14.45)	3.5 (1.03–11.91) **
2 children	25 (34.2)	30 (28.6)	4.58 (1.65–12.70)	3.94 (1.14–13.55) **
1child	6 (8.2)	33 (31.4)	1	1
Ever heard about IUCD (234)				
Yes	76 (97.4)	103 (66)	19.55 (4.62–82.74)	14.15 (2.82–71.18)**
No	2 (2.6)	53 (22.6)	1	1
Have you ever seen IUCD (234)				
Yes	70 (89.7	54 (34.6)	16.53 (7.41–36.87)	10.4 (4.0–27.17) **
No	8 (10.3)	102 (65.4)	1	1
Information on availability of IUCD in PHCU				
Yes	73 (93.6)	120 (76.9)	4.38 (1.65–11.67)*	6.11 (0.55–68.02)
No	5 (6.4)	36 (23.1)	1	1
Information on availability of HCP that insert IUCD				
Yes	67 (85.9)	84 (53.8)	5.22 (2.56–10.63)	3.9 (1.5–9.7) **
No	11 (14.1)	72 (46.2)	1	1
Information on IUCD protect pregnancy for about 12 years				
Yes	60 (76.9)	66 (42.6)	4.49 (2.43–8.32) *	1.42(.33–6.15)
No	18 (23.1)	89 (57.4)	1	1
Information on IUCD requires less follow up				
Yes	35 (44.9)	105 (68.2)	2.63 (1.53–4.61) *	1.26(.36–4.39)
No	43 (55.1)	49 (31.8)	1	1

*Significant $p < 0.25$, and ** Significant $p < 0.05$

not possess adequate knowledge about the IUD as a LARC method and consequently, provide incomplete information to potential clients or do not offer the IUD as a reliable method.

Visual exposure to IUCD is another independent predictor of IUCD utilization. Women who had ever seen IUCD are more than ten times to use IUCD than those with no visual exposure [AOR (95%CI) =10.4(4.0–27.17). This might be a result of health care providers neglect ion in counseling each option of contraception or lacking enough knowledge on counseling which is crucial step that helps clients to make a decision regarding voluntarily using a kind of most suitable, effective and safest contraceptive method. Or it can be due to a problem with promotion if IUCD through locally available audio-visual medias [15, 16].

One of the strength of this study was data was directly collected from respondents so there is no lost variable which determine IUCD use and no possible recall bias. As this is Case-control study compares those factors in each group (cases and control), so that cause-effect relation can be estimated. Although the readers should consider limitations like exclusion of private health care facilities, small sample size and lack of qualitative part which are recommended for further studies and innervations.

Conclusion

The result of this study showed that being married, number of pregnancy, number of living children, awareness about IUCD, information given about the availability of health care provider able to insert IUCD and visual exposure of IUCD have positive association with IUCD utilization. Therefore stake holders like Tigray Regional health bureau, health care facilities and others should work for improvement in service quality and providers performance to increase the utilization of this effective and safe modern contraceptive method IUCD.

Abbreviations

CPR: Contraceptive prevalence rate; FMOH: Federal Ministry of Health; IUCD: Inra uterine contraceptive device; LARC: Long acting and reversible contraceptives; OCP: Oral contraceptive pills; PPHC: Public primary health care; TFR: Total fertility rate

Acknowledgments

We would like to thank all the study participants for their participation and information they provided us. We would also like to extend our gratitude to Mekele University for all support and opportunity provided for us to conduct this study.

Authors' contributions

GT conceived and designed the study, developed data collection instruments and supervised data collection. GT, HG, BH, GA, NB, MS and SH participated in the testing and finalization of the data collection instruments and coordinated the study progress. GT and SH performed the statistical analysis and wrote all versions of the manuscript. All authors read and approved the final manuscript.

Author details

[1]Department of Midwifery, College of Medicine & Health Sciences, Arba Minch University, Arba Minch, Ethiopia. [2]Department of Midwifery, College of Health Sciences, Mekele University, Mekele, Ethiopia. [3]Department of Public Health, College of Medicine & Health Sciences, Arba Minch University, Arba Minch, Ethiopia. [4]Department of Midwifery, College of Medicine & Health Sciences, Dilla Minch University, Arba Minch, Ethiopia. [5]Department of Midwifery, College of Medicine & Health Sciences, Wolkite University, Wolkite, Ethiopia.

References

1. National Statistical Office (NSO) and ICF Macro. Malawi Demographic and Health Survey 2010. Zomba, Malawi, and Calverton: NSO and ICF Macro; 2011.
2. Shimels Wudie, Gudaynhe. Factors affecting the use of long-acting reversible contraceptive methods among married women in DebreMarkos town, Northwest Ethiopia 2013Global journal of medical research 2014. Issue V Volume XIV Version I.
3. Mauldin WP, Segal SJ. IUD use throughout the world: past, present, and future. Proc. Int. Conf. 1994. Boston: Butterworth-Heinemann IUDs, 4th, ed. WCBardin, DR MishellJr, pp. 1–10.
4. United Nations, Department of Economic and Social Affairs, population division (2015).
5. World Health Organization, UNICEF, UNFPA and the World Bank. Trends in Maternal Mortality: 1990 to 2015. Estimates developed by WHO, UNICEF, UNFPA and the World Bank. Geneva: World Health Organization; 2016.
6. Care. Addressing Unmet Need for Family Planning in Developing Countries: The Case for IUD. FP 2012 IUCD fact sheet.2014;4..
7. Earsido A, Gebeyehu A, Kisi T. Determinants of long acting and permanent contraceptive methods utilization among married women in Hossana town, Southern Ethiopia: A Case - Control Study. J Preg Child Health. 2015;2:165.
8. EDHS 2016, Ethiop-cmyp. 2015 projection estimate based on 2007 population census. Latest revised-may-12-2015; pdf page viii.
9. Alemayehu, et al. Factors associated with utilization of long acting and permanent contraceptive methods among married women of reproductive age in Mekelle town, Tigray region, north Ethiopia. BMC Pregnancy Childbirth. 2012;12:6.
10. Crosignani PG. Intra uterine devices and intra uterine system. Hum Reprod Update. 2008;14(3):197–208.
11. Joshi, et al. Determinants of intrauterine contraceptraceptive device use among womens of Nepal Urban areas. NJOG. 2013;8(20):16–20.
12. FMOH, National Guideline for Family Planning Services in Ethiopia. Federal Democratic Republic of Ethiopia Ministry of Health; 2011. p. 14. Available at: www.moh.gov.et
13. Central Statistical Agency (CSA) [Ethiopia] and ICF. Ethiopia Demographic and Health Survey 2016. Addis Ababa and Rockville: CSA and ICF; 2016.
14. Parvathy Mini P. Assessment of Factors Influencing the Choice and Use of Temporary Contraceptive Methods for Birth Spacing among Married Women in Rural Trivandrum (Doctoral dissertation, SCTIMST). 2014;3–4.
15. Asmamaw Wondifraw: Determinants of Long Acting Contraceptive Use among Reproductive Age Women in Ethiopia: Evidence from EDHS 2011. AsmamawW,2015.
16. Gebremichael H, Haile F, Dessie A, Birhane A, Alemayehu M, Yebyo H. Acceptance of long acting contraceptive methods and associated factors among women in Mekelle City, Northern Ethiopia. Sci J Public Health. 2014; 2(4):349–55. https://doi.org/10.11648/j.sjph.20140204.27.
17. ArunaSubha Shree RaoYellayi, Aruna S, SaradaBai K. "A Study on Acceptance and Discontinuation of Intrauterine Contraceptive Device and its Determinants in a Tertiary Care Centre". J Evid Based Med Healthcare. 2015. 2;26:3804–3811.
18. Hameed W, et al. Determinants of Method Switching among Social Franchise Clients Who Discontinued the Use of Intrauterine Contraceptive Device. Int J Reprod Med. 2015;Article ID 941708:8.

12

Level of knowledge, attitude and practice of family planning and associated factors among disabled persons, north-shewa zone, Amhara regional state, Ethiopia

Alemayehu Gonie Mekonnen[1*], Alebachew Demelash Bayleyegn[1], Yared Asmare Aynalem[1], Tigist Demssew Adane[1], Mikyas Arega Muluneh[2] and Meaza Asefa[3]

Abstract

Background: In Ethiopia, people with disabilities face socioeconomic disadvantages and they have a limited access to sexual and reproductive health information including family planning service. At present, however, there is a scarcity of research on the association between disability and family planning, and only limited data is available for disabled people in Ethiopia. Hence, this study assessed the level of knowledge, attitude, and practice of family planning and associated factors among disabled persons in North-shewa zone, Amhara regional state, Ethiopia.

Methods: A cross-sectional survey was conducted from June to October 2019. A total of 397 study participants were interviewed using a structured and pre-tested questionnaire. A multistage systematic sampling technique was employed to select study participants. Data were entered into Epi data and exported into Statistical Package for the Social Sciences (SPSS) version 21 for analysis. Logistic regression was performed to analyze the data. A significant association was declared at a *p*-value of less than 0.05.

Results: Forty-six percent of study participants were knowledgeable about family planning methods. The injectable was the most known method of modern contraception (74.8%) while withdrawal (18.1%) was the least known traditional family planning method. Fifty-five percent of our study participants had a good attitude about family planning methods and one-fourth (24.5%) of disabled persons currently utilized any method of family planning. Those having a good knowledge of family planning were 1.6 times more likely to utilize family planning methods than those having poor knowledge of family planning methods (AOR = 1.61, CI = 1.27, 16.24). Moreover, participants who completed college education were 7 times more likely to have a good knowledge of family planning methods than uneducated participants (AOR = 7.23; 95% CI = 2.28, 22.06).

Conclusions: In this study, the knowledge, attitude, and practice of disabled people about family planning methods were relatively low. Due attention should be given to ensure that disabled people are well informed about family planning methods through information, education, and communication activities.

Keywords: Family Planning, Contraceptive, Disability, Debre Berhan

* Correspondence: alemayehugonie19@gmail.com
[1]Department of Nursing, College of Health Science, Debre Berhan University, Po. Box 445, Debre Berhan, Ethiopia

Introduction

Family planning (FP) is an effective way of controlling fertility within a human rights framework by giving couples the ability to have their desired family size [1, 2]. Family planning has a significant role in improving the health of the mother and the child by avoiding undesired pregnancies and abortions, thus reducing the maternal and child mortality rate [3, 4]. However, social inequality, religious/cultural barriers, weak coordination across sectors, inadequate quality assurance actions, and misconceptions about modern contraceptives were reported as the challenges for family planning implementation [1, 5–7].

Specifically, persons with disabilities are marginalized groups of the populations and they frequently marginalized from FP education due to misconceptions that they are not sexually active [8–10]. Furthermore, disabled people may be subjected to unsafe abortion due to long-standing stigmatization [11]. They have poorer health outcomes than non-disabled people as a result of less access to reproductive health information. Healthcare services also lack sign language interpreters and other information formats such as Braille, audio, or plain language which can provide advice on sexual health-related issues including FP methods [12]. Remarkably, they were often unable to access community meetings about FP services [13]. Moreover, their disabilities may limit their chances to interact with non-disabled peers that can be the best opportunity for informal learning about sexual health and family planning [14].

Although disabled people have the same reproductive health needs as the abled people and they want to space and limit the number of children to their economic capacity [15], they are notably absent from equitable reproductive health access [16] and face barriers to information [17]. Health facilities lack physical infrastructure, suitable and affordable transportation, and assistive devices for persons with disabilities [11, 18]. As such, disabled people face unique barriers to accessing family planning services and are often treated as a low priority for those services. They are often socially isolated and abused which creates obstacles to obtaining FP services [12]. Stigma and negative attitudes by healthcare providers towards disabilities have been commonly cited as the barriers to access and uptake of family planning for disabled people [11, 19]. The previous study also reported a variety of factors that affect access to and uptake of family planning among people with disabilities. For example, research from four African countries found a lack of knowledge about FP methods and fear of side-effects are issues affecting access to and uptake of family planning among people with disabilities [20].

In Ethiopia, people with disabilities face socioeconomic disadvantages and they have a limited access to sexual and reproductive health information including family planning services. They have an increased risk of SRH-related problems and have become the main focus in recent years. At present, however, there is a scarcity of research on the association between disability and family planning, and only limited data is available for disabled people in Ethiopia. Hence, this study assessed the level of knowledge, attitude, and practice of family planning and associated factors among disabled persons in North-shewa zone, Amhara regional state, Ethiopia. An examination of the knowledge and attitude towards FP and the factors which influence their attitude will guide the effective usage of FP services for disabled people who are marginalized groups of the populations.

Methods and materials

Study design, setting and period

A cross-sectional survey was conducted from June to October 2019 in the North-shewa zone, Amhara regional state, Ethiopia. The Debre Berhan town (the zone city) is located at 130-k meter far from Addis Ababa (the capital city of Ethiopia). An estimated 214,595 people with any form of disability are estimated to live in the North-shewa zone. The zone has 10 functional disability-support organizations: one is found in Debre Berhan town and nine are found in the other nine districts of the zone. The rest 15 districts have no functional disability support-organization. Overall, these disability-support organizations comprised a total number of 1500 disabled persons. These organizations support all disabled peoples (physically handicapped, hearing impairment, partial mental impairment, visual impairment, multiple impairments). The support organizations provide advocacy service, provide life skill training and support to live in the community, get involved in work (*unpublished zonal health department report, 2019).*

Study population

All the reproductive-age groups of disabled people who enrolled in the disability-support organizations in the north-shewa zone were the study participants. Those who were ill and unable to communicate due to being ill were excluded from the study. Dual disabilities such as unable to see plus unable to hear were also excluded from the study.

Sample size and sampling technique

The sample size was calculated using a single population proportion formula. The assumptions were: the proportion of disabled persons who had reproductive health knowledge as 79.6% ($p = 0.796$) taken from Tanzania [16], with 95% confidence interval (CI) to be 1.96, and margin of error to be 5%. Adding a non-response rate of

5% and the design effect of 1.5, a total sample size of 412 persons with disabilities were selected.

A multistage systematic random sampling technique was employed. In the first sampling unit, five disability-support organizations were selected randomly. In the second sampling unit, the lists of disabled people (registry) were used as the sampling frame. The registry contained the contact addresses of disabled people. The calculated sample size was proportionally allocated to disability-support organizations and the required numbers of participants were selected using a systematic random sampling technique.

Data collection

A pre-tested and structured questionnaire was used to collect the data. The questionnaire was designed in English then translated into Amharic (native language) and back into English to ensure consistency. The data were collected by trained enumerators through a face-to-face interview. Five data collectors and five supervisors participated in the study. One of the data collector was a certified sign language interpreter who could collect data from participants who have a hearing impairment. Data completeness were checked by the investigators and supervisors.

Measurements

Most of the questions were taken from the Ethiopian demographic health survey 2016 [21] and peer-reviewed literature [14, 22]. The questions comprise the following sections; socio-demographic characteristics and questions which examined the participant's knowledge, attitude, and practice of FP methods. Knowledge questions were: what is family planning? Which FP methods did you know? What are the side effects of using family planning? Respondents answered either *"Yes"* or *"No"* or *"Do not know"* from the listed options. The attitude of respondents towards FP methods was assessed with seven attitudinal questions. All attitudinal statements were stated positively. The participants could choose one of the three possible response categories (1 = yes (agree), 2 = no (disagree), 3 = do not know). The practice of the FP was assessed with two statements: do you currently utilize any of the FP methods? Which type of FP methods do you utilize?

Mean scores of knowledge and attitude about FP were calculated to classify the respondents into two groups (knowledgeable and not knowledgeable, good attitude and poor attitude). To calculate the mean score of knowledge, participants who answered *"Yes"* were considered as correctly answered and those who answered *"No"* and *"I do not know"* were considered as not answered correctly. Respondents who scored the mean and above the mean score of the correctly answered questions were classified as knowledgeable, less than the mean score of correct answers were classified as not knowledgeable. To calculate the mean score of attitude, participants who answered "yes/agree" were considered as correctly answered and those who answered "no/disagree" and "I do not know" were considered as not answered correctly. Respondents who scored the mean and above the mean score of attitudinal statements were considered as having a good attitude and less than the mean score as a poor attitude. Concerning family planning practice, it was measured by calculating the percentage of disabled people who currently utilized any of family planning methods. If a married man whose wife was using FP of her choice and he could report that her FP utilization, then he was considered as the current FP user.

Data processing and analysis

Data was checked for completeness and inconsistencies. Epi-data version 3.1 was used for data entry and data were exported to SPSS version 21. Descriptive statistics were computed. Logistic regression was performed to analyze the data. The bivariate logistic regression analyses were performed between independent and the outcome variables. Those independent variables which were statistically significant in the bivariate model (*p-value* < *0.05*) were entered into the multivariable analysis. In the final model, a significant association was declared at a p-value of less than 0.05. And finally, the results were presented in texts and tables with an adjusted odds ratio (AOR) and the corresponding 95% CI.

Results

Socio-demographic characteristics

A total of 397 disabled persons were interviewed with a response rate of 96.4%. The mean age of the respondents was 27.7(±7.1SD) years. Most of the respondents (45.2%) had impaired mobility. Fifty-six percent of respondents were female and 48.1% of participants were single. The highest number of study participants were Orthodox Christians (93.0%). A quarter of participants were living alone and 41.1% of disabled persons had no job. Regarding the educational level of the respondents, 48 % (48.5%) of respondents had completed primary education (Table 1).

Knowledge and practice of participants about FP methods

As indicated in Table 2, about 85 % of disabled persons had ever heard about FP methods. The most common source of information was the media (television/radio (69.1%). The mean number of FP methods known by respondents was 44.6%. About three-fourth (74.8%) of the respondents knew injectable while withdrawal (18.1%) was the least known traditional FP method. The mean score of side effects reported by participants was 31.5%. Heavy bleeding or irregular bleeding was the most

Table 1 Sociodemographic characteristics of respondents in North-shewa zone, Ethiopia, 2019

Socio-demographic characteristics (***N*** = 397)	Categories	N (%)
Form of disability of respondents	Partial mental impairment	13(3.3)
	Hearing impairment	57(14.4)
	Visual impairment	94(23.7)
	Impaired mobility	197(45.2)
	Multiple impairments	53(13.3)
Age	18–30	271(68.1)
	31–40	47(11.9)
	41–50	79(20.0)
Sex	Female	173(43.7)
	Male	224(56.3)
Marital status	Married	142(35.9)
	Single	191(48.1)
	Divorced/widowed	64(15.9)
Religion	Orthodox	369(93.0)
	Muslim	19(4.8)
	Protestant/Catholic	9(2.3)
Educational status	No education	94(23.7)
	Primary education	194(48.9)
	Secondary education	52(13.0)
	College education	57(14.4)
Work status	Had no job	163(41.1)
	Student	63(15.9)
	Employed	57(14.4)
	Lottery seller	41(10.3)
	Others (merchants, daily laborer, beggar, tailor)	73(18.3)
Living condition	With parents	105(26.3)
	With relatives	21(5.2)
	With friends/peers	124(31.4)
	With partner	93(23.5)
	Alone	54(13.6)

reported side effect of modern contraceptives (35.9%). Overall, 46 % of study participants were knowledgeable about family planning methods. Only a quarter (24.4%) of disabled persons currently utilized any of family planning methods. Of these family planning users, 76(77.6%) of them were females (Table 2).

Attitude of participants towards FP methods

In this study, the calculated mean score of the attitudinal statements was 1.83(±0.39 SD). Forty-four percent (44.4%) of the respondents were above the mean score and they were considered as having a poor attitude towards FP methods (Table 3).

Table 2 The respondents' knowledge and practice of FP methods in North-shewa zone, Ethiopia, 2019

Variables	Categories	
Have you ever heard about FP methods? (*n* = 337)	Yes	337(84.9)
	No	60(15.1)
What was the source of information for FP? (n = 337)	Television/radio	233(69.1)
	School teachers	134(39.8)
	Health professionals	196(58.2)
	Associations	67(19.8)
	Training	116(34.6)
	Others[a]	99(29.6)
What is FP (N = 337)	**Yes**	**No**
Limiting of number of children	174(51.5)	163(48.5)
The spacing of birth intervals	288(85.5)	44(13.2)
Stopping births	85(25.0)	250(74.4)
Do not know	11(3.2)	
Which type of FP methods did you know? (*n* = 337)	**Yes**	**No**
Oral contraceptive pills	212(62.8)	125(37.2)
Condoms	183(54.4)	154(45.6)
Injectable	252(74.8)	85(25.2)
Implants	191(56.6)	146(43.4)
Intrauterine contraceptive devices	131(38.9)	206(61.1)
Sterilization (male and female)	92(27.4)	245(72.6)
Calendar method	97(28.8)	240(71.2)
Periodic abstinence	132(39.4)	205(60.6)
Withdrawal (coitus interruptus)	61(18.1)	276(81.9)
Lactational amenorrhea method	81(24.1)	256(75.9)
Mean number of methods known	204(60.6)	
What are the side effects of using family planning?	**Yes**	**No**
Heavy bleeding or irregular bleeding	121(35.9)	216(64.1)
Absence of menstrual cycle	72(21.3)	265(78.7)
Abdominal cramp	59(17.4)	278(82.6)
Do not know	148(43.8)	189(56.2)
Mean score of side effects known	106(31.52)	
Do you currently utilize any of family planning methods?	98(24.5)	299(75.5)
Overall FP knowledge level	**Not knowledgeable**	**Knowledgeable**
	182(54.0)	**155(46.0)**

[a]*Parent, friends, magazine, books*

Factors associated with knowledge, attitude, and practice of FP methods

In the bivariate model, the sex of the respondents and level of education were statistically significant with the knowledge of FP methods. Besides, age, marital status,

Table 3 The respondents' attitude towards FP methods in North-shewa zone, Ethiopia, 2019

Variables	Agree	Disagree	Do not know
Do you think using FP makes women unhealthy?	143(35.9)	187(47.0)	67(17.0)
Do you think pregnancy must be properly planned?	316(79.6)	37(9.3)	44(11.1)
Do you think pregnancy spaced < 2 years should be avoided by using family planning methods?	214(54.1)	104(26.3)	78(19.6)
Do you think the use of FP methods interfere sexual relationship between husband and wife?	88(22.2)	232(58.5)	77(19.3)
Do you think using modern FP methods causes anger from God?	198(50.0)	150(37.8)	48(12.2)
Do you think FP methods result in infertility to get pregnant later on?	118(29.6)	194(48.9)	85(21.5)
Do you think women are more responsible than men for using modern FP methods?	131(58.1)	114(28.9)	52(13.0)
Overall family planning attitude level	**Poor attitude**	**Good attitude**	
	176(44.4)	**221(55.6)**	

and knowledge of FP methods were associated with the utilization of any type of FP methods in the bivariate model. As indicated in Table 4, the results of the multivariate analysis showed that respondents who completed the primary education were three times more likely to have a good knowledge of FP methods than uneducated participants (AOR = 3.31; 95% CI = 1.37, 7.59). Moreover, participants who completed college education were 7 times more likely to have a good knowledge of FP methods than participants who were uneducated (AOR = 7.23; 95% CI = 2.28, 22.06). Moreover, participants who had a good knowledge of FP methods was 1.6 times (AOR = 1.61, CI = 1.27, 16.24) more likely to utilize any type of FP methods than those having poor knowledge of FP methods (Table 4).

Discussions

This study highlights interesting insights into the knowledge, attitude, and practice of family planning methods among persons with disabilities in North-shewa zone, Amhara regional state, Ethiopia, unfortunately, there is very limited data and unclear understanding of the knowledge has been problematic. The current study reported the level of knowledge, attitude, and practice of family planning methods among disabled persons who are marginalized groups of the populations. Accordingly, 46 % of study participants were knowledgeable about family planning methods. Likewise, the mean number of family planning methods known by respondents was 44.6%. The injectable was the most known method of modern contraception (74.8%) while withdrawal (18.1%)

Table 4 The analyses of factors associated with the knowledge and the current FP methods utilization among respondents in the North-shewa zone, Ethiopia, 2019

Variables associated with knowledge of FP methods (n = 337)		**Poor knowledge**	**Good knowledge**	**COR (95% CI)**	**AOR (95% CI)**
Sex	Female	58.4	35.6	1.00	1.00
	Male	41.8	64.4	2.54(1.03,2.77)*	3.12(0.76,8.11)
Educational status	No education	24.6	8.7	1.00	1.00
	Primary education	46.7	54.8	3.21(1.45,7.65)	3.31(1.37,7.59)*
	Secondary education	18.9	11.5	1.71(0.63, 4.83)	1.83(0.65,5.12)
	College education	9.8	25.0	6.96(2.63,19.85)	7.23(2.28,22.06)*
Variables associated with the current FP utilization (n = 337)		**Not utilized FP methods**	**Utilized FP methods**		
Age	18–30	68.5	66.7	1.00	1.00
	31–40	10.8	15.2	1.48(1.02,7.65)*	1.71(0.93,3.91)
	41–50	20.7	18.1	0.91(0.51,1.58)	0.80(0.56,2.13)
Marital status	Single	53.2	33.3	1.00	1.00
	Married	30.5	51.5	2.71(1.45,5.00)*	3.41(1.74,6.68)*
	Divorced/widowed	16.3	15.2	1.9(0.64,3.46)	2.11(0.86,5.71)
Respondent's knowledge on FP	Poor knowledge	77.0	23.0	1.00	1.00
	Good knowledge	68.3	31.7	1.54(1.11,12.50)*	1.61(1.27,16.24)*

1 = Reference, * p-value < 0.05

was the least known traditional FP method. This figure was slightly lower than the study reported in Kampala-Uganda [23]. Even though the knowledge of contraceptive methods among disabled people was not comparable with the general population, findings from the EDHS data also revealed that disabled people's knowledge on family planning methods was much lower than our result [21]. In Senegal, people with disabilities had very low knowledge about contraception [24]. Women with intellectual disabilities lacked basic knowledge of contraception in Southeast England [25]. This could be due to persons with disabilities commonly have a restricted access to the use of family planning methods, and they are often socially isolated in obtaining FP services.

Although 55 % of our study participants had favorable attitude about modern contraception, only one-fourth (24.5%) of participants currently utilized any method of contraceptives. In line with our finding, the majority of disabled women had a favorable attitude, but the utilization of FP methods by respondents was poor [26–28]. However, our finding was lower than the study conducted in Addis Ababa where 35% of persons with disabilities utilized modern contraceptives [24]. In Nigeria, 34% of physically disabled adolescents utilized modern contraceptive methods [29]. The utilization of FP methods was 39% among people with disabilities in Kampala district, Uganda [23]. This difference is probably because disabled people are discouraged from discussing sexual-related issues in the study area due to some cultural influences.

In the multivariate analysis, participants who had a good knowledge of FP methods were more likely to utilize any type of FP methods than those having poor knowledge. This agreed with a study reported by E Smith et al. [30] where awareness of family planning determined the utilization of modern contraception. Moreover, participants who completed college education were 7 times more likely to have a good knowledge of FP methods than none-educated participants. Similarly, lower education level was associated with lower utilization of family planning among disabilities [27, 28]. This is plausible finding in that education is a foundation for utilization of FP methods among disabled people through developing their knowledge. Moreover, our finding suggested that knowledge of FP have a positive impact on the utilization of FP methods among disabled people. It could be also explained that as the level of education increased, the person's level of seeking health information also increased which again improves the practice of FP utilization and services.

Despite its strengths, this study has some limitations that must be acknowledged. Although our study had a diverse set of participants, the study focused on disability-support organizations that may miss some people with disabilities in the community. The authors also acknowledge the possibility of information bias created by the sign language interpreters to interpret for respondents who had a hearing impairment, and the limitations associated with self-reported data.

Conclusions

In this study, the knowledge, attitude, and practice of disabled people about FP methods were relatively low. Due attention should be given to ensure that disabled people are well informed about FP methods through information, education and communication activities.

Abbreviations

AOR: Adjusted Odds Ratio; CI: Confidence Interval; COR: Crude Odds Ratio; FP: Family Planning; SD: Standard Deviation; SPSS: Statistical Package for the Social Sciences; SRH: Sexual and Reproductive Health

Acknowledgements

We would like to thank Debre Berhan University for financial grants to carry out this study. We are grateful to Debre Berhan zone social affairs office for providing us disability-related data. We would also like to acknowledge our study participants, data collectors, and district social experts who kindly participated in this study.

Authors' contributions

AG, AD, YA, TD, MA[5] and MA[6] participated in the design of the study, supervised the data collection. AG analyzed and interpreted the data, drafted and edited the manuscript. All authors read and approved the final manuscript.

Author details

[1]Department of Nursing, College of Health Science, Debre Berhan University, Po. Box 445, Debre Berhan, Ethiopia. [2]Department of Midwifery, College of Health Science, Debre Berhan University, Po. Box 445, Debre Berhan, Ethiopia. [3]Department of Medical Laboratory, College of Medicine, Debre Berhan University, Po. Box 445, Debre Berhan, Ethiopia.

References

1. Eliason S, Awoonor-Williams JK, Eliason C, Novignon J, Nonvignon J, Aikins M. Determinants of modern family planning use among women of reproductive age in the Nkwanta district of Ghana: a case-control study. Reprod Health. 2014;11(1):65.
2. Kasa AS, Tarekegn M, Embiale N. Knowledge, attitude and practice towards family planning among reproductive-age women in resource-limited settings of Northwest Ethiopia. BMC Res Notes. 2018;11(1):1–6.
3. Takele A, Degu G, Yitayal M. Demand for long-acting and permanent methods of contraceptives and factors for non-use among married women of Goba town, bale zone, South East Ethiopia. BMC Reprod Health. 2012; 9(1):26.
4. Choi Y, Fabic MS, Hounton S, Koroma D. Meeting demand for family planning within a generation: prospects and implications at country level. Glob Health Action. 2015;8(1):29734.
5. Gonie A, Wudneh A, Nigatu D, Dendir Z. Determinants of family planning use among married women in bale eco-region, Southeast Ethiopia: a community-based study. BMC Womens Health. 2018;18(1):50.
6. Family Planning 2020 Country Action: Opportunities, Challenges, and Priorities in Ethiopia. https://www.familyplanning2020.org/sites/default/files/Country_Action_Opportunities-Challenges-and-Priorities_ETHIOPIA_FINAL.pdf. Accessed 15 Mar 2020.
7. Tilahun T, Coene G, Luchters S, Kassahun W, Leye E, Temmerman M, Degomme O. Family planning knowledge, attitude and practice among married couples in Jimma Zone, Ethiopia. PLoS One. 2013;8(4):1–7.

8. Fabic MS, Choi Y, Bongaarts J, Darroch JE, Ross JA, Stover J, Tsui AO, Upadhyay J, Starbird E. Meeting demand for family planning within a generation: the post-2015 agenda. Lancet. 2015;385(9981):1928–31.
9. Obasi M, Manortey S, Kyei KA, Addo MK, Talboys S, Gay L, Baiden F. Sexual and reproductive health of adolescents in schools for people with disabilities. Pan Afr Med J. 2019;33:299.
10. Shakespeare T, Iezzoni LI, Groce NE. Disability and the training of health professionals. Lancet. 2009;374(9704):1815–6.
11. Tanabe M, Nagujjah Y, Rimal N, Bukania F, Krause S. Intersecting sexual and reproductive health and disability in humanitarian settings: risks, needs, and capacities of refugees with disabilities in Kenya, Nepal, and Uganda. Sex Disabil. 2015;33(4):411–27.
12. Kassa TA, Luck T, Bekele A, Riedel-Heller SG. Sexual and reproductive health of young people with disabilities in Ethiopia: a study on knowledge, attitude, and practice: a cross-sectional study. Glob Health. 2016;12(1):5.
13. Milligan MS, Neufeldt AH. The myth of asexuality: a survey of social and empirical evidence. Sex Disabil. 2001;19(2):91–109.
14. Mprah WK. Knowledge and use of contraceptive methods amongst deaf people in Ghana. Afr J Disabil. 2013;2(1):43.
15. Anderson P, Kitchin R. Disability, space and sexuality: access to family planning services. Soc Sci Med. 2000;51(8):1163–73.
16. Devkota HR, Murray E, Kett M, Groce N. Healthcare provider's attitude towards disability and experience of women with disabilities in the use of maternal healthcare service in rural Nepal. Reprod Health. 2017;14(1):79.
17. Promoting sexual and reproductive health for persons with disabilities WHO/UNFPA guidance note. 2009. https://apps.who.int/iris/bitstream/handle/10665/44207/9789241598682_eng.pdf. Accessed 15 Mar 2020.
18. Abdul KA. Exploring the sexual and reproductive health issues of visually impaired women in Ghana. Reprod Health Matters. 2017;25(50):128–33.
19. Fraser E, Corby N. Family Planning for women and girls with disabilities, Disability Inclusion Helpdesk Research Report No. 2 (pilot). London: Disability Inclusion Helpdesk; 2019.
20. Eide AH, Mannan H, Khogali M, Van Rooy G, Swartz L, Munthali A, Hem KG, MacLachlan M, Dyrstad K. Perceived barriers for accessing health services among individuals with a disability in four African countries. PLoS One. 2015;10(5):e0125915. https://doi.org/10.1371/journal.pone.0125915.
21. Central Statistical Agency (CSA) [Ethiopia] and ICF. Ethiopia Demographic and Health Survey 2016. Addis Ababa, Ethiopia, and Rockville: CSA and ICF; 2016.
22. Van Schrojenstein Lantman-de Valk HM, Rook F, Maaskant MA. The use of contraception by women with intellectual disabilities. J Intellect Disabil Res. 2011;55(4):434–40.
23. Mulindwa IN. Study on reproductive health and HIV/AIDS among persons with disabilities in Kampala, Katakwi and Rakai districts. Kampala: Disabled Women's Network and Resource Organization; 2003. https://asksource.info/resources/study-reproductive-health-and-hivaids-among-persons-disabilities-kampala-katakwi-and-rakai.
24. Kassa TA, Luck T, Birru SK, Riedel-Heller SG. Sexuality and sexual reproductive health of disabled young people in Ethiopia. Sex Transm Dis. 2014;41(10):583–8.
25. McCarthy M. Contraception and women with intellectual disabilities. J Appl Res Intellect Disabil. 2009;22(4):363–9.
26. Gürel R, Yılmaz DV. Examining the attitude towards family Planning of women with disability in Turkey. Sex Disabil. 2018;36(3):265–75.
27. DeBeaudrap P, Mouté C, Pasquier E, Mac-Seing M, Mukangwije PU, Beninguisse G. Disability and access to sexual and reproductive health services in Cameroon: a mediation analysis of the role of socioeconomic factors. Int J Environ Res Public Health. 2019;16(3):417.
28. Ngilangwa DP, Rajesh S, Kawala M, Mbeba R, Sambili B, Mkuwa S, Noronha R, Meremo AJ, Nyagero J. Accessibility to sexual and reproductive health and rights education among marginalized youth in selected districts of Tanzania. Pan Afr Med J. 2016;25(2):1–7.
29. Olajide FO, Omisore AG, Arije OO, Afolabi OT, Olajide AO. Awareness and use of modern contraceptives among physically challenged in-school adolescents in Osun state, Nigeria. Afr J Reprod Health. 2014;18(2):87–96.
30. Smith E, Murray SF, Yousafzai AK, Kasonka L. Barriers to accessing safe motherhood and reproductive health services: the situation of women with disabilities in Lusaka. Zambia Disabil Rehabil. 2004;26(2):121–7.

13

Prevalence and factors associated with postpartum use of long-acting reversible contraception in Bukombe District, Geita Region, Tanzania

Kiondo Solomon Kiondo[1], Eusebious Maro[1,2], Sophia Kiwango[1], Julius Pius Alloyce[2], Benjamin C. Shayo[1,2] and Michael Johnson Mahande[1,3*]

Abstract

Background: Globally, approximately half of all pregnancies occur before 24 months after child birth. In Sub Saharan Africa the unmet need for family planning is highest among postpartum women. There is a dearth of information regarding factors associated with postpartum use of long acting reversible contraception (LARC) in Tanzania particularly in the Lake zone. This study aimed to determine the prevalence and factors associated with postpartum use of LARC (< 24 months) in Bukombe District, Geita Region in the Lake zone, in 2018.

Methodology: Community based analytical cross-sectional study was conducted between May and June 2018 among women with less than 24 months since delivery. Multistage sampling technique was used to recruit participants. Face to face interviews with 768 postpartum women was conducted using standardized questionnaire. Data were analyzed using Stata Version 13.0. Multivariable logistic regression model was used to determine factors associated with postpartum use of LARC.

Results: Prevalence of postpartum use of LARC was 10.4%. Urban residence (AOR = 2.94, 95% CI: 1.07–8.06), having formal employment (AOR = 4.81, 95% CI: 1.85–12.57) and receiving family planning counseling (AOR = 4.39, 95% CI: 1.89–10.20) were significantly associated with postpartum LARC use.

Conclusion: The postpartum use of LARC was low in the studied population with implants being the most commonly used method. Urban residency, formal employment and receiving family planning counseling were associated with postpartum LARC use. Improving prenatal and quality of family planning counseling is warranted to increase postpartum LARC utilization in Bukombe.

Keywords: Long-acting reversible contraception, Postpartum, Determinants, Tanzania

* Correspondence: jmmahande@gmail.com
[1]Kilimanjaro Christian Medical University College, Moshi, Tanzania
[3]Department of Epidemiology and Biostatistics, Institute of Public Health, Kilimanjaro Christian Medical University College, Moshi, Tanzania

Introduction

Postpartum Family Planning (PPFP) is defined as the prevention of unintended pregnancy and closely spaced pregnancies through the first 12 months post-delivery [1]. Postpartum women have highest unmet need for family planning which increases their risk for mistimed and unintended pregnancies [1]. PPFP help couples to space pregnancies and achieve desired family size [1]. Postpartum contraceptives options include: short term methods such as condoms, injectables, oral contraceptives pills (OCP), long acting reversible contraception (LARC) [which includes subdermal implants and intra-uterine devices (IUDs)], where as permanent methods include vasectomy and female sterilization [2].

LARC can avert early unplanned pregnancies during an extended postpartum period better than any other contraceptions [2]. LARC has been reported to be as much as 20 times more effective than oral contraceptions, transdermal patches and vaginal rings [3], with a failure rate of 1 per 100 [2]. It is most effective than any form of contraception, cost effective, long-lasting and convenient [2].

Finding fromDemographic and Health Surveys from 27 countries revealed that 95% of women within 12 months postpartum needed to prevent pregnancy in the next 24 months after birth, but majority (70%) of these women were not using contraception [4]. This reflects high unmet need for postpartum contraception among this high risk group. Findings from 21 low—and middle—income countries (LMICS) regarding pregnancy risk and postpartum contraceptive method use showed that, 61% of postpartum women who were within 24 months postpartum had an unmet need for modern contraceptives [5]. Moreover, in LMICS less than 15% of postpartum women use LARC [6] but majority (50 – 96%) of them relies on use of short acting contraceptives which are less effective in preventing unwanted pregnancies [5].

Majority (61%) of women in Tanzania have been reported to have unmet needs for family planning within 2 years postpartum, with only 31% were using the family planning methods [7]. Again, family planning method mix shows that only 10% of the women reported using highly effective methods including long acting reversible contraceptives [5] while 1% and 7% of the women of reproductive age reported using IUDs and implants respectively [8]. As a consequences of high unmet need for modern contraceptives during this period, 36% of pregnancies are unwanted [9] and 19% of all births have short birth intervals, with nearly half (47%) of all pregnancies occurring within recommended optimal inter-pregnancy interval [24 months] [8]. In addition Tanzania has maternal mortality ratio of 556/100,000 per live birth, which is unacceptably high [8]. Geita region has 35% unmet need for modern contraceptives among all women of reproductive age with total fertility rate (TFR) of 5.5%; these figures are above the national estimates of 22% and 5.2 for unmet need for FP and total fertility rate respectively [8].

Despite the fact that Geita region has the highest unmet need for modern contraceptives use in the country, little has been documented about factors influencing postpartum family planning use particularly long acting reversible contraceptives in this region. In addition there is paucity of data in postpartum family planning use in Tanzania, coupled with low utilization of LARC methods.

Different studies in the literature have shown predictors of postpartum LARC use such as occupation [10], secondary or tertiary education [11], high parity [12] and mode of delivery [13]. This study aimed to determine the prevalence and factors associated with postpartum use of long acting reversible contraceptives (< 24 months) in Bukombe District, Geita Region in the Lake zone.

Methods and materials

Study design and settings

A community-based analytical cross sectional study was conducted from May to June 2018, in Bukombe District, Geita region. Bukombe district has 3 divisions, 17 wards, 52 villages and 184 sub-villages, and it has an estimated population of 224,542. Of these, 19.1% comprise Women of reproductive age [15–49]. Bukombe district is among the districts with highest population growth rate and birth rates in Tanzania (5.9% and 4.6% respectively) [14]. The main source of income generating activities include; agriculture, animal husbandry, gold mining, petty business and formal sector employment.

The district has one hospital and two health centers which are government-owned. There are also fifteen, dispensaries where by six belong to the government and the remaining nine belongs to private sector. Only ten [10] healthcare facilities in this district provide family planning services.

Study population, sample size and sampling techniques

This study included postpartum women [15–49 years] who were less than 24 months post-delivery from nine villages in Bukombe District. We estimated the sample size using single population proportion formula taking in consideration the following assumptions; standard deviation of 1.96 corresponding to 95% confidence interval (CI), proportion of 13 [8], marginal error of 3.5% and design effect of 2. After adding 10% for non-response rate the, estimated sample size was 780 postpartum women. However during the field work we could recruit 768 postpartum women.

Multi-stage sampling technique was used to obtain 768 postpartum women. The 1st stage involved purposeful selection of 2 out of 3 divisions based on their large population size. The 2nd stage involved selection of 3 wards after stratification of wards from 2 division into rural and urban, using proportion to size, 1 ward from urban settings and 2 wards from rural settings were selected. The 3rd stage involved selection of 9 villages whereby in each ward 3 villages were randomly selected. At the lowest level of local administration in Bukombe district (hamlets), 3 hamlets were randomly selected in each of selected villages and postpartum mothers who were less than 24 months since delivery at the time of data collection were identified through door to door approach with the help of local leaders and those who fulfilled study inclusion criteria were invited to participate in our study.

Study variables

The dependent variable in this study was use of long acting reversible contraceptives (Implants and IUD) during postpartum period and independent variable were socio-demographic characteristics (Age, marital status, education level, residence, occupation, income per month and Partner's level of education), others were reproductive characteristics (Number of living children, mode of index delivery, place of index delivery, menstrual resumption, duration of postpartum period, counseling on FP and discussing FP use with the partner).

Data collection methods and quality assurance

Due to the sensitive nature of this study, we used only female research assistants who were medical doctors in data collection process. All our research assistants were trained on key technical terminologies used in data collection tool as well as research ethical issues. Face to face interviews were used to collect data using structured questionnaires which was adopted from Tanzania Demographic health survey with slight modification to suit for cultural context. Information on socio-demographic characteristics, reproductive health characteristics, contraceptives use and contraceptive preference as well as children status. Principle investigator visited field sites frequently to supervise data collection activities and field staff convened with the principle investigator during the evenings to counter-check completeness of data captured before submission to data server.

Data analysis

Data were coded, entered, cleaned and transferred to Stata Version 13.0 for the analysis purposes. Descriptive statistics were summarized using proportion for categorical data, means, standard deviation (SD) median and interquartile range (IQR) for numerical data. Multivariable logistic regression model was used to determine odds ratio and 95% confidence intervals for factors associated with postpartum LARC use. A p-value of less than 5% was considered statistically significant.

Results

Socio-demographic Characteristics of the participants

A total of 768 women within 24 months postpartum were invited to participate in this study, whereby all agreed and were enrolled into the study, making a 100% response rate. Two participants were excluded in the analysis due to incomplete information. The mean age of respondents was 26.9 ± 6.7 SD years. Majority, [652 (85.1%)], of participants were married, [714 (93.2%)] had primary education/below while at least two thirds were residents of rural areas. Regarding partners' characteristics, [557 (86.2%)] of participants' partners had primary education (Table 1).

Reproductive characteristics of the participants

The median number of living children was 3 (IQR: 2—5). With regard to number of living children, slightly higher than two fifth [336 (43.9%)] of the postpartum women had 1–2 children. In the current delivery, most of the participants [735 (96%)] had vaginal delivery and nearly half [371 (48.4%)] of the postpartum women had delivered at home. Nearly two-thirds [428 (58.5%)] of

Table 1 Socio-demographic Characteristics of study participants ($N = 766$)

Variables	n	%
Age, years		
15–24	326	42.6
25–34	318	41.5
35–49	122	15.9
Age[a]	(26.9; 6.7)	
Marital status		
Married	652	85.1
Unmarried	114	14.9
Level of education		
Primary/below	714	93.2
Secondary/above	52	6.8
Occupation		
Unemployed	740	96.6
Employed	26	3.4
Estimated income per month (Tsh)		
< 100,000	618	80.7
> 100,000	148	19.3
Residence		
Rural	523	68.3
Urban	243	31.7
Partner's level of education (n = 731)[b]		
Primary/below	557	86.2
Secondary and above	174	23.8

Notes [a]Mean standard deviation [b]$n = 731$ those with partners participants reported to discuss family planning issues with their partners, whereas, at least half of the participants [425 (55.5%)] had menstrual resumption (Tables 2 and 3).

Prevalence of LARC use among postpartum women

Of the 766 postpartum women, 80 were using LARC, corresponding to a prevalence of 10.4%. Only eight percent reported to be using short methods, (Fig. 1). The most frequently used contraceptive methods were implants 76 (53.9%) and injectables 37 (26.2%). Other methods such as hormonal pills 13(9.2%), condoms 11(7.8%) and intrauterine devices 4 (2.8%) were infrequently used, (Fig. 2).

Socio-demographic and reproductive characteristics associated with postpartum LARC use

Bivariate and multivariable logistic regression models were used to identify factors associated with postpartum LARC use. Bivariate analyses showed that, women with secondary education or above had two fold higher odds of LARC use compared to their counterparts with primary/below education (COR = 2.37, 95% CI:1.05–4.57), women with formal employment were almost five times more likely to use LARC compared to those who were unemployed (COR = 4.99, 95% CI: 2.12–11.72). Women who reported to reside in urban had 4-folds (COR = 3.78, (95% CI): 2.32–6.15) higher odds of using LARC compared with their rural counterparts. In addition, partners education level, partner 's occupation, couples discussion about FP, mode of delivery, place of delivery during the index pregnancy, menstrual resumption, postpartum duration and counseling on FP-methods were also significantly associated with postpartum LARC use.

Variables which showed significance in the bivariate analysis and those with p value less than 0.25 were selected and included in the multivariable analysis to control for possible confounders on LARC use. The multivariable logistic regression model showed that postpartum women who were residents of urban areas and those who had formal employment were almost three times more (AOR = 2.94, 95% CI: 1.07–8.06) and five times more (AOR = 4.82, 95% CI: 1.85–12.57) likely to use postpartum LARC compared to their counterparts, respectively. Furthermore, postpartum women who were counseled on FP methods were four times more (AOR = 4.39, 95% CI: 1.89–10.20) likely to use LARC than those who were not counseled about FP use.

Table 2 Reproductive characteristics of the study participants (*N* = 766)

Variable	n	%
Living children		
1–2	336	43.9
3–4	228	29.8
5 +	202	26.4
Median (IQR)	3 [2–5]	
Mode of index delivery		
Vaginal delivery	735	96.0
Caesarean delivery	31	4.0
Place of index delivery		
Home	371	48.4
Health facility	395	51.6
Discuss FP with partner (n = 731)[a]		
No	303	41.5
Yes	428	58.5
Menstrual resumption		
No	341	44.5
Yes	425	55.5
Duration of postpartum period (months)		
< 6	241	31.5
6–12	270	35.2
> 12—< 24	255	33.3
Counseled on FP (n = 141)[b]		
No	57	40.4
Yes	84	59.6

Notes: [a]Those with partners; [b]*n* = 141 variable limited to users only " were you councelled on family planning methods before starting using current method"
Abbreviations: *FP* Family planning, *IQR* Interquantile range

Discussion

In this study, we found the prevalence of postpartum use of LARC methods was as low as 10.4%. Factors such as mother's occupation, mother's residence and being counseled on family planning use were important predictors for postpartum use of LARC.

The prevalence of postpartum LARC use estimated in our study is consistent with the national average estimate of 10% [8]. The similarity between these findings could be explained by comparability in population characteristics studied, as majority of women prefer short methods of contraceptive than the LARC. The present finding is also in congruent with previous studies conducted within and outside Africa. For example, in a community based study in rural Uganda by Anguzu et al., the authors reported the postpartum LARC prevalence of 8.5%, [12]. Similar finding was also reported in rural China where the authors reported postpartum LARC prevalence of 9.9% [13]. In contrast, higher prevalence of postpartum LARC use (34.3%) has been reported in Ethiopia [15], Kenya (38.3%) [16] and Ethiopia (36.7%), [17]. The possible reasons for difference in findings between our study and Ethiopian studies could be due to nature of the studied population. Our population was mainly rural while participants in the Ethiopian studies were mainly from urban area where majority of

Table 3 Factors associated with postpartum LARC use, Multivariable analysis (*N* = 766)

Variable	LARC use		COR (95% CI)	AOR (95% CI)	*P*-value
	No	Yes n (%)			
Sociodemographics					
Age (years)					
15–24	326	33 (10.1)	1		
25–34	318	39 (12.3)	1.24 (0.76–2.03)	0.76 (0.28–2.07)	0.592
35–49	122	8 (6.6)	0.62 (0.28–1.39)	0.40 (0.08–1.98)	0.261
Marital status					
Married	652	63 (9.7)	1		
Unmarried	114	17 (14.9)	1.64 (0.92- 2.92)	0.85 (0.25–2.81)	0.785
maternal education					
Primary/below	714	70 (9.8)	1		
Secondary/ above	52	10 (19.2)	2.19 (1.05–4.57)	0.82 (0.20–3.33)	0.784
Occupation					
Unemployed	740	71 (9.6)	1		
Employed	26	9 (34.6)	4.99 (2.12–11.72)	4.82 (1.85–12.57)	0.0004
Income per month					
< 100,000	618	65 (10.5)	1		
> 100,000	148	15 (10.1)	0.96 (0.53–1.74)	0.59 (0.22–1.57)	0.290
Residence					
Rural	523	32 (6.1)	1		
Urban	243	48 (19.8)	3.78 (2.32–6.15)	2.94 (1.07–8.06)	0.036
Partner's education (n = 731)					
Primary/below	557	48 (8.6)	1		
Secondary and above	174	27 (15.5)	1.95 (1.17–3.24)	1.81 (0.69–4.73)	0.226
Reproductive factors					
Discussing FP with partner (n = 731)					
No	303	5 (1.7)	1		
Yes	428	70 (16.4)	11.65 (4.51–30.08)	3.23 (0.8412.41)	0.088
Living children					
1–2	336	36 (10.7)	1		
3–4	228	28 (12.3)	1.17 (0.69–1.97)	1.45 (0.51–4.11)	0.489
5 +	202	16 (7.9)	1.13 (0.39–1.33)	0.79 (0.20–3.03)	0.727
Mode of index delivery					
Vaginal delivery	735	71 (9.7)	1		
C/S delivery	31	9 (29.0)	3.82 (1.68–8.67)	2.12 (0.32–14.12)	0.435
Place of index delivery					
Home	371	18 (4.9)	1		
Health facility	395	62 (15.7)	3.65 (2.09–6.36)	0.59 (0.21–1.64)	0.314
Menstrual resumption					
No	341	16 (4.7)	1		
Yes	425	64 (15.1)	21.71 (2.02–6.41)	0.61 (0.21–1.81)	0.375
Postpartum period					
< 6 months	241	17 (7.1)	1		
6–12 months	270	17 (6.3)	0.89 (0.44–1.78)	0.74 (0.20–2.73)	0.654

Table 3 Factors associated with postpartum LARC use, Multivariable analysis ($N = 766$) *(Continued)*

Variable	LARC use		COR (95% CI)	AOR (95% CI)	*P*-value
	No	Yes n (%)			
> 12- < 24 months	255	46 (18.0)	2.9 (1.60–5.26)	0.98 (0.31–3.13)	0.973
Counseled on FP (n = 141)					
No	57	20 (35.16)	1		
Yes	84	60 (71.4)	4.63 (2.13–10.05)	4.39 (1.89–10.20)	0.001

COR Crude odds ratio, *AOR* Adjusted odds ratio, *CI* Confidence interval

women have access to information regarding the importance of FP including LARC. However, this also could be due to the fact that most of the health facilities in previous studies have high health services coverages including family planning services [17]. The difference between our study and the Kenyan counterparts could be due to the fact that, the Kenya study was a hospital based study which might provide women with better access to information regarding reproductive and sexual education including FP as compared to women in the present study whose majority (68%) were rural dwellers with poor contact with the health care providers especially those from the pastoral communities whereby nearly 50% of postpartum mothers reported to have had home delivery in during their index delivery.

In the present study, most (82%) of postpartum women were not using any form of modern contraceptives during 2 years post-delivery. Consequently this predisposes a large proportion of women in the studied communities to unplanned pregnancies, short interpregnancy intervals and their associated complications. Planning and spacing of children especially with the use of modern contraceptives especially LARC is important for the general well-being of the family and community at large.

In this study, majority of mothers who reported to be using LARC, were using hormonal implants. Our findings form a concordance with the national estimate which revealed that only 7% and 1% of the women of reproductive age use hormonal implants and IUDs, respectively [8]. Likewise, previous studies in Ethiopia [11, 17] and Kenya [18] showed observed that majority of women reported using hormonal implants. Findings from 12 countries in sub-Saharan African including Tanzania reported that hormonal implants were the first or second most widely used in 10 out of 12 countries studied compared with IUDs, pills and injectables [19]. The low use of IUDs could be explained by perceived misconceptions such as fear of abdomen pain, discomfort during sex and myth that IUDs can move into the abdomen during sexual intercourse [20]. Our finding is in contrast with previous study in rural China where the authors found that majority reported using IUDs than implants [13].

In this study, urban residence was an important predictor for postpartum LARC use. Postpartum women in the urban settings were more likely to use LARC as compared to their rural counterparts. This finding is consistent with previous studies conducted in northwest Ethiopia [21]. The possible explanation could be that postpartum women in urban areas have been reported to have better access to information regarding family planning and general reproductive and sexual health matters than women who reside in rural setting with poor health services [22]. This might be the case for the

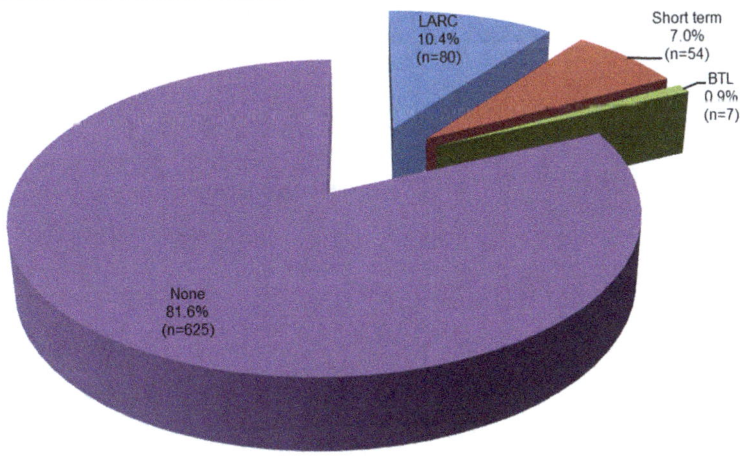

Fig. 1 Prevalence of modern contraceptives use by method type among postpartum women

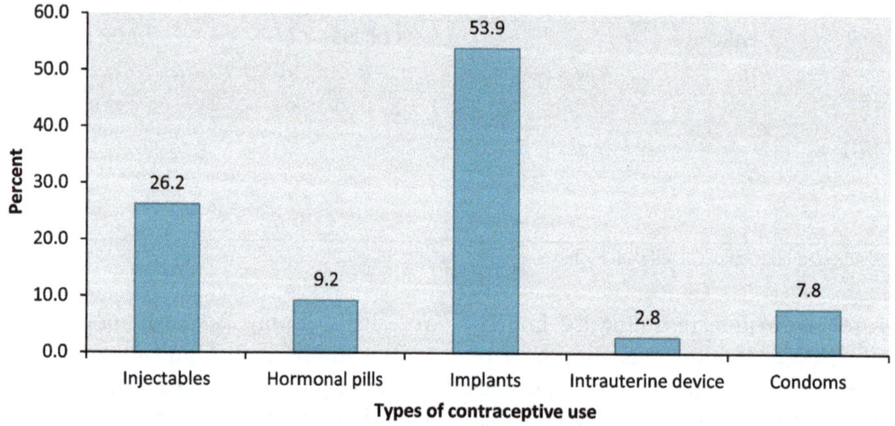

Fig. 2 Types of Modern contraceptives used by postpartum women

women in the studied population. Our findings imply that postpartum family planning services are no different, therefore there is a need for more efforts to increase utilization of modern family planning use among women in rural areas.

We also established that the occupation of the postpartum mother was associated with LARC use, particularly the formal employment. Similar relationship was reported among Kenyan women [16]. This could be explained by the fact that women with formal employment are more likely to be knowledgeable and well informed on family planning matters, have higher desire for fertility control and possibly have better access to family planning services.

Postpartum family planning counseling increased women's likelihood of using LARC methods. Even though current study didn 't assess the timing of family planning counseling, but previous studies in Ethiopia [17] and Thailand [23] revealed that contraceptive counseling was associated with an increased LARC use especially when done during immediate postpartum period. Previous authors also have demonstrated that, anticipatory counseling regarding side effects and bleeding profile can help in improving acceptability and continuation rate to postpartum contraceptive use [24]. Therefore, this should be offered upon initiation of contraceptive method.

Study limitations

The study design was a cross-section in nature which make difficult to establish the causal effect relationship. This study was done in a district where majority belong to the pastoral communities, this limit the generalization of findings whole country, but may reflect the situation in similar settings.

Conclusion

The postpartum use of LARC was low in the studied population with implants being the most commonly used method. Postpartum women from urban residence, with formal employment, and who were counseled about LARC were more likely to use LARC.

Our finding highlights the importance of family planning counseling, particularly client should be empowered with knowledge to make informed choice, to understand common side effects of LARC and should understand the management of side effects in case needs arises. Quality counseling will help to dispel community myths and misconception towards LARC method which will help to scale up the utilization of postpartum family planning. Furthermore we call for more efforts to increase LARC use in rural areas.

Abbreviations

AOR: Adjusted odds ratio; COR: Crude odds ratio; CI: Confidence Interval; CRERC: College Research Ethics and Review Committee; DELTAS: Developing Excellence in Leadership, Training and Science; IQR: Median and interquartile range; IUDs: Intrauterine devices; FP: Family Planning; LMICS: Low—and middle—income countries; LARC: Long acting reversible contraception; PPFP: Postpartum Family Planning; OCP: Oral contraceptives pills; SD: Standard deviation

Acknowledgements

Our sincere gratitude goes to research assistants, participants, Geita Regional medical officer, Bukombe District Medical officer and local village leaders. Lastly, we would like to appreciate Endulen. eV of Germany and MoHCDGEC for studies Scholarship at KCMUCo.

Author' contributions

KSK, MJM: designed the study, participated in data collection and played part in manuscript writing. EM: participated in study design and manuscript writing. SK and BCS participated in manuscript writing. JPA: performed statistical analysis. All authors read and approved the manuscript.

Author details

[1]Kilimanjaro Christian Medical University College, Moshi, Tanzania. [2]Department of Obstetrics and Gynecology, Kilimanjaro Christian Medical Centre, Moshi, Tanzania. [3]Department of Epidemiology and Biostatistics, Institute of Public Health, Kilimanjaro Christian Medical University College, Moshi, Tanzania.

References

1. WHO. Programming Strategies for Postpartum Family Planning. Geneva: WHO Press; 2013.
2. RCOG. Best practice in postpartum family planning. 2015 [Cited 7 May 2020]. Available from: https://www.google.com/search?q=Best+practice+in+postpartum+family+planning%2C+rcog+2015&oq=Best+practice+in+postpartum+family+planning%2C+rcog+2015&aqs=chrome..69i57.106 88j0j7&sourceid=chrome&ie=UTF-8.
3. Winner B, Peipert JF, Zhao Q, Buckel C, Madden T, Allsworth JE, et al. Effectiveness of long-acting reversible contraception. N Engl J Med. 2012; 366(21):1998–2007.
4. Ross JA, Winfrey WL. Contraceptive Use, Intention to Use and Unmet Need During the Extended Postpartum Period. International Family Planning Perspectives. 2001;27(1):20–7.
5. Moore Z, Pfitzer A, Gubin R, Charurat E, Elliott L, Croft T. Missed opportunities for family planning : an analysis of pregnancy risk and contraceptive method use among postpartum women in 21 low- and middle-income countries. Contraception. 2015;92(1):31–9.
6. Harrison MS, Goldenberg RL. Immediate postpartum use of long-acting reversible contraceptives in low- and middle-income countries. Maternal Health Neonatology Perinatology. 2017;3:24.
7. National Bureau of Statistics (NBS) [Tanzania] and ICF Macro. Tanzania Demographic and Health Survey 2010. Dar es Salaam: NBS and ICF Macro; 2011.
8. Ministry of Health, Community Development, Gender, Elderly and Children (MoHCDGEC) [Tanzania Mainland], Ministry of Health (MoH) [Zanzibar], National Bureau of Statistics (NBS), Office of the Chief Government Statistician (OCGS), and ICF 2016 Tanzania Demographic and Health Survey and Malaria Indicator Survey (TDHS MIS) 2015-16 Dar es Salaam Rockville MoHCDGEC, MoH, NBS, OCGS, and ICF.
9. Keogh SC, Urassa M, Kumogola Y, Kalongoji S, Kimaro D, Zaba B. Postpartum Contraception in Northern Tanzania: Patterns of Use, Relationship to Antenatal Intentions, and Impact of Antenatal Counseling. Stud FamPlann. 2015;46(4):405–22.
10. Chansin W, Jittima M, Wattanayingcharoenchai R, Aimjirakul K. Postpartum Use of Long-Acting Reversible Contraception in Primiparous Women: RamathibodiHospital' s Experiences. Thai J ObstetGynaecol. 2014;22(1):29–36.
11. Abraha TH, Teferra AS, Gelagay AA. Postpartum modern contraceptive use in northern Ethiopia: prevalence and associated factors. Epidemiol Health. 2017;39:e201701.
12. Anguzu R, Sempeera H, Sekandi JN. High parity predicts use of long-acting reversible contraceptives in the extended postpartum period among women in rural Uganda. Contraception and Reproductive Medicine. 2018;3:6.
13. Kang C, Li P, Liu X, Ding Y, Wang X, Zhou H. Use of contraceptives and uptake of long-acting reversible contraception among postpartum women in rural China. BMJ Sex Reprod Health. 2018;0:1–6.
14. PO-RALG. Bukombe district councils strategic plan for the period of 2016 - 2021. Bukombe, Geita; 2016.
15. Gebremedhin AY, Kebede Y, Gelagay AA, Habitu YA. Family planning use and its associated factors among women in the extended postpartum period in Addis Ababa. Ethiopia Contraception and Reproductive Medicine. 2018;3:1.
16. Jalang'o R, Thuita F, Barasa SO, Njoroge P. Determinants of contraceptive use among postpartum women in a county hospital in rural KENYA. BMC Public Health. 2017;17:604.
17. Tamrie YE, Hanna EG, Argaw MD. Determinants of Long Acting Reversible Contraception Method Use among Mothers in Extended Postpartum Period, Durame Town, Southern Ethiopia : A Cross Sectional Community Based Survey. Health. 2015;7:1315–26.
18. Ontiri S, Ndirangu G, Kabue M, Biesma R, Stekelenburg J, Ouma C. Long-Acting Reversible Contraception Uptake and Associated Factors among Women of Reproductive Age in Rural Kenya. Int J Environ Res Public Health. 2019;16:1543.
19. Jacobstein R. Liftoff : The Blossoming of Contraceptive Implant Use in Africa. Global Health: Science and Practise. 2018;6(1):17–39.
20. Mwafulirwa T, Shea MSO, Hamela G, Samuel E, Chipangula V, Hosseinipour MC, et al. Family Planning Providers ' Experiences and Perceptions of Long - Acting Reversible Contraception in Lilongwe. Malawi African Journal of Reproductive Health. 2016;20(2):62–71.
21. Mengesha ZB, Worku AG, Feleke SA. Contraceptive adoption in the extended postpartum period is low in Northwest Ethiopia. BMC Pregnancy and Childbirth. 2015;15:60.
22. Sultan S. The Effects of Education, Poverty, and Resources on Family Planning in Developing Countries Clinics in Mother and Child Health. Clinics Mother Child Health. 2018;15:289.
23. Kaewkiattikun K. Effects of immediate postpartum contraceptive counseling on long-acting reversible contraceptive use in adolescents. Adolescent Health Medicine and Therapeutics. 2017;8:115–23.
24. Villavicencio J, Allen RH. Unscheduled bleeding and contraceptive choice: increasing satisfaction and continuation rates. Open Access Journal of Contraception. 2016;7:43–52.

14

Use and discontinuation of intrauterine contraceptive device in the Greater Accra Region of Ghana

Fred Yao Gbagbo[1*] and Esinam Afi Kayi[2]

Abstract

Background: The intrauterine contraceptive device is one of the modern long-acting and reversible contraception that is very safe and effective. Yet, less than 2 % of women are using intrauterine devices in Ghana. This study therefore explored the experiences and barriers to intrauterine contraceptive device use and discontinuation in Greater Accra Region, Ghana.

Methods: Intrauterine contraceptive device users and providers were purposively selected from eight private family planning clinics in the Greater Accra Region. Semi-structured interview guides were used for in-depth interviews during data collection. The interviews were audio-taped to ascertain accurate accounts of the interviews and recordings replayed for analytical responses. Field assistants transcribed the interviews conducted themselves and read through the transcripts produced twice to increase familiarity with the dataset. A list of code labels was created and a series of categories for the main themes that emerged from the transcripts were developed. The transcribed data was organized, coded and manually thematically analysed in word. Study results were presented in tables and quotes from respondents.

Results: Results showed that key motivations for intrauterine contraceptive device use include effectiveness, benefits, and efficacy of the device, fertility regulation, peace of mind, contraceptive method switching, health provider effects, desire for long-acting contraceptive method, and partner characteristics. Intrauterine contraceptive device discontinuation was due to bleeding irregularities, vaginal infections, desire to increase fertility, physical features of the intrauterine device, and partner disapproval of use. Other reasons in both cases pertained to non-hormonal aspects of the intrauterine device, partner characteristics, and provider encouragement and influence.

Conclusions: Several factors influence the use and discontinuation of intrauterine device in Ghana. Comprehensive contraceptive counselling on the intrauterine device is essential in promoting uptake and knowledge of the intrauterine device at the health facility level. Various targeted messages are also needed to dispel misconceptions at the community level.

Keywords: Use, Discontinuation, Intrauterine contraceptive device, Greater Accra Region, Ghana

* Correspondence: gbagbofredyao2002@yahoo.co.uk; fygbagbo@uew.edu.gh
[1]University of Education Winneba, Box 25, Winneba, Ghana

Background

Globally, the intrauterine contraceptive device (IUD) has been recognised as one of the modern long-term reversible contraceptive methods suitable for women of all reproductive ages [1]. It represents the most cost effective reversible method for preventing unwanted pregnancies [2]. Scientifically proven for its safety, efficacy and cost-effectiveness [3], the copper T380A and Levonorgestrel releasing IUD is known to be more effective and longer lasting in preventing pregnancy than tubal sterilization, pills, patches and contraceptive rings [4, 5].

A number of studies show that several factors account for the poor IUD use among women [6–8]. These factors relate to healthcare provider characteristics, health system and individual or user factors [9, 10]. While these may be enough, sociocultural norms, beliefs and practices may serve to regulate IUD use even among high risk women or sub-groups particularly in Africa where there are entrenched sociocultural norms, beliefs and practices on childbirth [10].

Health provider characteristics that contribute to low IUD utilisation include misperception that IUD is associated with an ongoing risk of pelvic inflammatory disease (PID) and resultant infertility which particularly hinder IUD use among nulliparous women, especially if they are single or have several sexual partners [11]. In addition, few health care providers are shown to be hesitant to insert an IUD into nulliparous women because of perceived technical challenges [12].

Individual factors which prevent IUD uptake are often accentuated by misconceptions, beliefs and myths. Whilst women report conceptual concerns and fears about having a foreign body placed inside their womb, a lack of counselling and adequate information about IUDs from healthcare providers to enable them make informed decisions [13], fear of painful insertion [14, 15] and the perception of IUDs as abortifacients, risks of PID and ectopic pregnancy [16] deterred IUD use.

Although IUDs are considered as one of the most popular long acting and reversible contraceptive methods worldwide [17], they are used by less than 2% of Ghanaian women in their reproductive age [18]. Ghana's Demographic and Health Surveys (GDHS) have all shown very low IUD usage among both married and unmarried women [19]. Whilst reasons for low IUD use are poorly understood, the DHS does not provide an in-depth understanding of the factors or reasons associated with low use because the methodology is purely quantitative. This study therefore aimed to explore women's knowledge and perception about IUD, reasons for IUD use, barriers facing IUD uptake and provider characteristics influencing IUD using a qualitative method to provide in-depth information that will complement the GDHS data on IUD to inform policy and programme interventions aimed at increasing IUD uptake in Ghana.

Methods

Study design

The study employed a retrospective and cross-sectional qualitative design with an in-depth interview to obtain, analyze, interpret and report data. This was adapted from a previous study that used a cross-sectional designed [20]. The purpose of using this qualitative design in this study was to explore a range of opinions and its different interpretations with the aim of maximizing the opportunity to understand the different positions taken by different members of the social milieu. This design therefore enabled an in-depth exploration of women's experiences with the IUDs as represented differently from their own perspective.

Study population

Women in their reproductive ages (15–49 years) who had ever received family planning (FP) services, and particularly, IUD from the study facilities were selected to participate in the study. Women who were eligible to partake in the study were: Non-IUD users, current IUD users and women who had ever used IUD. The justification for choosing these women was because their experiences for not using, using or discontinuing the IUD use helped to answer the research questions. They were also most appropriate individuals to provide rich detailed information on IUD use. Trained and practicing IUD service providers (midwives and medical doctors) from the family planning units of public, private and NGO health facilities were also purposively interviewed to obtain divergent opinions on their experiences with FP choices including IUDs.

Study setting

The study was conducted in six renowned health facilities (2 public, 2 private and 2 NGO) that provide family planning services within the Greater Accra Region. The selection of these facilities was purposive. This was based on complete family planning data availability from the regional health directorate and the facilities client information management systems from 2008 to 2015. These facilities so far have not examined factors affecting uptake, satisfaction and acceptability of reversible family planning methods, hence creating a gap between client demand and provider supply which justifies the need to conduct the study in this setting to inform FP decisions.

Ethical considerations

Written informed consent was obtained from all interviewees for their participation and for the audio-recording of the interviews. Interviews were conducted in private places such as consulting rooms, respondents' homes and offices as recommended by respondents to protect the confidentiality of responses and enhance the comfort of respondents. This study received ethical approval from the Ghana Health Service (GHS) Ethical Review Committee (ERC). Permission was also sought from the various health facilities and respondents used in this study.

Data collection procedure

Data collection began using a sample frame. A list of women who had visited the identified health facilities for IUD insertion or removal during the past six months were obtained from the client information system after several unsuccessful attempts to directly recruit the required number of participants at the study sites. Considering the general low patronage of IUDs at the study site during the period of data collection, it was very challenging obtaining the required number of respondents for a meaningful analysis hence the need to fall on client records for retrospective interview of current and previous IUD users from the indicated facilities. Clients using other modern contraceptive methods were also interviewed to explore why they are not using IUDs but other methods. Family planning providers offering modern family planning methods, including IUD insertions and removal in the selected facilities were also interviewed to examine their experiences about clients concerns with providing IUD services.

Participants were recruited either by face-face or through phone calls after they were informed about the nature, benefits, risks, and purpose of the study and consented to participate. Information on voluntary participation, rights to withdraw and consent was made known to study respondents. Half of the in-depth interviews (IDIs) were conducted at health facilities, whilst the remaining were held at respondent's home, and at places deemed convenient and comfortable for respondents.

Data were collected using modified research instruments to build upon previous literature. In line with the study objectives and issues identified in the literature reviewed, four (4) different semi-structured interview guides were developed to address the research questions. The interview guides contained questions on participants' socio-demographic data (such as age, educational level, current FP use, previous FP method use, and parity); FP knowledge, and knowledge about IUD, and factors/reasons for IUD use. Questions for IUD users' differed slightly from questions asked of women who had ever used the IUD. For instance, whilst IUD users were questioned on their perception about the IUD when they initially began using it, women who had removed the IUD were asked to report on reasons for their removal of the IUD, side-effects, and future intentions to use the IUD. Thus, although questions differed slightly on some respects, a few similar questions were asked to answer the research objectives. Family planning providers were interviewed on the nature of their relationship with clients, clients' knowledge on the IUD and clients reasons for discontinuation of the IUD.

Three female research assistants were trained by the lead investigator to administer the interview guides. Although they were encouraged to be flexible during data collection, strict adherence to the study guide was discouraged if new topics in relation to originally stated questions emerged during the discussions. This flexibility was to encourage capturing of emerging issues which are different from the order given in the interview guides [21]. The field research assistants were also oriented on key ethical issues regarding research ethics involving humans as research subjects and were encouraged to be nonjudgmental in their responses to the experiences of the study participants. Face to face in-depth interviews were conducted in the local language 'Twi' or in English. Nine (9) study participants were interviewed in 'Twi' and the rest were in English. The In-depth Interviews lasted for an average of 40 min.

The interviews were audio-taped with permission from participants to ascertain accurate accounts of the interviews. The recordings were then replayed for analytical responses. Interviews were transcribed immediately thereafter while 'Twi' interviews were translated to English and later transcribed. Field assistants transcribed the interviews they conducted themselves. As the transcripts were produced, they were read through to increase familiarity with the data. Data was manually analysed by the researchers using the thematic analysis approach. To do this, a list of code labels was created and a series of categories for the main themes that emerged from the transcripts were developed. The transcribed data was then organized, coded and manually thematically analysed in word. Results of the study were then presented using descriptive statistics and quotes from respondents.

Results

Table 1 presents the socio-demographic characteristics of respondents excluding FP providers. For IUD users, six (6) were aged between 40 and 49 years, and the remaining were between 25 and 29 years. Two (2) out of the ten participants had no formal education. Only one woman was unmarried but she had two (2) children. Majority (8) had been using the IUD for more than six (6) months; only two (2) women had used it for two months and five months respectively. Twelve (12) women had ever used the IUD for duration of two weeks to thirteen (13) years. Their current FP methods comprised of both modern and traditional FP methods such as, implants, injectable, condom, withdrawal and the calendar method. Two (2) were not using a method; one was pregnant, and three were trying to get pregnant.

Table 1 Socio-demographic characteristics of study respondents

Characteristic	IUD users	Ever IUD users	Non-IUD users	Total
	n = 10	*n* = 12	*n* = 7	*N* = 29
Age				
20–25	2		2	4
26–30	2	3	3	8
31–35		3	2	5
36–40	1	3		4
41–45	3	1		4
46–50	2	2		4
Educational status				
No education	2			2
Primary	1	1	3	5
Secondary	3	2	4	9
Tertiary	4	9		13
Marital status				
Unmarried	1	2	1	4
Married	9	9	6	24
Divorced/separated				
Widowed		1		1
Occupation				
Unemployed			1	1
Self-employed	7	4	4	15
Public worker	1	3		4
Private formal worker	2	5	2	9
Parity				
1	1			1
2	2	3	1	6
3	3	4	3	10
4	2	3		5
5	2			2
6+				
Current FP method				
None		2	2	4
Trying to get pregnant/ pregnant		4	2	6
IUD	10			10
Implant		1	2	3
Injectables		1	1	2
Male Condom		1		1
Female condom				
Withdrawal		1		1
Calendar method		2		2
Tubal ligation				
Number of years using current FP				
Less than 6 months	5	3	3	11
6 months –1 year	3	3		6
2 years- 5 years	2			2
6 years–10 years				
More than 10 years				
Previous FP method				
None	3		1	4
IUD	2	11		13
IUS		1		1
Implant	1		2	3
Injectables	1		1	2
Pills	2		1	3
Male Condom				
Female condom				
Male condom				
Calendar method	1			1
Tubal ligation				
Number of years used previous FP method				
Less than 6 months	1	3		4
6 months –1 year	2	5	1	8
2 years- 5 years		3		3
6 years–10 years			2	2
More than 10 years	1			1
Total				28

Amongst these women, one didn't complete primary education, two had completed senior high school, and the rest had tertiary education. Two (2) participants worked in the public service, six (6) worked in private organizations, and four (4) were self-employed.

From the total IDIs conducted, seven (7) respondents had never used IUD as an FP method. Their ages ranged between 25 years to 32 years. Only one (1) was not married. Two (2) were currently using the implants; one (1) was using injectables; two (2) were trying to get pregnant, and the remaining two (2) were not using any FP method. The highest educational status attained by respondents in this group was secondary, (four respondents) and three (3) had completed junior high school. Almost all women had at least two (2) children, except two women who were trying to get pregnant.

Seven (7) IUD providers participated in the IDIs. Three out of the seven from NGO facilities whilst the remaining four (4) were from private (2) and public (2) facilities. The professional qualifications of FP providers ranged from Health assistant, Midwife, Nursing officer, Obstetrician and gynaecologist. There was a sole male FP provider in the study who worked as an Obstetrician. All providers have been providing FP services for more than 5 years except the health assistant who was not professionally trained and specialized to offer IUD insertions for women. Her responses are therefore not included in the analysis.

A total of thirty-six (36) IDIs were conducted. Out of this number, ten (10) women were currently using IUD, twelve (12) had ever used the IUD, and seven (7) had never used the IUD. The remaining seven (7) were family planning (FP) providers. Majority (12) of interviewees were selected from NGO facilities. Of the FP providers interviewed, only one was not providing IUD services. Her responses are therefore not included in the analysis. The number of IDIs conducted at each study setting is presented in Table 2.

Knowledge of family planning

Findings showed that all women had good knowledge about FP methods. Each study participant knew of at least, three FP methods and how it works. The commonly mentioned FP methods were injectables, implants, and pills. However, half of the women could not provide the name of the implants by themselves, but were able to describe where and how it was inserted. Very few (three) respondents mentioned sterilization (vasectomy and tubal ligation), diaphragm. One woman mentioned IUS. Furthermore, the interviews showed that IUD users and ever IUD users had adequate knowledge of the IUD compared to women who were not using IUD. Study respondents' level of knowledge about the mechanism of action (i.e. how the IUD works) of the IUD, description of its physical features, and who can use it was comparatively the same among current and previous IUD users.

Findings from current IUD users

From the IDIs, only ten (10) women were currently using the IUD. Out of the ten women, five (5) voluntarily decided to use the IUD whilst the remaining were given the IUD as a post-abortion contraception method. Three women who voluntarily preferred to use the IUD stated it was their personal decision; they were not encouraged or motivated by family, friends or staff, whilst the other two admitted being motivated by their friends, and health providers. A respondent categorically reported that her desire to use the IUD was out of a strong personal volition irrespective of her partner's consent. A respondent said:

> *"Nobody encouraged me to use the IUD. My husband, mum and siblings even did not want me to do the FP since they were all afraid of the side effects. So it was my own decision. I just got up one day and decided to go and do it because my children have very short intervals in relation to age. So even my husband doesn't know I've done FP unless I tell them" (29 year old married woman currently on copper-T IUD for 1 year).*

Although the walked-in clients reported to have voluntarily consented for IUD based on the counselling they received, clients who had the IUD following post-abortion care reported to have been coerced/forced/encouraged/influenced to have an IUD as post abortion contraception to avoid repeat unwanted pregnancy and abortion. Two respondents mentioned that they were respectively encouraged and influenced to use the IUD by the provider after having undergone an induced abortion. A respondent stated that:

> *"I refused an immediate family planning uptake despite the in-depth counselling given me after the previous abortion. So when I went and got pregnant and came again for another abortion, she said by force she will do one for me so I agreed for her to do it for me although it was against my wish" (40 year old married woman on Copper-T, IUD for1 year).*

Half of the participants reported no side effects after switching from injectables to having the IUD inserted. Again, another half felt slight abdominal pains soon after insertion of the IUD which was relieved after ingesting pain killers given by the provider. One respondent stated:

> *"I went back to the IUD because for me it was very successful. I never had any problems with the IUD compared to when I was using the injectables. I didn't*

Table 2 Number of IDIs conducted at each study setting

Study group	Facility 1	Facility 2	Facility 3	Facility 4	Facility 5	Facility 6	Total
IUD users	3	2	2	1	1	1	10
Ever IUD users	4	1	1	2	1	3	12
Non-IUD users	2	–	1	1	2	1	7
FP providers	3	1	1	1	–	1	7
Total	12	4	5	5	4	6	36

have any problems with my period, I didn't have any weight issues and headaches compared to the injectables that I previously used" (43 year old unmarried woman using Copper –T 380A for 2years)

Another respondent indicated that:

"my experience so far is that my menstrual flow has reduced from 5 days to 4 days since using the IUD for six months now after I delivered my last baby. I decided to ask a doctor friend and he said nothing is wrong with me. I also realized, comparing this with the injectables that I used to be on, the severe heart beat and headache I used to have disappeared. Initially, I was a bit tensed, that maybe my husband will find out. So one day, I asked him about it whether he can feel anything. And he said no. So he asked is it like the other ones? I said no, your menstrual cycle is it normal? I said normal, regular 28days cycle. I said I'm ok. I don't know; I'm not worried. I feel normal. I feel ok. So I've been encouraging some of my colleagues to do the IUD" (29year old married woman on Copper T 380 A for 2years)

In another instance, one participant indicated having prolonged menstrual flow and offensive vaginal discharges. According to her, the duration of menstruation is slightly longer and heavier compared to when she had not inserted the IUD. She narrated her experiences as follows:

"You are just there and then you get a discharge. It's not too comfortable, but then, I initially tried to cope until the discharge became offensive which compelled me to seek medical help that advised me to remove it after two months of unsuccessful treatment.

I realize that, even though it is just about two months since removing the IUD, It's a little better. Now the discharges come at the time of ovulating. Although I realize that there are more discharges it's no longer offensive. I learnt it's going to go back to normal after a while" (42 year old married woman wo used Copper-T 380A for 2months but currently on combined oral contraceptive pills).

Another respondent asserted that her menstrual flow is now irregular compared to when she hadn't inserted the IUD. Also, she initially experienced some brief periods of vaginal discharge, which did not smell but currently doesn't have any discharge. She indicated that:

"......I later realized that some 'water (referring to discharge) comes from my vagina. But they told me that when we see some water and we don't like it we should come back. But I didn't go back and the water stopped. Since then I have not experienced any major problem just that my menses is not flowing like it should be." (46 year old married woman on Copper-T 30A for 1year).*

Two respondents reported that this was their second time of using the IUD. Both of them reported no side effects on both occasions. According to one participant, she removed the IUD to test her fertility and continued usage after childbirth as encouraged by her doctor's explanation and counselling. She narrated her story as follows:

"....So he said that IUD will be the best solution so I went into that. I used that for about 6 years, I met this guy we talked about marriage and he was like the thing that people are telling him is that if you take it off you won't get pregnant again. He insisted that before we get married I should get pregnant for him first. So I took it off and became pregnant the following month and got married but aborted the pregnancy on health grounds after which I had another replaced for 3years. I took it out again and I got pregnant again (laugh) after I gave birth, I read about LNG-IUS and I went to the hospital requesting for it because of its advantages. But I was told it is not available in Ghana yet. I was like okay am not going to have any babies any time soon so let me go back to my Copper IUD. So I had it again for almost 10years now." (43year old unmarried woman on Copper-T 380A for 10years).

Factors that influence IUD uptake

Table 3 presents an illustrative summary of factors influencing IUD uptake in order of most frequently mentioned

Table 3 Illustrative summary of factors influencing IUD use among current IUD users

No.	Factors influencing IUD uptake	Frequency	Percentage (%)
1	Prevention of unwanted pregnancy	20	21
2	Reduce births	17	18
3	Space births	15	16
4	Prevent abortion	11	11
5	Contraceptive failure	10	10
6	Avoid forgetfulness in taking pill	6	9
7	Substitute to other FP methods due to unpleasant experiences	5	5
8	Desire for a long lasting permanent method	4	4
9	Concentrate on work, or business	3	3
10	Non-hormonal method	2	2
11	Concentrate on academics	1	1
Total		94	100

factors. Respondents gave varied reasons for current use of IUD compared to other methods. The main reasons reported to have determined IUD uptake pertained to protection against unwanted pregnancy, to reduce births or space childbearing.

Other factors that influenced IUD uptake were centred on the characteristics and benefits of the IUD over implants, pills and injectables. Half of respondents' decision for using the IUD was premised on past contraceptive failure and a desire for a long lasting family planning method. In a narrative account, a study participant's decision to adopt the IUD was due to ineffectiveness of traditional natural FP method; to avoid unpleasant previous experiences with other FP methods; fear of partner's reaction to successive pregnancy, and desire for a different FP method other than implants, injectables or pills in order to avoid another repeated abortion. She admits being encouraged by the provider to use IUD during post-abortion counselling. The need to avoid unpleasant side effects with the pills, injectables as well as forgetting to take the pills and ease of use influenced IUD uptake. Two women reported:

> *"I had issues with the tablet because I kept forgetting yes and your menstrual cycle change with it and all that. That is why I went for the IUD" (39year old unmarried woman on Copper-T IUD for, 2years)*

Another respondent indicated that:

> *"I had wanted to do the 5years type of IUD but it wasn't available. I was told the 5years type of IUD, the implants and 3 months injectables are almost the same. Since I had done the 3 months and felt dizzy, I decided to do the 10 years IUD because that one isn't medicine but just something to close the vagina" (29year old married woman, using copper-T 380A for 2years)*

Two respondents were convinced about the efficacy of the IUD influenced their choice of the IUD as a method to prevent pregnancy. One said: *"It was effective for me previously and it's still the best for me" (23 year old married woman on Copper-T 380A for 1 year).*

Another also said: *"I was more convinced about the efficacy of it the choice" (43 year old unmarried woman, on Copper-T 380A for 2 years).*

In furtherance to the reasons for IUD use, two women also decided to use IUD because of its non-hormonal nature which does not affect their hormonal system. In their view, the IUD was the best method. One noted in the following:

> *"IUD is the best method because, I think it does not have any hormonal thing when you do it unlike the one that you inject or has something to do with your blood. Those ones I hear people have complications, hormonal disturbances, I think IUD is best because it just blocks your womb and no sperm enters to have an egg fertilized" (23year old married woman, on Copper-380A for 2years.*

Partner characteristics also determined preference for IUD use in a few cases. For one woman, the decision to use the IUD was fear of partner's reaction to successive pregnancy, and to avoid problems with partner. Narrating her story she said:

> *"I became pregnant for the fourth time and I fear my husband will complain and refuse my education. My husband suggested an abortion and IUD. He encouraged me this is the best after the abortion which I did" (29year old married woman, on Copper-T 380A for 3 year).*

Another respondents indicated that:

> *"I already have four kids and my husband is giving me problems to have more. if I tell him about family planning he would not allow me to do so I came to do this on my own secretly" (44year old married woman on Copper-T 380A for 2years).*

The insistence and encouragement of some health providers led to IUD uptake for some women. A respondent categorically admitted being encouraged by providers to use IUD after post-abortion counselling. They claimed providers did not directly influence their choice, but rather advised on the need for adopting an effective method to prevent repeated abortions. A respondent asserted in the following:

> *"——So when I went and got pregnant and came again and she said by force she will do one for me so I agreed for her to do it for me"....(40year old married woman, 3 children on Copper T 380A for 3years).*

Another respondent indicated that:

> *" —midwife insisted on me taking an IUD after doing the abortion else she will not help me again. Because of the respect I had for her, I had the IUD soon after the abortion for free" (28year old widow, 2 children on Copper T 380A for 1year).*

Perceptions about IUD

Study participants' indicated to have had mixed reactions when first introduced to the IUD. Majority (8) of the respondents said they were scared when they first heard about the IUD. The insertion procedure created fear amongst them hence did not opt for an IUD as FP method. Two respondents explained:

"I have heard about FP before. They say some FP is put in the arms, some too were injections and some too were inserted in the womb. But I didn't know how it looks like. So when I came and it was explained to me I was scared so I didn't do it but opted for the injection" (40 year old married woman on injectables).

The other respondent indicated:

"Yes, I was very afraid; because I had not done some before. I'm a person full of fear. I taught of something different. But the provider took time to counsel me and even used models for demonstrations on how it is done. Despite my fears, I tried it. I taught it will be painful for months but nothing of that sort happened" (25 year old married woman, on Copper-T 380A for 3years).

Women's perception of the IUD was also associated with myths and negative reactions from friends. They raised concerns about some myths that they had heard about the IUD getting stuck in the womb, and potential health risks in later years. For respondents who associated myths and misconceptions about the IUD, they affirmed that their perceptions had now changed. A respondent reported that her lack of knowledge about how the IUD works, and how it looked like made her afraid. The fact that "something" was going to be inserted in the womb created fear, because her understanding of the procedure is similar to undergoing a D & C. However, her perception changed after explanations from the provider. She explained:

"Oh in the beginning when they were about to fix it and it scared me a bit because I didn't know how it will work or how it is. Ehee, but they made us understand that it wasn't anything scary. Something that they said they will put in your womb, you will be a bit scared" (46year old married woman on Copper – T 380A for 5months)

Other respondents who did not discuss their FP choices with their partners, feared that their partners might find out about having the IUD since the strings were likely to be visible. One respondents indicated that:

"Initially, I was a bit tensed, that maybe my husband will find out. So one day, I asked him about it whether he can feel anything in me during sex. And he said no. I then became comfortable keeping it all these years without him knowing" (29year old married woman on copper-T 380A for 5 years).

Some respondents were just curious and desirous to try a longer lasting FP method when initially informed about the IUD by a health provider. Other respondents were further motivated to use the IUD with positive assurances and encouragement from friends. Further, another woman also expressed indifference when initially informed about it. She said: *'I just wanted to protect myself, I didn't have any attitude towards it' (29 year old married woman, on Copper-T 380A for 2 months).*

Perception of health risks associated with using the IUD

In Ghana, knowledge about Family Planning methods is generally acquired though formal and informal public education. Whereas the educated population read about family planning methods when the need arises, the less educated obtain family planning information in health facilities, friends and significant others including television, radio and social media adverts. When respondents were asked whether using the IUD was associated with health risks, seven (7) reported no health risks associated with using the IUD, while one (1) respondent couldn't tell whether or not the IUD posed a health risk. She indicated:

"I was not scared of any risk, because I didn't think there will be any. But there was one thing that was at the back of my mind, that if I am not comfortable with it, I will take it out. Do you know, if I am not comfortable I didn't think that they could do something, you know negative, but all I was thinking is that, if I am not comfortable, I will take it out" (42year old married woman, on Copper–T 380A for 5 years)

A respondent admitted that no health risks were possible except risk of getting infected through usage of unsterilized equipment. However, one woman feared being sterilized after using the IUD. Another participant had no knowledge about whether IUD usage could harm her in future. She explained:

'If there is a development that it affects something because the copper something scared me, because I didn't understand why you should have metal in you but I googled and read about it and I think its ok, it doesn't have any health risks' (23year old unmarried woman on Copper-T 380A for 3 months).

Although majority (7) of the women interviewed felt safe with using the IUD, a few (five) disliked the uncomfortable feeling of the strings hanging in vagina during menses, bathing and somehow wished the string will be 'cut off'. Three of them had this to say:

"Yeah the little thing that I don't like about it is that, when you are having your menses the bleeding brings the strings out. They put the "T" thing in the womb, and then they leave this (referring to the string) to hang out into the vagina. So as you, you know, if, mensuration stops it sort of goes in to... "Aha", When you are taking shower and your hand just goes there, you can feel it. I would have wished they will even cut my string out" (42year old married woman, on Copper –T 380A for 5 years).

Another respondent explained:

"oh the first time I fixed it, the thread was lying around my vagina so I was afraid so I was pushing it in, then I later went there to complain about it. They removed it for me and then fixed another IUD for me but still there's some thread lying around my vagina. Anytime I wash that area, I feel it but now I don't care" (23 year old married woman, on LNG-IUS for 1 year).

Another respondent was of the view that:

"the previous IUD I inserted, I don't know what happened maybe I had a heavy flow in a particular month and it came out and you know it has a string attached to it, so I think it was choking me around my cervix and when I was sitting, it was so down, I was feeling a little pain that's why I went to change it; but apart from that, I'm ok with the current one as its very comfortable" (29year old married woman, on Copper –T 380A for 2 years).

Findings from women who have ever used the IUD as post abortion contraception

Four respondents previously used the IUD as a post-abortion contraception after repeated abortions. A respondent exclaimed: *"They rather gave it to me because of the abortion and they didn't sell it to me. It was free after I did the abortion to protect me" (39 year old widow, on Copper-T 380A for 4 years).* The other respondents however paid for the IUD separately.

Problems or side-effects experienced with using IUD

Generally, findings showed that at least, each woman (study participant) suffered from one of several side effects of the IUD after a few weeks of insertion. For some, the side-effects was severe and sufficient to warrant a removal of the IUD. An illustrative summary of the reported side-effects and reasons for IUD removal is outlined in Table 4.

The results indicate that reasons for removal of the IUD do not differ substantially from the side-effects experienced by respondents. Other reasons that led respondents to remove the IUD involve partner disapproval with the use of a FP method. One of the respondents explained that her partner disapproves of FP and so she was scared that although she has the IUD, the partner might notice the IUD and there might be a problem with that. She states:

*"My fear is maybe what if you are making love with your husband one day and the IUD gets remove by itself. Sometimes it bothers my mind and I'm scared when having sex" (*31year old married woman on Copper-T 380A for 8 months).

The physical features of the IUD also deterred some participant from continued use of the method. A respondents indicated that:

"I think the uneasiness of that thread thing makes me dislike it. You know, once you're cleaning it wants to come out and you have to push it there, you know... it has to be in there, it doesn't need to stick out so that brings uneasiness" (47year old married woman on Copper-T 380A for 2 years).

Another respondent said:

'Why should I allow that nasty thing to be put in my body? The shape of it alone puts me off so I will always go for another decent method and certainly not the IUD' (25 year old unmarried woman using the injectable for 3years)

Table 4 Summary of side-effects of IUD and reasons for removal

Reported Side-effects with IUD experienced	Reported reasons for removal of IUD
• Heavy bleeding	• Heavy prolonged bleeding
• Foul vaginal discharge (sometimes coloured)	• Vaginal discharge
• Infections	• To give birth
• Abdominal cramps	• Abdominal cramps
• Spotting bleeding	• Spotting or irregular bleeding
• Prolonged bleeding	• Infections
• Irregular bleeding	• Feeling of device removing
	• Discomfort with strings
	• Partner disapproval of FP method

Three respondents removed the IUD to give birth, but two of them categorically expressed their intentions of inserting the IUD again after birth. They both indicated their intentions as follows:

> *"I removed the IUD to have another baby, but right after the pregnancy, I will wear the IUD again to protect myself from unplanned pregnancy because it is good for me" (39year old widow, who previously used Copper –T 380A for 4years).*

The other respondents said:

> *"—even this when I was coming to remove it, the nurse asked me [laughing] 'why do you want to remove it' and I said I want to give birth again to two children. I think my partner is okay with the IUD and I will have it again after delivery" (38year old married woman, who previously used copper –T 380A for 2 years).*

Reasons for IUD use among ever IUD users

Many reasons were noted for the use of IUD among the respondents who have ever used an IUD. Key among the reasons for women's use of the IUD however pertained to a desire for a long acting FP method compared to short term FP methods. Summary of reasons given are arranged in order of most frequently mentioned in (Table 5).

To satisfy a desire for long acting family planning method, some respondents went out at all lengths to ensure that they had their desired FP method of choice. A respondent explained that:

Table 5 Illustrative summary of reasons for IUD use among ever IUD users

No.	Reasons for IUD use among ever IUD users	Frequency	Percentages (%)
1	Desire for long acting family planning method	18	24
2	Avoid unpleasant side effects with other FP types	15	20
3	Avoid forgetfulness to take pill	12	16
4	No hormonal influence	9	12
5	Perception of no side effects	7	9
6	Protect against pregnancy	5	7
7	Provider influence	4	5
8	Preference for an 'obscure' FP ('obscure = hidden')	3	4
9	Health reasons	2	2
10	Prevent worry	1	1
Total		76	100

> *"I first went to a public hospital in Kumasi which had only short term FP methods. I wasn't really convinced so I heard about the IUD from a NGO facility which I visited just for something more permanent. So I just walked in she took me through all the methods and after my last baby I was advised on that as the best option based on being hypertensive" (47 year old married woman on Copper-T 380A for 8 years).*

Another respondent said:

> *'I actually brought the LNG-IUS from the USA to be inserted for me here in Ghana because I really love it but very expensive to be inserted in the USA' (23 year old unmarried woman on LNG-IUS for 2 years)*

Other respondents also mentioned avoidance of side effects with other FP methods and reduced forgetfulness in taking the pill. One respondent reported:

> *"Oh yeah I love the IUD because there was nothing like I have forgotten to take my pills, I have forgotten to do this or that. It was just convenient I didn't have to worry about anything. I didn't have to worry. Once it was there and I was assured that it was 99% safe. So I didn't worry" (....38 year old married woman, on copper-T 380A for 2 years).*

Two accounts from two women which capture their decision to use the IUD is presented in the following:

> *"The fact that it's inside makes me satisfied. I don't have to see it, apart from the little pain I will experience over the months, I'm done. I can't be faithful to that, taking the pill" (....26year old single woman ever used Copper-T 380A)*

The other respondent indicated that:

> *"Because I was told it has nothing to do with the hormones and cells in me I think it is normal" (32year old married woman, ever used Copper-T 380A).*

Perception of health risks associated with using the IUD

Mixed responses were obtained when the question on perception of health risk was asked. One woman feared that the IUD could cause cancer. According to her:

> *"When I was going I didn't know what to do and you know I was asking a lot of questions so I was going on the internet and my elder sister who passed away last year was telling me "Don't do it!. Don't do these things, they give cancer. "She died out of cancer but she said*

"don't do it again". They give cancers, the one...that thing insert here two things affect your blood and you get bloated up. You know, there were lot of fears" (.47year old woman on LNG IUS for 3 years).

Another woman believed that though the IUD was effective in preventing pregnancy but the risk of contracting infections through the IUD makes it not to be totally safe. She explained that:

"When it comes to health risks, I don't know how you want me to; .oh you will still get STIs, you will still have seamen coming into you. You will still get the STIs" (....30 year old woman on Copper-T 380A).

Another risk as mentioned by a 26 year old woman pertained more to a misconception about the IUD moving around the body into other organs by itself after insertion. She also mentioned the probability of experiencing perforation in the uterus when IUD is inserted. Although a rear occurrence with trained and competent providers the probability of perforation has been reported in clinical incidents relating to IUD insertion due to provider errors and use of rigid instruments among others. In the respondents own words she indicated that:

"With the health risk you know when you put it on, when you insert they have this nylon thread, that they wrap it, sometimes it comes off as it helps the IUD to move around. You may not know, sometimes there may be some perforation or something. It may hurt u. I think that is, that makes it the only problem but aside that, it's not a problem".

However, this same woman maintains that *"I don't think there are any health risks, if u have an IUD inserted u don't let everybody play around that part because if their fingers are...., I think the health risk is more about us and how you take care of yourself".*

One respondent experiencing vaginal discharges was concerned that the discharges were due to the Copper IUD she had used for the past 2 years and might be risky to her health. She said:

"Yeah, as I was saying about the discharges, I fear it could lead to something else" (...32year old single woman on Copper-T 380A)

According to another woman, she was of the view that women risk having an ectopic pregnancy after using the IUD as a FP method. She explained saying:

"Obviously yeah. You risk ectopic. You risk ectopic pregnancy I know that. I may say it has been argued with the LNG-IUS because of the hormone they can cause issues of the hormone imbalance things like that. I didn't experience it anyway" (40year old married woman, on LNG-IUS for 3 years)

In contrast to some respondents' stated fears about the IUD, two other women could not certainly tell whether using the IUD was risky to their health. One said:

"health risk? Not as I know" (....38 year old woman on Copper-T380A).

Similarly, two other women believed since they didn't experience any side effects or problems with the IUD, and upon the recommendation of health providers, then there was no health risks associated with it. One of them indicated that:

"I don't know much but so far, no. I've been to two midwives and they themselves said they used that one. That's what makes me go in for that one" (....31year old woman, o Copper-T 380A for 2 years).

Future intention to use IUD

Women were asked about their future intention to use the IUD, and from their responses, only five (5) declared their intention to use it again because it was good, useful and effective for them. One respondent said:

"I will come for the same thing when God willing I give birth"...38year old married woman, 2 children

Another woman also reported

"Yes, but right after the pregnancy, I will wear the IUD again to protect myself because it is good for me"... 39year old widow, 4 children

It was clear from the IDIs that some women wished the IUD would have worked for them because they preferred a longer acting method, and also since it was recommended by a provider. Unfortunately some respondents experienced heavy/painful menses and frequent expulsion when given the IUD hence had to have it removed two months after insertion. Two women reported:

"It's not all that safe since I had heavy and painful menses when I was on IUD. I mean I wish it had worked for me, honestly. I really wished it had worked for me, I mean I was really counting on it. The fact that I mean it will be there for the next 5 years, for the next 10 years, you are protected and all that, u don't

have a problem. I really hoped it worked"....(30year old unmarried woman ever used Copper-T 380A)

The other said:

"I was quite unfortunate to have had the IUD falling off by its self on three occasions so I had to discontinue its use. But if it was working for me, I would have loved it. Why? Because it doesn't let me grow fat or anything. You know, you stay your normal and you know that after five years which is quite a long time, you can change it. Five or ten years I think for you to change it. If you feel some uneasiness, you just walk into the facility and you just take it off" (47year old woman, on Copper-T IUD for 4 years).

Women's knowledge about the IUD

All family planning providers reported that women (also clients) have very little knowledge of the IUD pertaining to its mechanism of action, its physical features, how it feels, and the essence of the copper around it. They attributed women's knowledge of the IUD from shared experiences of friends, and which is represented negatively. Thus, when they asked clients knowledge of the IUD, clients primarily stated their misconceptions, side-effects and myths neglecting the usefulness and efficacy. On provider said:

"Sometimes, they can be influenced by their friends. If I'm giving it percentage wise, it's about 30percent of them who know depo, IUD, secure and all those stuffs from their friends" (IUD provider)

Another provider reported that:

"When you ask them, they tell you yes, I've heard it, but I've not seen it so you let them touch it and feel how it is before you do it for them. They will ask you so what is it, the wire that we are seeing there, it is just plastic. So they hold it to see how flexible it is. This is just a copper that is wound around it and is nothing that is going to hurt them, or touch anything" (IUD provider).

Two providers asserted that among women who had visited them for contraceptive counselling and uptake, less educated women tended to have no knowledge about the IUD compared to educated clients who sometimes search the internet to read and obtain knowledge of the IUD prior to their visit to the FP clinic. The availability of internet services on smart phones provides quick information to users in areas that have good reception. This enable clients seeking information on contraception to browse quickly for knowledge. The observation made however is, clients who don't have such facilities regardless of their educational levels tend to rely on service providers and/or significant others for information on family planning services. On this same issue, three providers also mentioned that only few clients have heard of IUD, and out of this number, very few have ever seen or touched it before. A provider narrated her experience as follows:

"Yes, have you heard about IUD? You ask. You came in here we do family planning, which one do you like? The person if she's ... She will tell you that, I don't have any idea about family planning" (IUD provider).

On the other hand, a male provider strongly professed that because clients have little knowledge of modern FP methods particularly, IUD, he mostly provided it for them based on their past medical history, parity and the number of previous deliveries. Thus, he directly influenced clients' use of the IUD. He indicated that:

"Well over there, if they come, most of them don't know about the IUD. Theirs is that they are here to protect themselves against pregnancy or are here for FP. So I take them through all the methods and then I ask how many children they have. And most of them too they gave birth at my place so I already know their history. After the counselling they will ask me, out of the whole lot which one am I choosing for them? You see, they are such that they have that trust and belief in me, so anything I say they comply" (IUD provider).

Women's reasons for not using the IUD

From the interviews, providers stated that women's reasons for not using the IUD is mainly because of the fear of inserting the IUD in the uterus, and fears about the IUD. Fears about the IUD pertain to myths and misconceptions, as well as fears that the IUD will affect their health in the long term.. A respondent narrated some misconceptions and fears as follows:

"I learnt the IUD can walk to the heart. I also learnt a woman had a baby and the baby was carrying IUD in her hand. If you get IUD, you won't have children again. They have been saying all these things. So I tell them, it is not true."

Other reasons such as male partners' disapproval of IUD use, (and any other FP method); fear of male partners' knowledge about the IUD, and the uncomfortable feeling of the strings during sexual intercourse. Poor knowledge base of the IUD, a strong mind-set and resistance to the IUD also deterred uptake.

Concerning fears about the procedure for inserting the IUD, a female provider explained that unlike the short term FP methods like injectables or pills which are unobtrusive, IUD is noticeable and can be felt by the partner through the strings which lie in the vagina during intercourse. There is therefore a greater chance of it been detected or felt by the partner even when the partner has no knowledge about it.

Providers' reasons for clients IUD removals

The main reasons for clients' removal of the IUD from providers view is the side effects evident through bleeding, cramps, vaginal infection, and abnormal menstrual cycle. The second key reason is for reproduction. Other reasons providers cited are to prevent feuds with their partners in circumstances where the IUD was inserted without partners' knowledge and approval; fear of IUD from moving to other parts of the body; fear of IUD causing fibroid and cancer after prolonged use and for other health reasons.

> *"The reason for them taking it out, some of them they bleed even after. Some can bleed for the whole 28days. They become very anaemic, fatigued and weak. For some, it's not all, but as soon as you take it off and put them on medication for a week, that thing ceases and you monitor that client for about three cycles, you see that the client will be happy; and have the normal menstrual flow. The second thing too is that, she will come with that problem, you will take it off and this will go and interfere with her normal menstrual cycle, then she will be having abnormal menstrual cycle; instead of 28 days, at times they can go 26, 40." (IUD Provider)*

Another provider said:

> *"Some of them they come in for it without the consent from their partners. So along the way, their partners find out. And it tends to bring a quarrel among them so they quickly come for it to be removed" (IUD provider).*

A female provider categorically maintained that some women who came to remove the IUD did so for no obvious reason; neither were they experiencing complications except to change to a different FP method. She indicated that:

> *"There are instances they don't come with any complaint, they feel it has been there for quite a long time, so they feel they should take it off and change to another method to see the best. Somebody who has been on the IUD for 7 years will come and take it off. Why do you want to take it off, and she tells you, I want to change it. It has been there for long so I want to change it. Just take it off and do something else for me" (IUD Provider).*

It was also noted that other women also wanted to test their fertility or reproducibility after prolonged IUD use. According to an IUD provider's account:

> *"They think once is been there for long without them getting pregnant, they should remove it and see if they are still fertile. And so they will remove, they will get pregnant and then they will come for help" (IUD Provider).*

Client- provider- relationship in health facilities during FP counselling

All FP providers unanimously agreed having a good positive relationship with clients during contraceptive counselling. They described the counselling sessions as cordial and open to allow clients to freely discuss their concerns, and ask questions about the IUD, as well as other FP methods. Counselling is done in an open manner in a language which clients understand to facilitate communication.

Ways to encourage IUD uptake among women

Currently, education on family planning services is integrated into general sexual and reproductive health promotion and education programmes at the local, regional and national levels. The scope of the sexual education at the public level is basic information on human reproduction and mechanism of how contraceptives work. Although there is a national family planning standards and protocols guiding family planning educational activities, the implementation of this protocol is determined by who is doing the education, the target population, mode of education and the level of theoretical and practical experience of the educator. In this regard, comprehensive education on long acting and reversible contraceptives as well as permanent methods looking at medical eligibility, side effects and complications are usually reserved for clinical trainings of providers and not the general public. Consequently, the limited scope of IUD education compels potential clients' new users or adopters of IUD to rely on self-education by reading or information from significant others some of whom have limited knowledge shrouded with some of the identified myths and misconceptions that prevents IUD use and encourages discontinuation when side effects occur among users.

To encourage IUD use among women, all the FP providers suggested a holistic education and public sensitization. The holistic education as reported encompasses information on eligibility, side effects and complications for women on the IUD, as well as other long term FP methods for informed decisions on choice. Comprehensive education in this regard, should be carried out through the media (print and electronic) and mobile information vans particularly in rural communities. Additionally, messages should be targeted at dispelling the myths and misconceptions about the IUD. Sexually active young individuals should also be educated at the junior high school level on IUDs for future decision making. FP providers also recommended the use of text messages to promote IUDs on social media as a medium for reaching out to young people most of whom appears to frequent social media in recent times.

The sole male provider interviewed in the study stressed that public education aimed at promoting IUD adoption should consider the social context within which services are provided to encourage positive community attitudes, especially in areas where there is strong resistance or opposition to contraceptive practices. This will involve working with key opinion leaders on values clarification and satisfied clients in these communities to share experiences with IUDs. A female provider working at one of Marie Stopes centre however lamented that measures put in place by the organization to increase awareness and knowledge of long acting FP methods was inadequate. This she further explained that the activities being implanted to increase awareness and knowledge of long acting FP methods are 'above the line marketing strategies' which do not necessarily translate into uptake of services since there are issues of behavioural change and modification that must equally be addressed to compliment the efforts being made in the area of education and awareness creation at the community level to ensure high uptake.

The need for effective counselling that focuses on the positive aspects of the IUD was recommended to encourage interest and uptake among women. According to an IUD provider she indicated that:

"for counselling to be effective, we need to tell them the benefits of IUD, it saves time, it saves your money, it makes you do your house chores. There's always peace at home, family are happy. Economic situation, because now the economy, when you insert IUD, is for long term. It doesn't prevent you from doing your normal duties. The time that you waste here to come and do the 3 months, sometimes you tend to forget. When you insert IUD, you are at peace. You get time to do your real job" (IUD provider).

On the contrary a provider indicated the relevance of informing clients about side effects and possible complications of IUDs as well. The provider stated that:

"some IUD providers don't tell the clients everything about the method they only tell them the benefits without informing them about the side effects and complications. So when the clients leave and have any bad effect they lose trust in the method and provider and rush back to have it remove. They won't remove it if well informed" (IUD provider)

Discussion

This study aimed to explore determinants of IUD use among women currently using the IUD, and women who had ever used the IUD; explore women's experiences with the IUD pertaining to perceptions, side effects; reasons for removal; health risks, and future intention to use the IUD. Also, another objective was to explore level of knowledge of IUD among all women using a modern family planning (FP) method.

Findings show that women's reactions and perceptions of the IUD was shaped by and associated with prior knowledge on the device, myths, fears and misinformation that they had heard about the IUD from their friends despite their full awareness of the importance of contraceptive use. Two-thirds of IUD users and few past IUD users were scared to consider the IUD as a FP method upon initially hearing of it. To a large extent, inadequate knowledge of the IUD, reinforced by general myths surrounding use of modern FP methods accounts for low uptake of the IUD. Some studies also show that misinformation, and lack of correct knowledge results in low uptake of LARC [22]. Women's perceptions and knowledge are therefore shaped by these myths which further discourage contraceptive use and lead to open and incessant negative expressions of contraception.

Women's negative perceptions about the IUD corroborate with providers responses. Providers stated that the fear of how IUD was inserted, misconceptions and fears about the IUD based on myths deterred women from accepting the IUD as a FP method. Yet, women who wanted to space, limit or stop childbearing had positive perceptions of the IUD. Similarly, women who preferred the IUD as FP method after being encouraged by providers held positive attitudes about it, in contrast to those who expressed side effects with it. Proper and effective counselling focusing on the benefits/ advantages of the IUD should be provided to women desiring to use a long acting reversible, and possibly, non-hormonal contraception to prevent pregnancies.

Lack of adequate knowledge may prevent IUD use; however, when women believe that FP providers are knowledgeable and can be trusted to maintain confidentiality, advice on method use, side effects and potential health risks. Women will be more receptive and convinced to take up the IUD as a first choice FP method.

FP providers therefore have a major role to play in encouraging positive attitudes towards using the IUD through counselling.

On the contrary, some findings from the study show that because some clients are ignorant about family planning methods, there are elements of provider biases during counselling which leads to some providers either advising clients to use IUD based on their personal experiences or preference for IUD. In some reported instances the providers 'forced' clients to have an IUD as a post abortion contraception. This observation defeats the purpose of family planning counselling as it does not encourage choice and medical eligibility for IUD. Unannounced continuous supportive supervision of family planning service providers in their facilities will provide a valuable opportunity to identify gaps and provider biases during family planning counselling for further provider refresher education and updates on family planning counselling and decision making.

Women's reasons for using the IUD varied slightly among current and ever users. Among current IUD users, preventing unwanted pregnancy emerged as the most important motivating factor, whilst the desire for a long acting FP was mentioned most often among ever IUD users. Although the ever IUD users would have loved to continue using the IUD, unbearable side effects of heavy menses and cramps lead to discontinuation. A further probe on this assertion shows that the type of IUD being referred to is the Cupper T 380^{A}. There were few reported instance were clients opted for LNG-IUS but was not available in the facility. Perhaps, the availability of LNG-IUS (hormonal IUD) in facilities would have been preferred over Copper-T 380A which might have increased IUD usage in the study area. This suggests that among ever IUD users, there is an unmet need for LNG-IUS (hormonal IUD) which calls for programming and contraceptive security. The observation that IUDs have shown no or minimal reported side effects is an opportunity to use such satisfied clients for public education on IUDs to ensure continuity and increasing patronage since clients will really choose an IUD due to their understanding on the duration and perceived benefits over other methods.

Two-thirds of women expressed desire for a long acting method of protection for convenience purposes, ease of use, and avoid contraception failure. Post abortion women currently using the IUD, including women who removed it to give birth expressed immense usefulness and satisfaction since using it. They considered it to be very effective in serving the purpose they desired without side effects. There is evidence demonstrating the efficacy, safety, and cost-effectiveness of the IUD in pregnancy prevention [23, 24]. Other determinants of IUD use include: to prevent abortions; preference for an 'obscure' FP method; non-hormonal benefits; provider influence and encouragement; health reasons; protection from contraceptive failure; freedom from emotional worries; ease of use in order to focus on work and school.

The side effects of using IUD were reported as heavy prolonged bleeding, vaginal discharges, infections, spotting or irregular bleeding, and abdominal cramps. These are consistent with empirical evidence that IUDS are associated with irregular bleeding in some women [25].

Participants reported that continuous experience of these side effects for more than four months led to removal of the IUD. Findings are supported by providers who also attributed women's removal of the IUD to mainly side effects. Women's continuous experiences of side effects served as a barrier to future intention to IUD use. Among these women, some wished that the IUD worked for them, but felt that the side effects were indications of negative reactions, and the bodily system's rejection of the IUD, as well as potential health risks with continued use.

Although none of the women suffering infections from using the IUD associated it with lack of personal hygiene, cross infection from partner infidelity, or poor insanitary lavatory conditions as common potential triggers of infections, there are other known causes of vaginal infections following IUD insertion among women which is important for providers to hint clients so that post IUD infections are not unnecessarily associated with these or the method. Similarly, understanding pre-exposure history of women regarding infections could enhance pre and post-method counselling.

Partners' disapproval of FP use also contributed to removal of the IUD. Although this revelation is not new in our context through anecdotal evidence, it should be useful and practical to informing providers to find ways to encourage and educate male partners' in contraception uptake. Few women who had ever used the IUD pointed out that, due to fear of negatively impacting their marriages decided to remove the IUD clandestinely. Some however noted that their partners were not informed about it, hence their decision to have it removed. In their view, the 'strings' heightened their dislike for the IUD, and to which their partners might notice.

Mixed views on perceptions of health risks associated with using the IUD were reported. Study participants thought having the IUD inserted might cause cancer, ectopic pregnancy, STIs, and uterine perforation. Although two-thirds of women thought otherwise, it is important that women are given appropriate and accurate information on all health complications that accompany each modern FP use. They should also be made to understand that individual differences, hormonal balance, and specific criteria pertain to the uptake of one modern FP method over the other.

The women in the study (a sample predisposed to knowing about FP by having visited a FP clinic before) knew of at least one modern method. This finding is consistent with previous findings in Ghana's Demographic and Health Surveys (2008, 2014) which report universal contraceptive knowledge among all women. At least, all women mentioned three contraception types with the injectables and implants most frequently mentioned, followed by pills, condoms, and IUD. Less than one-third of the women interviewed mentioned male and female sterilization, and diaphragm. One study respondent mentioned the IUS as her current contraceptive method. Nine (9) out of the total selected women were currently not using any contraception. Social and cultural norms governing fertility, in addition to fear of contraceptive side effects, myths, and health risks may hinder contraceptive use. Demand creation through mass education with FP providers needs to be intensified and promoted among women in reproductive ages. Interventions should also focus on couples counselling to increase positive attitudes towards contraception for both partners.

It is also important to mention that from non-IUD users' socio-demographic data, there is a high propensity for these women to increase their fertility since they are within active reproductive ages (20–35) but are not using any contraceptives due to unpleasant past experiences with IUD use. Although they all reported fears with using IUD again or any contraceptive, it is important that FP providers provide effective counselling for this group of women on other available and accessible alternatives of contraceptives to meet their FP needs.

Past IUD users who have switched from IUD to other FP methods are also highly susceptible to becoming pregnant should their contraceptive use become inconsistent/ irregular, or in the case of method failure. Only one woman out of the previous IUD users is currently using a LARC. Amongst the remaining, one-third is trying to become pregnant, while the rest are using a mix of short term and traditional methods due to the unavailability of preferred FP choice of implants (implanon NXT). In sum, the contraceptive history patterns of past IUD users are risky and raise concerns over unmet need for implants (implanon NXT) in the FP facilities.

Implications

Results from this study has several programmatic and policy implications for improving uptake of LARC, especially IUD for women in all reproductive ages. Programs should:

- Focus on using social media to debunk myths and misconceptions that people have about LARC, particularly, IUD. Use of social media should be sensitive about the mode of communication. It should be in a language that people can understand and relate to, whiles considering the social context and social exchange systems.
- Design interventions (for instance, community interventions) to promote uptake of LARC methods and enhance existing service provision channels to provide accurate information and services on IUD in order to make it accessible, and available to young women desirous of LARC. Community interventions should be sensitive to the social context and appropriate medium of communication.
- Sensitize all persons visiting MSI centres on FP methods and post-abortion contraception through distribution of brochures and FP documentaries on video tapes. Documentaries should be comprehensive, and focus on advantages of IUD use, safety, efficacy and side effects to increase and sustain positive attitudes.
- Ensure the provision of comprehensive sexuality education for young girls and boys at senior high schools to equip them with appropriate information on family planning, contraception, and birth control methods as means of regulating fertility, spacing and reducing births. The resent positive outcome of the advocacy drive on sexuality education in schools resulting in the inclusion of sexuality education in schools curriculum in Ghana is timely as this provides a good entry point for this policy implementation in schools for the desired results

A key policy implication is task sharing IUD insertion and removal with mid-level providers in Ghana to ensure greater provider availability in all health facilities to improve uptake. This is a fall out from table1 indicating few numbers of FP providers in the study facilities. The researchers believed there would have been higher provider numbers if an IUD task sharing policy is in place and being implemented.

Conclusion

A number of factors influence the use or discontinuation of IUD in Ghana. Provider capacity building for in-depth client counselling is required to make informed decisions at the facility level. Various targeted messages and use of satisfied clients are also needed to dispel IUD related myths and misconceptions at the community level. A future large scale study is also required to investigate if there are any seasonal, socio-economic and demographic variations in FP uptake within health facilities in Ghana. This when done will provide further information to informed national FP programme and policy decisions.

Abbreviations

ERC: Ethical review committee; FP: Family planning; GDHS: Ghana demographic and health survey; GHS: Ghana health service; IDI: In-depth interview; IUD: Intra uterine device; IUS: Intra uterine system; LARC: Long acting and reversible contraceptive; LNG: Levongesterol

Acknowledgments

The authors are grateful to all the facilities and respondents that participated in the study. Many thanks also to Marie Stopes International Ghana for the logistical support during data collection.

Authors' contributions

GFY conceptualized the study, provided guidance to the field work and the report. EAK supervised the field work, analyzed the data and drafted the initial report. Both authors have all approved the final submission.

Author details

[1]University of Education Winneba, Box 25, Winneba, Ghana. [2]Regional Institute for Population Studies, University of Ghana, Box LG 96, Accra, Ghana.

References

1. World Health Organization. Medical eligibility criteria for contraceptive use. 4th ed. Geneva: World Health Organization; 2009.
2. Trussell J, Lalla AM, Doan QV, Reyes E, Pinto L, Gricar J. Cost effectiveness of contraceptives in the United States. Contraception. 2009;79(1):5–14.
3. Chiou CF, Trussell J, Reyes E, et al. Economic analysis of contraceptives for women. Contraception. 2003;68:3–10.
4. Grimes D, Jones KP, Knutson CC, Wysocki S. Use of intrauterine contraception in the United States: Association of Reproductive Health Professionals. Washington, DC: Elsevier Inc.; 2004.
5. Yoost J. Understanding benefits and addressing misperceptions and barriers to intrauterine device access among populations in the United States. Patient Preference Adherence. 2014;8:947–57.
6. Sanfield A. Popularity disparity: attitudes about the IUD in Europe and the United States. Guttmacher Policy Rev. 2007;10:19–24.
7. Black K, Lotke P, Kai J, Buhling N, Zite B. A review of barriers and myths preventing the more widespread use of intrauterine contraception in nulliparous women. Eur J Contracept Reprod Health Care. 2012;17:340–50.
8. Stanwood NL, Garrett JM, Konrad TR. Obstetrician-gynecologists and the intrauterine device: a survey of attitudes and practice. Obstet Gynecol. 2002; 99:275–80.
9. Postlethwaite D, Trussell J, Zoolakis A, Shabear R, Petitti D. A comparison of contraceptive procurement pre- and post- benefit change. Contraception. 2007;76:360–5.
10. Goodman S, Hendlish SK, Benedict C, Reeves MF, Pera-Floyd M, Foster-Rosales A. Increasing intrauterine contraception use by reducing barriers to post-abortal and interval insertion. Contraception. 2008;78:136–42.
11. Middleton AJ, Naish J, Singer N. General practitioners' views on the use of the levonorgestrel-releasing intrauterine system in young, nulligravid women, in London, UK. Eur J Contracept Reprod Health Care. 2011;16:311–8.
12. Allen RH, Goldberg AB, Grimes DA. Expanding access to intrauterine contraception. Am J Obstet Gynecol. 2009;4(56):1–5.
13. Lyus R, Lohr P, Prager S. Board of the Society of family planning. Use of the Mirena LNG-IUS and Paragard CuT380A intrauterine devices in nulliparous women. Contraception. 2010;81:367–71.
14. Harper CC, Blum M, de Bocanegra HT, et al. Challenges in translating evidence to practice: the provision of intrauterine contraception. Obstet Gynecol. 2008;111:1359–69.
15. Hubacher D, Lara-Ricalde R, Taylor DJ, et al. Use of copper intrauterine devices and the risk of tubal infertility among nulligravid women. N Engl J Med. 2001;345:561–7.
16. Allen RH, Bartz D, Grimes DA, et al. Interventions for pain with intrauterine device insertion. Cochrane Database Syst Rev. 2009;3:CD007373.
17. Mishell D, Sulak P. The IUD: dispelling the myths and assessing the potential. Dialogues Contraception. 1997;5(2):1–4.
18. Ghana Statistical Service (GSS), Ghana Health Service (GHS), and ICF Macro. Ghana demographic and health survey 2014. Accra: GSS, GHS, and ICF Macro; 2014.
19. Ghana Statistical Service (GSS), Ghana Health Service (GHS), and ICF Macro. Ghana demographic and health survey (1993, 1998, 2003, 2008, 2014). Accra: GSS, GHS, and ICF Macro.
20. Schwandt HM, Creanga AA, Adanu RM, Danso KA, Agbenyega T, Hindin MJ. Pathways to unsafe abortion in Ghana: the role of male partners, women and health care providers. Contraception. 2013;88(4):509–17.
21. Speidel JJ, Harper CC, Shields WC. The potential of long-acting reversible contraception to decrease unintended pregnancy. Contraception. 2008;78: 197–200.
22. Wickstrom J, Jacobstein R. Contraceptive security: incomplete without long-acting and permanent methods of family planning. Stud Fam Plan. 2011;42: 291–8.
23. Weston MR, Martins SL, Neustadt AB, Gilliam ML. Factors influencing uptake of intrauterine devices among postpartum adolescents: a qualitative study. Am J Obstet Gynecol. 2012;206:40.e1–7.
24. Mohamed AM, Rachael SK, Cleland JN, Thoai D, Shah IH. Long-term contraceptive protection, discontinuation and switching behaviour: intrauterine device (IUD) use dynamics in 14 developing countries. London: World Health Organization and Marie Stopes International; 2011.
25. Hatcher R, Trussell J, Nelson A, Cates W, Stewart F. Contraception technology. 19th ed. New York: Ardent Media; 2008.

Abortion attitudes, training and experience among medical students in Jamaica, West Indies

Glenmarie Matthews[1*], Jessica Atrio[1], Horace Fletcher[2], Nathalie Medley[2], Leo Walker[2] and Nerys Benfield[1]

Abstract

Objective: To define abortion attitudes, training and experience among medical students in Jamaica, a restricted environment for legal abortion.

Method: From September to November 2017 we conducted an anonymous online cross-sectional survey among medical students enrolled at the University of West Indies (UWI) in Jamaica. An abortion attitudes sum score was used for analysis. Multivariate regression was applied to evaluate the impact of characteristics and experiences on abortion attitudes.

Results: The primary outcome was a validated composite abortion attitudes sum score, ranging from zero to forty-five. 1404 students completed the survey for a response rate of 88%. 64% had a positive attitude towards abortion. In multivariate analysis, medical students' attitudes were favorably impacted by a prior personal or family experience with abortion, identifying as non-religious, being older in age and mixed raced. 1321 (94%) agreed that abortion training should be included in the medical school curriculum. 78.8% reported no abortion training and only 17.9% reported miscarriage management training.

Conclusion: Medical students at UWI had favorable attitudes towards abortion, despite their limited training in a restrictive environment. Prior personal experience with abortion and being non-religious were the strongest predictor of favorable attitudes. Increased training and clinical exposure may prove to be crucial in improving access of safe abortion.

Keywords: Abortion, Abortion attitude sum score (AbAs), Medical students, Abortion training, And Jamaica abortion

Background

Unsafe abortion contributes to maternal mortality in the Caribbean and Latin America. These regions also have the highest estimated annual abortion rates in the world, at 65 per 1000 women of childbearing age in 2014 [1]. In Jamaica, abortion is legally restricted and unsafe abortion is prevalent. According to the World Health Organization more than 22,000 abortions occurred in Jamaica in 2011 and complications ranked as the eighth leading cause of maternal mortality in country [2].

The abortion law in Jamaica originates from the "Offences against the Person Act of 1861" modified by the decision in the Rex v. Bourne case of 1938 to permit abortion for health reasons [3, 4]. Current interpretation of the law cites that abortion is indicated to preserve the physical and mental health of the mother; but does not include rape or incest, fetal impairment, economic or social indications, or contraceptive failure [2]. In order to obtain a legal abortion two physicians must agree that

* Correspondence: glenmariem@hotmail.com
[1]Department of Obstetrics and Gynecology, Montefiore Hospital & Albert Einstein College of Medicine, 1695 Eastchester Road, Bronx 10461, NY, USA

the abortion is necessary. In the face of these restrictions, illegal or unsafe abortions are prevalent [5]. Previous research has demonstrated the majority of practicing Jamaican physicians (72%) felt that they did not have adequate training in abortion care [6]. However, the majority of Jamaican general practitioners (GPs) and obstetrician-gynecologists (obgyns) report there should be greater availability of induced abortions, which would reduce maternal mortality.

In settings where abortion is legally protected research among medical students has demonstrated favorable attitudes, which may in turn correlate with intentions to provide abortion care and advocate for women. A study of students at the University of Washington found that 70% supported legal abortion under any circumstances. Thirty-one percent intended to provide medical abortion in their practice, and 18% planned to offer surgical abortion [7]. A study in South Africa found that 70% of students believed women should have access to abortion [8]. Additionally, studies have found that abortion education, training, and care can influence student's attitudes towards abortion [9–11].

There is no published data regarding the attitudes of Caribbean medical students towards abortion. Our research sought to assess attitudes, training, exposure, intentions to provide, and legal knowledge regarding abortion access and care among University of the West Indies (UWI) medical students in Kingston, Jamaica. UWI is the largest medical school in the Caribbean, with approximately 315 students enrolled annually, the majority of graduates practice in the Caribbean. The medical school consists of five years of training, the first three years are basic science course-work, and the last two years are clinical clerkships. Approximately 60% of graduates go on to complete one year of postgraduate internship before becoming general practitioners [12].

Methods

From September to November 2017, we conducted an anonymous online cross-sectional survey of medical students enrolled at UWI. The UWI Institutional Review Board (IRB) and Einstein IRB approved the research. The UWI registrar's office distributed electronic survey invitations and electronic consent was obtained. Research Electronic Database Capture (REDCap) was used to administer questions and compile data in an online portal. Duplicated questionaries' where identified and deleted. As a descriptive survey, no power calculations were conducted and a sample of convenience was utilized.

The survey consisted of six domains: social and demographic characteristics, knowledge of the country's abortion law, attitudes and beliefs about abortion provision, medical curriculum and training in abortion services, future abortion advocacy, and intention to provide abortion. The survey included questions from previously validated surveys, which have been described in the literature as well as new questions developed by the investigators [9]. The instrument was piloted among UWI faculty, and obgyn residents. In order to assess attitudes about abortion students were given a total of nine questions evaluating various reasons why a woman might seek and abortion. Student's attitudes were scored from 1 to 5, for each scenario (eg. 1 = strongly disagree; 5 = strongly agree) [9]. An abortion attitudes sum score (AbAS) was calculated by totaling the responses, ranges of possible SS were 1 to 45. A favorable attitude towards abortion, was defined as an abortion attitudes sum score (AbAS) > or equal to 27.

Descriptive statistics and bivariate analyses were conducted using chi-square and t-tests or ANOVA, or their non-parametric equivalents. For analysis, clinical years of training were dichotomized into preclinical (years 1–3) vs. clinical (years 4–5), and intended specialty was divided into three categories - those who planned on being women health providers (obgyns and GPs), other specialties, and undecided. A multivariate linear regression model was developed in a stepwise fashion to identify associations between AbAS and individual characteristics. Any bivariate associations with the strength of association of at least $p = 0.2$ were assessed for inclusion in the multivariate model. Once an inclusive model was created, all contributing co-variates were assessed in a sequential fashion, if a variable no longer contributed equal to or greater than $p < 0.05$ it was removed. Once the model was finalized, assumptions of the multivariate linear regression model were evaluated and influential data (outliers) were removed.

Results

Of the 1589 enrolled UWI medical students 1404 completed the survey for a response rate of 88%. The mean age was 22 and the majority identified as being single (61.9%), with only 4.3% being married. 597 (43%) identified as female, and 21% chose not to identify their gender (Table 1). Majority of the students were of African/Afro-Caribbean descent (44%) with second most common race being mixed (18.7%). 54.7% of participants identifying as very religious. The most common religion was Christianity (72%) and 75% of students reported regular attendance at religious services. 71% of students reported personal exposure or knowing someone who have had an abortion. Majority of students intended to practice medicine in Jamaica (53.7%) or surrounding Caribbean nation (41.9%).

The mean AbAS was 32, and the majority of participants believed abortion should be legal (88%). 74% agreed that abortion should be legal for rape or incest,

Table 1 Summary of Characteristics of Medical Students at University of West Indies ($n = 1404$)

Characteristics	N(%)
Age – mean (SD)	22.68 (2.87)
Gender	
Female	597 (42.52)
Male	509 (36.25)
Choose not to identify	298 (21.23)
Race	
Black/Afro Caribbean	621 (44.23)
Mixed	262 (18.66)
Other [a]	521 (37.11)
Martial status	
Single	858 (61.99)
Married	59 (4.26)
Partnered	467 (33.74)
Years of training	
Preclinical	892 (63.53)
Clinical	512 (36.47)
Intended Specialty	
Women health provider	345 (24.57)
Other specialties	793 (56.48)
Unsure	266 (18.95)
Intended place of practice	
Jamaica	755 (53.77)
Caribbean nation	589 (41.95)
Other [b]	60 (4.27)
Have you had or someone close to you had an abortion?	
Yes	998 (71.13)
No	405 (28.87)
Religion	
Christianity	1008 (72.31)
Other religions[c]	386 (27.69)
How often do you attend religious services?	
Never	344 (24.50)
≥ 1-2x a month	1060 (75.5)

[a] Other races included - East Indian (91), Hispanic (3), Asian (83), choose not to identify (303)
[b] Other intended place of practice – North America (52), Europe & United Kingdom (9)
[c] Other religion - Hindu, Buddhist, Islam, Atheist, undecided

Table 2 University of the West Indies Medical Student Attitudes Towards Abortion

	$N = 1404$	Agree N(%)	Disagree N(%)
Average Attitude Sum score (AbAS)[a]	31.59 ((±9.50)		
Would provide abortion in case of:			
Financial distress		677 (48.22)	727 (51.78)
Disruption of career or education goals		658 (46.90)	745 (53.10)
Family is complete		555 (39.56)	848 (60.44)
Rape/Incest		1039 (74)	365 (26)
Threat to maternal physical health		1326 (94.51)	77 (5.49)
Threat to maternal mental Health		1275 (91.01)	126 (8.99)
Preference for the different gender or fetal sex		456 (32.52)	946 (67.48)
Fetal anomalies		1274 (90.81)	129 (9.19)
Infection with Zika virus		1272 (90.66)	131 (9.34)

[a] abortion attitude sum score (AbAS) ranges from 1 to 45, with ≥27 representing favorable attitude

94% if pregnancy was a threat to a women's physical health, 91% if it was a threat to a women's mental health, 91% for fetal anomalies and 91% for a woman recently infected with zika virus (Table 2).

The majority of participants reported limited training or exposure to abortion care. 78.8% stated that abortion care has never been included in any portion of medical school, with only 13.6% participating in the care of a woman who has had an abortion. Among the 297 (22%) of students who reported some abortion training, lecture was the primary means of education (96.9%) (Table 3). For the limited students who participated in direct patient care, it typically consisted of the medical abortion (85.3%). Majority of the students denied any exposure to or involvement in the care of a patient with an illegal abortion 1326 (94.7%).

Knowledge of the abortion law in Jamaica was limited. Approximately 65% of participants were unable to accurately identify one of the reasons a woman could legally access a therapeutic abortion in Jamaica, which includes threat to mental or physical health of a women. Students in their clinical years were more likely to identify any of these indications (64.8%) compared to students in the preclinical years (40.9%) $p < 0.001$ (Table 4).

81% of students were willing to refer patients to other clinics and providers if a woman requested an abortion (Table 5). However, only 398 (28%) of medical students intended to incorporate medical or surgical abortion into their future practice. The most common reason for not intending to provide abortion was to not oppose the law (36.7%), and 659 (46%) of all medical students reported being willing to provide abortion if the legal restrictions were lifted. 345 (24.6%) of participants reported that they plan to practice as an obgyn or GP. Approximately

Table 3 Training on abortion among University of the West Indies Medical Students

	N(%)
Has abortion care been included in any portion of your medical school?	
Not at all	1106 (78.83)
Somewhat	160 (11.40)
Sufficiently	137 (9.47)
Have you participated in abortion care during your training?	
Yes	192 (13.68)
No	1211 (86.32)
What experiences with abortion care have you had throughout your medical training [a]	
Counseling on abortion	137 (71.73)
Medical abortion	163 (85.34)
Uterine aspiration	43 (22.51)
Management of complications	110 (57.59)
How many times have you participated in the care of a woman with a miscarriage	
Never	1148 (81.82)
> 1–5 times	255 (18.18)
How many times have you participated in the care of a woman who had a legal abortion	
Never	1329 (94.73)
> 1–5 times	74 (5.27)
How many times have you participated in the care of a woman who had an illegal abortion?	
Never	1326 (94.65)
> 1–5 times	75 (5.35)

*chi-square or fisher exact test
[a] of the 13.6% of student that participated in abortion training

Table 4 Knowledge about Abortion among University of the West Indies Medical Students

	N(%)	Preclinical years	Clinical years	P
In Jamaica abortion in is?				< 0.001
Always penalized	457 (32.57)	351 (39.39)	106 (20.70)	
Legal for the mental or physical health of the woman[a]	381 (27.16)	168 (18.86)	213 (41.60)	
Legal if the pregnancy is the result of a rape	92 (6.56)	54 (6.06)	38 (7.422	
Legal for fetal anomalies	112 (7.98)	60 (6.73)	52 (10.16)	
Legal when the mother has a disease that can worsen with pregnancy [a]	180 (12.83)	93 (10.44)	87 (16.99)	
Legal under certain circumstances [a]	406 (28.94)	232 (26.04)	174 (33.98)	
Legal in all cases	3 (0.21)	2 (0.22)	1 (0.20)	
I do not know	248 (17.68)	175 (19.64)	73 (14.26)	

[a] Indicates the reasons for which a woman can obtain a legal abortion in Jamaica

half of these future women's health providers intend to provide medical or surgical abortion care 159 (46%). 178 (52%) of future women's health providers reported they would be willing to provide abortion care if the legal restrictions were changed.

The majority of respondents ($N = 1113$, 80%) agree that they would be willing to advocate for women's health. However less than half of respondents (41%) stated they would be willing to advocate for abortion access and care in Jamaica. Slightly more students who intend to be women health providers are willing to advocate for change to the law to expand access to abortion care: 33% compared to 26% of persons pursuing other health specialties, $p < 0.001$.

The development of the model with sequential stepwise analysis of the cohort resulted in a more parsimonious model, which included a total of 13 characteristics. In the multivariate regression model co-variates that favorably impacted abortion attitudes sum score, included identifying as mixed raced, older age, not religious or reporting a personal or family history experience with abortion (Table 6). Covariates correlated with a lower score, and a more negative abortion attitude, included participants who identified as Afro-Caribbean, single, inaccurate knowledge of the abortion law, lack of abortion training, refusing to refer a patient for abortion care and a belief that abortion should not be legal.

Discussion

The majority of UWI medical students report favorable attitudes towards abortion in the setting of nationally restricted abortion access, and majority stated that abortion should be legal in Jamaica. These attitudes are comparable to those reported by medical students in the United States, where abortion is federally protected [13]. Internationally, favorable attitudes toward abortion have been noted among medical trainees at comparable levels in South Africa (70%), where abortion laws have changed in the last 22 years to be legally permissible for all indications up to 12 weeks [8]. Furthermore, acceptance and attitudes of students are comparable to the attitudes reported by Jamaican general practitioners surveyed in 2008 [6, 8, 14].

Comparable to previous research among general practitioners, current students report limited or absent exposure to or training in abortion care [6]. If students reported any training is was predominately in lecture format. This may not be the optimal format to engage in abortion education; pervious research among trainees and practitioners demonstrated that they would prefer, and stand to gain more impactful knowledge from,

Table 5 Intention to provide abortion by intended specialty among University of the West Indies Medical Students

	N (%)	Woman's health provider[a]	Other specialties	Unsure	P
Intention to provide medical or surgical abortion care					< 0.001
Yes	398 (20.35)	159 (46.09)	151 (19.04)	88 (33.08)	
No	740 (52.71)	132 (38.26)	474 (59.77)	134 (50.38)	
I don't know	266 (18.95)	54 (15.65)	168 (21.19)	44 (16.54)	
Would you be willing to refer patient for abortion services					0.004
Yes	1134 (81)	257 (74.49)	663 (83.92)	214 (80.75)	
No	162 (11.57)	57 (16.52)	77 (9.57)	28 (10.57)	
I don't know	104 (7.43)	31 (8.99)	50 (6.33)	23 (8.68)	
Would you be willing to provide abortion if the legal restrictions were lifted					0.078
Yes	659 (47.04)	178 (51.59)	352 (44.50)	129 (48.68)	
No	469 (33.48)	114 (33.04)	276 (34.89)	79 (29.81)	
I don't know	273 (19.49)	53 (15.36)	163 (20.61)	57 (21.51)	

[a]Women health providers include obgyn & family medicine

clinically applied and patient focused abortion care and management of complications through applied experiences [15].

The minority of students reported accurate knowledge of the legal status of abortion in Jamaica. Additionally, a third of participants though abortion was effectively illegal under any circumstances (including a threat to a mother's life) and subject to persecution in Jamaica, with the concomitant concern that physician are penalized and incarcerated for participating in abortion care (32.5%). Consistent with these perceptions the majority of respondents stated that they would not be willing to

Table 6 Multivariate Logistic Regression Model Regarding Abortion Attitude Sum Score and Associated Characteristics among University of the West Indies Medical Students

Dependent Variable	Independent variables with favorable impact	β coefficient (95% CI)	*P* value
Attitude			
	History of personal or family exposure to abortion	2.63 (1.92 to 3.34)	< 0.001
	I am not religious	2.74 (2.09 to 3.38)	< 0.001
	Race (Mixed)	2.58 (1.69 to 3.47)	< 0.001
	Would be willing to provide abortion if law was lifted	0.99 (0.34 to 1.66)	0.003
	Intend to become women health provider[$]	0.86 (0.12 to 1.60)	0.022
Dependent Variable	**Independent variables with negative impact**	**β coefficient (95% CI)**	***P* value**
Attitude	Abortion should not be legal in Jamaica	−15.65(−16.93 to −14.37)	< 0.001
	Inaccurate knowledge of abortion law	−5.60(−6.30 to −4.89)	< 0.001
	Afro-Caribbean Race	− 4.27(− 5.11 to −3.45)	< 0.001
	Not willing to refer patient for abortion	−3.85(− 4.95 to −2.74)	< 0.001
	No training in abortion	− 2.78(− 3.67 to − 1.89)	< 0.001
	Martial status (single)	−1.47(− 2.17 to - 0.77)	< 0.001
	Female gender	- 0.40(− 1.02 to 0.23)	0.22
	Older age (years)	−0.25(−0.39 to −0.13)	< 0.001

[a]Women health provider = General Practitioner and obstetric& gynecology

provide abortions for fear of violating the law. The law serves as a tremendous deterrent to provision, and effectively is a means to re-stigmatize reproductive health care, by causing reproductive health providers to make practice decisions and medical decisions based on a potentially flawed and imperfect understanding of the law. Erroneous knowledge of legal restrictions, with concern for possible incarceration could be a real contributor to inadequate access to abortion care, inadequate management of complications, or lack of referral to abortion care in a country that experiences tremendous maternal morbidity from unsafe abortion.

Opportunities for improved educational experiences or values clarification workshops on abortion and abortion training could impact student's readiness and willingness to engage in abortion related care. Furthermore education regarding the current legal indications for abortion may demystify, destigmitize, and decriminalize the scope of practice and engage students with evidence based, lifesaving, translatable skills related to abortion care as well as the medical management of septic abortion or miscarriage. Furthmore, students report that Jamaican women should have access to abortion through revision and changes in the laws. The majority of respondents have personal experience with abortion and the majority consider themselves to be women's health advocates which also harnesses the potential for this community to implement effective women's health policies and evidence-based care practices for the women of the Caribbean.

Religion is a potentially fixed and non-modifiable identity characteristic associated with medical professional abortion-related attitudes [8]. Previous research have suggested that health care providers recognize the distinction between personal and professional attitudes toward abortion, and believe that a personal religious objection does not impact on the provision of legal services to women, including nondirective counseling, referrals, and surgical and medication abortion [16, 17]. By contrast our research suggest that personal values impact attitudes and potentially practice because non- religious students (45.5%) had more favorable attitudes towards abortion ($p < 0.001$). Other research has demonstrated that personal experience and exposure to abortion impacts beliefs & perceptions, whereby "a broader understanding of the vagaries of existence that make abortions at times unavoidable" can impact attitudes toward abortion [8]. Our data demonstrate that personal experience with and or a family exposure to abortion were the most powerful and significant contributors to a favorable AbAS.

Strength

The strength of our research was the robust response rate, which in turn improved the fitness of our analysis and model development. We are confident that our results accurately represent the UWI medical student community, which comprise a diverse and international student body. We consider our findings to be representative of the attitudes of future Jamaican physicians and the surrounding West Indian Islands. We achieved a high level of response through the engagement of faculty and students, integration of the registrar and a collaborative stakeholder approach. Recruitment of medical students was done directly through course lectures, and other peer student's recruitment. An additional strength is the instrument itself, which was designed carefully, piloted extensively, and tested for internal reliability and consistency.

Limitation

As a survey this instrument was subjected to limitations related to self-reporting and recall bias. Researchers did not have the opportunity to longitudinally assess participants over time to see if these intentions and attitudes are reflective of practice patterns and abortion provision. Additionally, social desirability bias may have influenced people to identify more favourable intentions regarding reproductive rights. However, the confidential and de-identified nature of the survey was intended to minimize these concerns.

Conclusion

Medical students had favorable attitudes towards abortion. However, training in and exposure to abortion are extremely limited. Having prior personal experience with abortion was the most impactful predictor of favorable attitudes. Modifiable characteristics like training during medical school and an awareness of the current legal indications for abortion are opportunities to improve medical students awareness and attitudes regarding the public health impact abortion has on the women of Jamaica. These modifiable changes can combat unsafe abortion maternal mortality.

Abbreviations

AbAs: Abortion attitude sum score; GPs: General practitioners; obgyns: Obstetrician-gynecologists; UWI: University of the West Indies; IRB: UWI Institutional Review Board; REDCap: Research Electronic Database Capture

Acknowledgments

This research was funded by society of family planning. Funding for the use of REDCap was provided through the National Center for Research Resources, National Center for Advancing Translational Sciences through REDCap Grant 8UL1TR00086. Thanks to the UWI medical school and the students for participating in this study.

Authors' contributions

Glenmarie Matthews- primary investigator, main author of manuscript, design, conducts, data analysis. Jessica Atrio- design and manuscript. Horace

Fletcher – local aid in conducting study. Nathalie Medley – local aid in conducting study. Leo Walker – local aid in conducting study. Nerys Benfield- aid in design and analysis. All authors read and approved the final manuscript.

Author details

[1]Department of Obstetrics and Gynecology, Montefiore Hospital & Albert Einstein College of Medicine, 1695 Eastchester Road, Bronx 10461, NY, USA. [2]University of West Indies – Mona Campus, Kingston, West Indies, Jamaica.

References

1. Sedgh G, Bearak J, Singh S, et al. Abortion incidence between 1990 and 2014: global, regional, and subregional levels and trends. Lancet. 2016; 388(10041):258–67.
2. Singh S et al. Abortion Worldwide 2017: Uneven Progress and Unequal Access, New York: Guttmacher Institute; 2018. https://www.guttmacher.org/sites/default/files/462-369.png. Accessed 22 Jan 2020.
3. Aziza Ahmed CN, Maggie Schmeitz, Marsha Massiah. Maternal mortality, abortion,and health sector reform in four caribbean countries: Barbados,Jamaica,Suriname, and Trinidad and Tobago. Dawn Caribbean Aspire; 2005:82–84. (book).
4. Jamaica, Government of 1953, "Offenses Against the Person Act 1861, Article 65-66." In the law of Jamaica, volume 6. (revised edition). Kingston: Government Printer.
5. Boersma AA, de Bruijn JG. Contraception and induced abortion in the West Indies: a review. West Indian Med J. 2011;60(5):564–70.
6. Clark S, Blum J, Blanchard K, Galvao L, Fletcher H, Winikoff B. Misoprostol use in obstetrics and gynecology in Brazil, Jamaica, and the United States. Int J Gynaecol Obstet. 2002;76(1):65–74.
7. Fletcher H, Gordon-Strachan G, McFarlane S, Hamilton P, Frederick J. A survey of providers' knowledge, opinions, and practices regarding induced abortion in Jamaica. Int J Gynaecol Obstet. 2011;113(3):183–6.
8. Shotorbani S, Zimmerman FJ, Bell JF, Ward D, Assefi N. Attitudes and intentions of future health care providers toward abortion provision. Perspect Sex Reprod Health. 2004;36(2):58–63.
9. Wheeler SB, Zullig LL, Reeve BB, Buga GA, Morroni C. Attitudes and intentions regarding abortion provision among medical school students in South Africa. Int Perspect Sex Reprod Health. 2012;38(3):154–63.
10. Pace L, Sandahl Y, Backus L, Silveira M, Steinauer J. Medical students for Choice's reproductive health externships: impact on medical students' knowledge, attitudes and intention to provide abortions. Contraception. 2008;78(1):31–5.
11. Espey E, Ogburn T, Dorman F. Student attitudes about a clinical experience in abortion care during the obstetrics and gynecology clerkship. Acad Med. 2004;79(1):96–100.
12. Brock EN, Hardy-Fairbanks AJ, Stockdale CM. The effect of clinical clerkships on medical Students' attitudes toward abortion and contraception [181]. Obstet Gynecol. 2015;125.
13. Vaughan K, Samms-Vaughan M. The anatomy and physiology of the medical class of 1982a. West Indian Med J. 2008;57:621–6.
14. Rosenheck RE, Feigal C, Brown N, Barcellos T, Bender N. Attitudes on abortion. a cross-sectional analysis of medical students in their preclinical years [3F]. Obstet Gynecol. 2016;127.
15. Espey E, Ogburn T, Leeman L, Nguyen T, Gill G. Abortion education in the medical curriculum: a survey of student attitudes. Contraception. 2008;77(3): 205–8.
16. Emmons S, Sells CW, Eiff MP. A review of medical and allied health learners' satisfaction with their training in women's health. Am J Obstet Gynecol. 2002;186(6):1259–65 discussion 1265-1257.
17. Schwarz EB, Luetkemeyer A, Foster DG, Weitz TA, Lindes D, Stewart FH. Willing and able? Provision of medication for abortion by future internists. Women's Health Issues. 2005;15(1):39–44.

Prevalence of unintended pregnancy and associated factors among pregnant mothers in Jimma town, southwest Ethiopia

Girma Alemayehu Beyene

Abstract

Background: Unintended pregnancy is a pregnancy that occurred when no children were desired or earlier than desired. One in three births in Ethiopia were unintended, which is major contributor to maternal morbidity and mortality. The objective of this study was to assess prevalence of unintended pregnancy and associated factors among pregnant women in Jimma.

Methods: Community based cross-sectional study was conducted from May to June, 2016. Estimated sample size of 356 was allocated proportionally to the randomly selected kebeles based on number of pregnant women in their kebeles and simple random sampling technique was used in selecting participants. Data were collected by structured questionnaires with face to face interview, analyzed by SPSS and multivariate logistic regression was fitted to identify factors independently associated with unintended pregnancy.

Results: The prevalence of unintended pregnancy among the study participants was 36.5% (95% CI: 31–42%), of which 97 (27.2%) were unwanted and 33 (9.3%) were mistimed. The most common reasons for failure to avoid unintended pregnancy were because they believed they were not fertile 54 (41.5%) and 26 (20%) became pregnant despite the use of contraceptive methods. Age of the mother over 35 years, lower educational status of the partner, higher family size, smaller number of children desired and less knowledge of modern contraceptive methods were independent predictors of unintended pregnancy.

Conclusion: The prevalence of unintended pregnancy was high in the study area and programs aimed at reducing unintended pregnancy should target older couple. In addition, improving educational status of the partner and knowledge of modern contraceptive methods is demanded.

Keywords: Unintended, Mistimed, Unwanted, Unplanned, Pregnancy

Background

Unintended pregnancy is a pregnancy that is either unwanted or mistimed. Unwanted pregnancy is pregnancy that occurred when no children were desired and mistimed pregnancy is the one that occurred earlier than desired [1]. In spite of availability and widespread information how to use modern contraceptive methods, unintended pregnancy is one of the most common reproductive health problems faced by women of child bearing age.

Globally, there were an estimated 99.1 million unintended pregnancies per year, of which 21.6 million were in Africa and Eastern Africa alone encompasses 8.85 million. Worldwide, an estimated 44% of pregnancies and 23% of births were unintended and 56% of all unintended pregnancies ended in abortion. Likewise, 39% of all pregnancies in Africa and 46% of pregnancies in Eastern Africa were unintended. Similarly, 27% of births in Africa and 37% of births in Eastern Africa were unintended [2].

Despite decline of total fertility rate to 4.6 children per woman in 2016, there is high prevalence of unintended

Correspondence: gaglovely@gmail.com
Department of Public Health, College of Health Science and Medicine, Wolkite University, Wolkite, Ethiopia

childbirth in Ethiopia. Nearly one in three (32%) of births in Ethiopia were unintended; and about two-thirds of them were mistimed [3, 4]. Prevalence of unintended pregnancy among pregnant women in Oromia region ranges from 37.3% in Bale zone to 27.1% in Gelemso Hospital [5–8]. More than third of pregnant mothers in Southern Ethiopia reported that their most recent pregnancy was unintended [9–11].

Unintended pregnancy mainly results from not using contraception, or inconsistent or incorrect use of effective contraceptive methods [1]. Younger age at marriage, lower educational and occupational status of the mother, history of previous unintended pregnancy, low awareness and use of contraceptive methods, husband refusal to use family planning, less number of children desired, low awareness of the concept of unintended pregnancy is preventable, high parity were factors significantly associated with unintended pregnancy [7, 10, 12, 13].

Couples ability to have the number of children they want when they want them is central to the quality of their lives and has vital significance for the future of the family and the world. Planning the number and timing of pregnancy may give the time to be ready physically, economically and mentally for healthy pregnancy and childbirth, recover easily after giving birth. Women with unintended pregnancies are less likely to seek prenatal care during the first trimester, more likely to use substances like alcohol and tobacco during pregnancy, have low birth-weight infants or abortion. In countries where abortion is illegal and unsafe, unintended pregnancy is a major contributor to maternal morbidity and mortality [14–16].

Limited studies have described the magnitude of unintended pregnancy and associated factors among pregnant mothers; even those few studies were conducted in health facilities among mothers attending antenatal or post-natal care which by itself affected by intentional status of pregnancy. Hence, this study tried to fill the aforementioned gap by conducting the study in community setting. Therefore, the aim of this study was to determine the prevalence of unintended pregnancy and associated factors among pregnant mothers residing in Jimma town, southwest Ethiopia. The finding of this study aims to guide health professionals, reproductive health program planners and policy makers as well as other concerned bodies to understand tackle unintended pregnancy targeting factors having significant association and reduce the risk of maternal and infant morbidity and mortality.

Methods

Study area and period

The study was conducted in Jimma town of Oromia regional state which is located at 346 km to South West of the national capital, Addis Ababa. According to the data obtained from Jimma town vital statistics office the total population of the town is 189,733 of which 96,764 are females and the rest are males. The town consists 19 kebeles (administrative units in Ethiopia) of which 13 are urban and 6 of them are rural kebeles. There are two hospitals, four health centers, 34 drug store, 113 clinics including private and non-governmental organizations and 15 health posts in the town. The study was conducted from May to June, 2016.

Study design and population

Community based cross sectional study was conducted among pregnant women in Jimma town.

Sample size

The sample size for the study was calculated using Epi Info™ version 7 StatCalc function of Sample Size calculation for population survey at 95% confidence interval (CI), 5% marginal of error, considering 36.5% of pregnant women reported unintended pregnancy from related study in Ganji woreda of west Wollega zone [7] which gave the largest sample size and adding 10% non-response rate, a total of 356 study participants were estimated for this study.

Sampling technique

Six kebeles were selected randomly by lottery method. Total sample size was allocated proportionally to the selected kebeles based on number of pregnant women in their kebeles. Households with pregnant women were listed out from family folder of health extension workers (HEW) and the study participants were selected using simple random sampling technique specifically Excel generated random numbers.

Data collection techniques and procedures

Data relevant for the study was collected by using structured questionnaires adapted from related studies and incorporating additional potential variables with face to face interview of the respondents by three trained health extension workers. The questionnaire was developed in English and translated in to local language Afaan Oromo to facilitate communication. Pregnancy intention were measured using the standard approach, which probes women to recall their feelings at the time they became pregnant [1].

Data quality assurance

The quality of data collection was monitored by giving clear instruction to data collectors how to approach respondents and fill the questionnaire. Close supervision by Degree holder was made and filled formats and questionnaires were checked on daily basis for completeness and consistency. At the end of each day of data collection the completed questionnaire paper were checked for its consistency.

Data processing and analysis

The collected data were cleaned, coded and entered into Epi Info™ 7 statistical software package and exported to SPSS version 22 for statistical analysis. Frequency distribution for selected variables was performed. Bivariate logistic regression analyses were conducted to nominate candidate variables for multivariable analysis and those with $p \leq 0.25$ were included into the initial multiple logistic regression models, using backward fitting. Variables persisted to be associated with the outcome at $p \leq 0.05$ were used and displayed in the final model. Adjusted Odds ratio (AOR) with its 95% CI was considered to judge for precision and decide whether independent association between outcome and independent variables exist. Finally, the results of the study were presented using texts, tables and figures based on nature of the data obtained.

Operational definitions

Unintended pregnancy: pregnancy that occurred when no children were desired or that occurred earlier than desired [1].

Unwanted pregnancy: pregnancy that has occurred to the women who not wants to become pregnant neither at the time of conception nor in the future [16].

Mistimed pregnancy: pregnancy that occurred when a woman has a desire to be pregnant and have a child or children sometime in the future, but not now [7].

Knowledge of contraceptive methods: Ten knowledge questions about modern contraceptive methods were used and those who answered eight or more questions were categorized as more knowledgeable & those who answered less than eight were grouped as less knowledgeable [12].

Partner: A person with whom the woman had intimate sexual relationship and became pregnant with the index pregnancy.

Results

Sociodemographic characteristics

A total of 356 pregnant women responded to the questionnaire which makes the response rate of 100%. Most of the study participants, 167 (46.9%) of them were in age group of 26–35 years followed by those aged 36 years and more 108 (30.3%). The mean (Standard deviation (SD)) age of the study subjects was 30.89 (± 6.55) years. More than three fourth, 277 (77.8%) of the respondents were married and more than three fifth, 220 (61.8%) of them were followers of orthodox religion. Regarding educational status, 109 (30.6%) of the study participants attained primary education and 92 (25.8%) of them completed secondary education. More than half, 186 (52.2%) of the respondents were housewives. Concerning educational status and occupation of the partner 104 (29.2%) of them attained secondary education and 134 (37.6%) of them were self-employed (Table 1).

Reproductive history

The mean (SD) age the study subjects married was 25.03 (± 12.24) years. More than third, 127 (35.7%) of the participants were married at age of 20 or less. More than three fifth, 219 (61.5%) of mothers desired to have 4–6 number of children and only quarter 91 (25.6%) of them desired having more than six children. Among the study participants 127 (35.7%) of them had previously experienced unintended pregnancy and 91 (25.6%) of them had history of abortion (Table 2).

Prevalence of unintended pregnancy

Among the pregnant mothers included in the study 97 (27.2%) of them conceived when no more child was desired (unwanted pregnancy) and 33 (9.3%) of them became pregnant earlier than they desired to be (mistimed pregnancy). This makes the prevalence of unintended pregnancy among the study participants to be 36.5% (95% CI: 31–42%). The remaining were conceived either at the right time or later than desired, hence the pregnancy was intended (Table 3 & Fig. 1).

Perceived reasons for unintended pregnancy

Among those who reported to have unintended pregnancy, the most common reason incriminated for failure to avoid unintended pregnancy were because they believed that they were not fertile 54 (41.5%) and one in five 26 (20%) of the mothers with unintended pregnancy became pregnant despite the use of contraceptive method due to contraceptive method failure. Twenty-three (17.7%) of mothers with unintended pregnancy became pregnant with-out their will because their husband prefers to have more children (Fig. 2).

Factors associated with unintended pregnancy

From bivariate analysis age and educational status of the mother, educational status of the partner, family size, number of pregnancies, desired number of children, previous unintended pregnancy, history of abortion and knowledge of contraceptive methods were selected as a candidate variable for multivariate analysis so as to appreciate their independent effect. However, in multivariate analysis using multiple logistic regression age of the mother, educational status of the partner, family size, desired number of children and knowledge of modern contraceptive methods were found to be independently and significantly associated with unintended pregnancy.

After controlling for other independent factors maternal age was found to be significantly associated with unintended pregnancy. Mothers aged 36 years or

Table 1 Socio-demographic characteristics of study participants in Jimma, Ethiopia, 2016

Variables	Frequency	Percent
Age (Mean = 30.89 ± 6.55)		
≤ 25	81	22.8
26–35	167	46.9
≥ 36	108	30.3
Family size (Mean = 3.38 ± 2.17)		
0–3	189	53.1
4–6	136	38.2
> 6	31	8.7
Marital status		
Married	277	77.8
Single	8	2.2
Widowed	47	13.2
Divorced	24	6.7
Religion		
Orthodox	220	61.8
Muslim	85	23.9
Catholic	6	1.7
Protestant	45	12.6
Educational status of the respondent		
Can't read and write	31	8.7
Read and write	70	19.7
Primary	109	30.6
Secondary	92	25.8
College & above	54	15.2
Occupation of the respondent		
Housewife	186	52.2
Student	32	9
Self-employed	86	24.2
Employee	52	14.6
Educational status of the partner		
Can't read and write	35	9.8
Read and write	63	17.7
Primary	96	27
Secondary	104	29.2
College and above	58	16.3
Occupation of the partner		
Farmer	87	24.4
Student	4	1.1
Employee	117	32.9
Self-employed	148	41.6

more were nearly five times more likely to experience unintended pregnancy compared to mothers aged 25 years or less (AOR: 4.97; 95% CI: 2.53, 9.77).

Table 2 Reproductive history of study participants in Jimma, Ethiopia, 2016

Variables	Frequency	Percent
Age at marriage (Mean = 25.03 ± 12.24)		
≤ 20	127	35.7
21–24	110	30.9
> 25	119	33.4
Number of pregnancies (Mean = 4.92 ± 2.52)		
< 4	117	32.9
4–6	146	41
> 6	93	26.1
Number of children desired (Mean = 5.41 ± 1.47)		
< 4	46	12.9
4–6	219	61.5
> 6	91	25.6
Previous unintended pregnancy		
Yes	127	35.7
No	229	64.3
Think unintended pregnancy is preventable?		
Yes	222	62.4
No	134	37.6
Antenatal care visit		
Yes	182	51.1
No	174	48.9
History of abortion		
Yes	91	25.6
No	265	74.4
Knowledge of contraceptive methods		
Less knowledgeable	160	44.9
More knowledgeable	196	55.1

Mothers whose partner can't read and write were more than 14 times more likely to have unintended pregnancy when compared to those whose partner attained college and above (AOR: 14.59; 95% CI: 4.60, 46.31). Mothers with partner who can read and write (AOR: 3.62; 95% CI: 1.47, 8.93) and who attained primary education (AOR: 3.36; 95% CI: 1.42, 7.97) were more than three times more likely to experience unintended pregnancy compared to mothers whose partner attained college level or above.

Table 3 Magnitude of unintended pregnancy among study participants in Jimma, Ethiopia, 2016

Timing of current pregnancy	Frequency	Percent
Unwanted	97	27.2
Mistimed	33	9.3
Right time	167	46.9
Later than desired	59	16.6

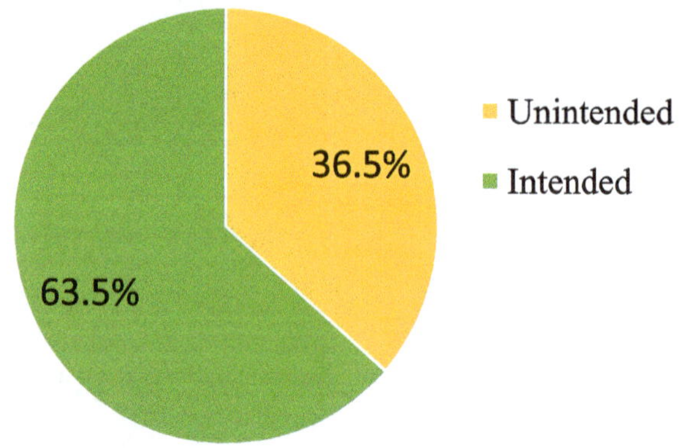

Fig. 1 Pregnancy intention among pregnant women in Jimma town, Southwest Ethiopia, 2016

Independent of other predictor variables, the higher the family size, the higher likely is the unintended pregnancy. Family having 4–6 members were four times more likely to have unintended pregnancy compared to those with three or less family members (AOR: 4.19; 95% CI: 2.01, 8.76). Family with more than six members were more than seven times more likely to have unintended pregnancy compared to family with three or less members (AOR: 7.63; 95% CI: 2.37, 24.52).

Those who desired to have less than four children were 2.89 times more likely to report unintended pregnancy compared to those who desired to have six or more number of children (AOR: 2.89; 95% CI: 1.25, 6.73). Those who desired to have 4–6 children were 2.11 times more likely to have unintended pregnancy compared to those who desired to have six or more number of children (AOR: 2.11; 95% CI: 1.34, 3.92).

Controlling for potential predictor factors, mothers who are less knowledgeable about contraceptive methods were nearly three times more likely to have unintended pregnancy compared to their counterparts (AOR: 2.92; 95% CI: 1.87, 4.56).

However, educational status of the mother, number of pregnancies, previous unintended pregnancy and history of abortion were not significantly associated with unintended pregnancy (Table 4).

Discussion

The prevalence of unintended pregnancy in this study was 36.5%: (95% CI: 31–42%), which is consistent with similar study conducted in Bale zone, Ganji, Duguna Fango, Debre-Markos, Hossana and Harar [5, 7, 8, 10, 11, 17]. But, higher than the study conducted in Arba-Minch [12], indicating higher rate of unintended pregnancy despite increased reproductive health services.

The most common reasons mentioned by women for failure to avoid unintended pregnancy are not considering oneself as fertile, 54 (41.5%) and contraceptive method failure 26 (20%). A similar finding was reported from a study in Gelemso, East Ethiopia [6]. Which indicated sustained gaps in creating awareness of reproductive aged women concerning appropriate utilization of modern contraceptives methods. Health education related to fertility has to be provided to reproductive age women, so that they understand the time they would be fertile.

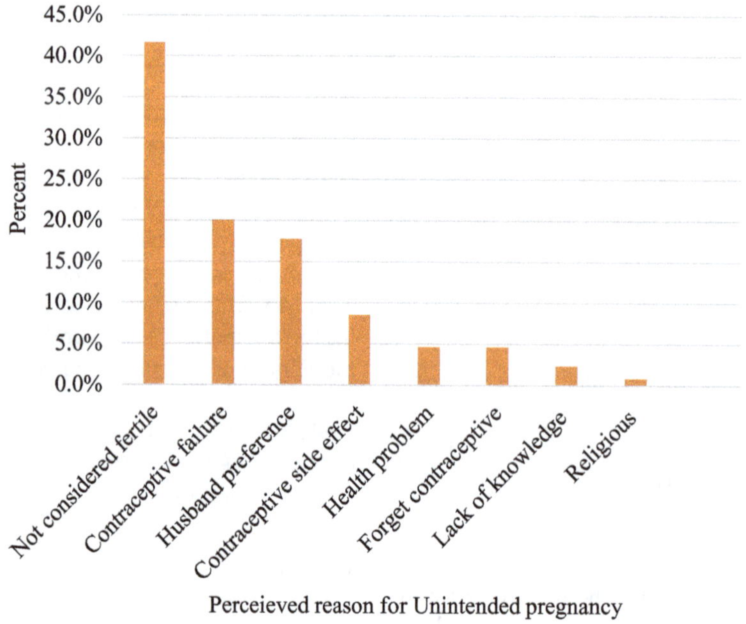

Fig. 2 Perceived reasons for unintended pregnancy among pregnant women in Jimma town, Southwest Ethiopia, 2016

Table 4 Bivariate and Multivariate analysis of factors associated with unintended pregnancy among pregnant mothers in Jimma, 2016

Characteristics	Categories	Unintended	Intended	COR (95% CI)	AOR (95% CI)	*P*-value
Age of the mother	≤25	22	59	1	1	
	26–35	34	133	0.68(0.37,1.27)	0.61(0.32,1.16)	0.13
	≥36	74	34	5.84(3.09,11.03)	**4.97(2.53,9.77)** **	0.00
Educational status of the mother	Can't read & write	18	13	5.41(2.05,14.33)	0.94 (0.10,8.42)	0.95
	Read and write	27	43	2.46(1.08,5.56)	0.54(0.07,4.23)	0.56
	Primary	43	66	2.55(1.18,5.48)	2.01(0.22,18.63)	0.54
	Secondary	31	61	1.98(0.90,4.38)	0.94(0.12,7.54)	0.96
	College & above	11	43	1	1	
Educational status of the partner	Can't read & write	28	7	17.09(5.94,49.18)	**14.59(4.60,46.31)** **	0.00
	Read and write	29	34	3.65(1.60,8.29)	**3.62(1.47,8.93)** **	0.00
	Primary	33	63	2.24(1.03,4.88)	**3.36(1.42,7.97)** **	0.00
	Secondary	29	75	1.65(0.75,3.62)	2.06(0.87,4.85)	0.10
	College & above	11	47	1	1	
Family size	0–3	37	152	1	1	
	4–6	71	65	4.49 (2.74,7.34)	**4.19(2.01,8.76)** **	0.00
	> 6	22	9	10.04(4.27,23.61)	**7.63(2.37,24.52)** **	0.00
Number of pregnancies	< 4	25	92	1	1	
	4–6	47	99	1.75(0.99,3.06)	0.68(0.31,1.47)	0.33
	> 6	58	35	6.09(3.32,11.22)	1.47(0.56,3.83)	0.44
Desired number of children	< 4	20	26	2.15(1.02,4.53)	**2.89(1.25,6.73)** *	0.01
	4–6	86	133	1.81(1.05,3.09)	**2.11(1.34,3.92)** *	0.02
	> 6	24	67	1	1	
Previous unintended pregnancy	No	65	164	1	1	
	Yes	65	62	2.65(1.68,4.15)	0.86(0.47,1.58)	0.63
Abortion history	Yes	40	51	1.53(0.94,2.48)	1.42(0.86,2.35)	0.17
	No	90	175	1	1	
Knowledge of contraceptive methods	More knowledgeable	50	146	1	1	
	Less knowledgeable	80	80	2.92(1.87,4.56)	**2.92(1.87,4.56)** **	0.00

**: significant at *p* value < 0.00
*: significant at *p* value < 0.05

Women who are less knowledgeable about modern contraceptive methods were more likely to have unintended pregnancy, which is consistent with the study done in Arba-Minch [12]. This might be explained by the fact that women with less knowledge about modern contraceptive methods were less likely to know the available, accessible and safe contraceptive methods and other reproductive health services. Therefore, less likely to utilize the method correctly and and hence more likely to have unintended pregnancy. As a result, it's important to improve reproductive age women knowledge about modern contraceptive methods in order to tackle unintended pregnancy.

Unintended pregnancy was found to be higher among women older than 35 years. Which is inconsistent with study conducted in Gelemso hospital, Bale zone, Hossana and Brazil [5, 6, 10, 18] but consistent with the study done in Kersa and Ganji Woreda of West Wollega that showed higher unintended pregnancy among older women [7, 19]. This might be due to the fact that older women will not consider themselves as fertile, less likely to be educated and hence less knowledgeable about modern contraceptive methods and also more likely to have partner with lower educational status. Hence, programs aiming to reduce unintended pregnancy should consider older women as potential target.

Women with partner of lower educational status is more likely to report unintended pregnancy possible explanation for this might be partner with no formal education or lower educational status disagree with mother's preference to use modern contraceptive methods and/ or less likely to encourage their wives to use family planning methods. Attitudes and behaviors of male partners may influence women's intentions, sexual behavior, contraceptive use and parenting [1].

The finding of the study depicted the higher the family size, the higher likely is the unintended pregnancy, this is in line with the study conducted in Damote Gale, Southern Ethiopia and Debre-Markos Town, North West Ethiopia [9, 17]. The rational for this might be families with a greater number of children already reached their desired number of children and hence, any more pregnancy is likely to be unintended.

The lower number of children desired, the higher the risk of unintended pregnancy, which is consistent with the study done in Hossana town, Southern Ethiopia [10]. This might be due to the fact that the lower the number of children the mother desired, higher order pregnancies are more likely to be unintended.

Conclusion and recommendation

The prevalence of unintended pregnancy was high in the study area being major reproductive health problems with all its adverse health outcomes to the mothers, children, families and societies at large. Age of the mother over 35 years, lower educational status of the partner, family size of more than four children, a smaller number of children desired and less knowledge of modern contraceptive methods were independent predictors of unintended pregnancy.

Teenagers and young adults were considered to be at higher risk of unintended pregnancy. As a result, unintended pregnancy was linked with teenage pregnancy. However, our finding indicated older women are at higher risk of unintended pregnancy and hence programs aimed at reducing unintended pregnancy should target the elders.

In addition to educating and empowering women, attention has to be given for educating male partner as most decisions in the household, including the timing of pregnancy and number of children desired, are strongly influenced by the male partner. Moreover, improving knowledge regarding the use of modern contraceptive methods is demanded.

Most women became pregnant because they did not consider themselves as fertile, so fertility education has to be provided to the older women so that they clearly understand the time in which they would be fertile. It is recommended that policy makers, health professionals, and health authorities should give due attention to the improvement in the provision of effective Information Education and Communication (IEC) and counseling and quality of care. Sexual and reproductive health education with more focus on fertility and contraceptive methods should be given for the couples, with more emphasis for the older as they are the less likely to achieve formal education.

Abbreviations

AOR: Adjusted odds ratio; CI: Confidence interval; HEW: Health extension workers; IEC: Information Education & Communication; NGO: Non-governmental organization; SD: Standard Deviation; SPSS: Statistical Package for Social Science

Acknowledgements

I would like to acknowledge the study participants, data collectors and supervisors who participated in the study. I'm very grateful for my family for their ever-increasing support and encouragement.

Authors' contributions

GA: involved from the inception to design of the study, acquisition of data, analysis and interpretation of results. **GA:** drafted, reviewed the manuscript and gave final approval of the version to be published. The author read and approved the final manuscript.

References

1. Santelli J, et al. The measurement and meaning of unintended Pregnancy. Perspect Sex Reprod Health. 2003;35(2):94–101.
2. Bearak J, et al. Global, regional, and subregional trends in unintended pregnancy and its outcomes from 1990 to 2014: estimates from a Bayesian hierarchical model. Lancet Glob Health. 2018;6(4):e380–9.
3. Ethiopian Central Statistical Agency, C. and ICF. *Ethiopia Demographic and Health Survey* 2016*: Key Indicators Report*. Addis Ababa, Ethiopia, and Rockville, Maryland, USA: CSA and ICF; 2016.
4. Tebekaw Y, Aemro B, Teller C. Prevalence and determinants of unintended childbirth in Ethiopia. BMC Pregnancy Childbirth. 2014;14:326.
5. Darega B, Dida N. Unplanned Pregnancy: Prevalence and associated factors among antenatal care attending women in bale zone, Oromiya region, Southeast Ethiopia: a facility - based cross sectional study. Glob J Med Res. 2015;15(4). https://medicalresearchjournal.org/index.php/GJMR/article/view/936/846.
6. Mohammed F, Musa A, Amano A. Prevalence and determinants of unintended pregnancy among pregnant woman attending ANC at Gelemso general hospital, Oromiya region, East Ethiopia: a facility based cross-sectional study. BMC Womens Health. 2016;16(1):56.
7. Teshome FT, Hailu AG, Teklehaymanot AN. Prevalence of unintended pregnancy and associated factors among married pregnant women in Ganji woreda, west Wollega Oromia region. Ethiop Sci J Public Health. 2014;2(2): 92–101.
8. Worku S, Fantahun M. Unintended pregnancy and induced abortion in a town with accessible family planning services: the case of Harar in eastern Ethiopia. Ethiop J Health Dev. 2006;20(2):79–83.
9. Geda NR, Lako TK. A population based study on unintended pregnancy among married women in a district in southern Ethiopia. J Geogr Reg Plan. 2011;4(7):417.
10. Hamdela B, G/mariam A, Tilahun T. Unwanted pregnancy and associated factors among pregnant married women in Hosanna Town, Southern Ethiopia. PLoS One. 2012;7(6):e39074. https://journals.plos.org/plosone/article?id=10.1371/journal.pone.0039074.
11. Getachew FD. Level of Unintended Pregnancy and its Associated Factors among Currently Pregnant Women in Duguna Fango District, Wolaita Zone, Southern Ethiopia. Malays. J Med Biol res. 2015;2:75–88.
12. Gite A, et al. Unintended Pregnancy: magnitude and associated factors among pregnant women in Arba Minch town, Gamo Gofa zone, Ethiopia, 2015. Reprod Syst Sex Disord. 2016;5(193). https://medicalresearchjournal.org/index.php/GJMR/article/view/936/846.
13. Abayu H, et al. Prevalence and associated factors of unintended Pregnancy in Welkaite Woreda, Tigray and North Ethiopia cross sectional study by 2012. J Pregnancy Child Health. 2015;(2):2.
14. Amo-Adjei J, Anamaale Tuoyire D. Effects of planned, mistimed and unwanted pregnancies on the use of prenatal health services in sub-Saharan Africa: a multicountry analysis of demographic and health survey data. Tropical Med Int Health. 2016;21(12):1552–61.
15. Dibaba Y, Fantahun M, Hindin MJ. The effects of pregnancy intention on the use of antenatal care services: systematic review and meta-analysis. Reprod Health. 2013;(10):50.

16. Wado YD, Afework MF, Hindin MJ. Unintended pregnancies and the use of maternal health services in southwestern Ethiopia. BMC Int Health Hum Rights. 2013;13:36.
17. Kibret, A., H. Bayu, and M. Merga, Prevalence of Unintended Pregnancy and Associated Factors among Pregnant Women Attending Antenatal Clinics in Debre-markos Town, *North West Ethiopia 2012*. Women's health care, 2015. 4(3).
18. Theme-Filha MM, et al. Factors associated with unintended pregnancy in Brazil: cross-sectional results from the birth in Brazil National Survey, 2011/2012. Reprod Health. 2016;13(Suppl 3):118.
19. Kassa N, Berhane Y, Worku A. Predictors of unintended pregnancy in Kersa, eastern Ethiopia, 2010. Reprod Health. 2012;9(1).

Factors associated with contraceptive use among sexually active Nepalese youths in the Kathmandu Valley

Laxmi Tamang[1*], Camille Raynes-Greenow[2], Kevin McGeechan[2] and Kirsten Black[3]

Abstract

Background: In Nepal, evidence is sparse regarding the use of contraception at first and current relationships among sexually active young people. This study examined the factors associated with modern contraceptive use at first and current sexual relationships.

Methods: A descriptive cross-sectional household survey conducted amongst young Nepalese men and women living in the urban areas of the Kathmandu valley. We used logistic regression to model the relationship between selected independent variables and outcome variables (use at first sexual intercourse and current use of modern contraception) among 492 ever sexually active youth aged 15–24 years.

Results: We found that the key factors associated with current non-use of modern contraceptives among sexually active youth age 15–24 were young age at first sexual contact and a relationship with someone other than a spouse, while significant factor associated with current use of contraception was religion, revealing that Hindu youths having lower odds of use compared to young people who belonged to other religions.

Conclusions: The findings suggest that contraception education should be intensified and directly towards those entering adolescence to encourage youths to adopt contraception at the time of their first sexual relationship. The influence of religion on use of modern contraception needs further exploration.

Keywords: Contraceptive, Nepal, Young people

Background

Access to safe and effective contraception is essential for optimal sexual and reproductive health [1, 2] and allows for the prevention of unintended pregnancies, improved pregnancy spacing and reduced transmission of sexually transmitted infections and HIV [3–5]. Although overall contraceptive use has increased worldwide, youth access to sexual and reproductive health services and comprehensive sexuality education, that are high-quality, youth-friendly and respect the right to confidentiality, privacy and informed consent remains a challenge in many countries [6–8]. Globally, from a public health perspective there is a widening gap between sexual debut and age of marriage, and increased sexual activity prior to marriage [9], which exposes young people to the risk of unplanned pregnancy [10–12].

The few studies that have been conducted in Nepal on young peoples' sexual behaviour have found that they experience a wide range of consensual and coercive sexual relationships and that the proportion of sexually experienced unmarried young people is rising [7, 13–17]. Early sexual experimentation, combined with low and irregular use of condoms in Nepalese society places young people at risk of HIV and other sexually transmitted infection [7, 13, 15–17]. Indeed the Nepal Adolescent and Youth Survey 2010/2011 reported that one in six young people aged 15–24 had been involved in risky sexual practices such as oral, anal and paid sex and almost 13% had premarital sex, of which only 46% had used contraception at the time of their first sexual intercourse [15]. The same study revealed that almost one-fifth of young people had their first sexual intercourse unwillingly and forcefully.

* Correspondence: laxtshering@yahoo.com
[1]APS Prasuti Tatha Prajanan Swasthya Kendra, Link Marg 1045, Kuleshwor, Kathmandu, Nepal

As well as being exposed to sexually transmitted infections, unsafe sex exposes young people to the risk of unplanned pregnancy. Across South Asia the uptake of modern contraceptive methods amongst sexually active young people has been poor and early childbearing is common [9, 18]. This is true of women in Nepal where almost one quarter of women give birth by age 18 and nearly half by age 20 [17]. While use of any contraceptive method, including modern contraceptive methods by reproductive aged women married or in a union, is around the average for South Asian countries at 49%, the incidence of unintended pregnancy is higher in Nepalese adolescents (32%) [19]. Furthermore, the 2011 Nepal Demographic Health Survey reported that unmet need for contraception is particularly high among young women aged 15–19 and 20–24, at 41% and 37% respectively compared to women in older age groups 30% or less.

In Nepal, family planning being one of the priority programs of the government modern contraceptive methods both short-acting and long acting reversible contraceptive services are freely available to all reproductive age men and women through public health system. The main aim of the national family planning program is to ensure that individuals and couples are able to fulfil their reproductive needs by using appropriate contraceptive methods based on informed choice.

Following the International Conference on Population and Development held in Cairo in 1994, the government of Nepal committed to promoting and protecting the sexual and reproductive rights of adolescents and youth [20]. Collaborating with national and international agencies the Nepalese government is striving to achieve the development goals that place considerable importance on increasing the use of contraception and reducing the fertility rate, as well as to address gender inequality and women's empowerment [21]. Understanding the key factors influencing contraceptive use among young sexually active youths who are at risk of unwanted pregnancies is key to the development of effective family planning programs. This study aims to examine the factors associated with contraceptive use at the first sexual intercourse and current relationships among Nepalese youth living in urban areas of the Kathmandu Valley.

Methods

Study setting and design

The data were collected from a field survey conducted in the urban areas of the Kathmandu Valley, comprising all five major cities: Kathmandu metropolitan city, Lalitpur sub-metropolitan city, Bhaktapur municipality, Kirtipur municipality, and Thimi municipality. The study was part of a larger study that employed mix-methods, and comprised a household survey, focus group discussions and in-depth interviews aiming to investigate how gendered power relations influence knowledge of SRH and access to, and utilisation of, SRH services among youth in the Kathmandu valley, Nepal. In this paper we present the cross-sectional household survey information. The data were collected using two-stage cluster sampling from the study area. In the first stage of sample selection, primary sampling units (clusters i.e. wards) were selected using a probability proportional-to-size from each study area. We randomly selected a total of 40 clusters from three district urban areas using household and population information from the 2011 Population Census developed by the Central Bureau of Statistics. In the second stage, 35 households in each cluster were selected using a systematic sampling technique. Thus, we needed to visit a total of 1400 households in order to interview the required number of youths.

Study population

This study was part of the large study among youth thus information was collected from 1400 urban youths, comprising 720 females and 680 males. The sample size for the study was calculated based on the 50% prevalence of young Nepalese women aged 15–24 who had ever had sexual intercourse with 95% confidence intervals, 5% margin of error, 1.6 design effect obtained from those who had had sexual intercourse before age 18 and 10% none response rate [15, 17]. However, for the purpose of this paper only 492 young men and women who had prior sexual experience were included to examine the use of contraceptives at their first and current sexual relationships.

Questionnaire

The questionnaire consisted of standard items that were adapted from previous studies and validated in similar settings including questions from the Nepal Demographic Health Surveys [15, 22–25]. Some items were modified and added to the questionnaire to suit the context of the study. The questionnaire was finalised after pilot-testing outside the study areas.

Two questionnaires were administered: the household questionnaire and the individual questionnaire. The household questionnaires were used to list all the usual members in the selected households and gathered basic information about the household and characteristics of individuals living there. The individual questionnaire was administered to all youth aged 15–24 by trained female research assistants. The respondents were interviewed face-to-face and provided with an explanation for question items.

Measures

Respondents were asked if they had ever had engaged in sexual intercourse in their life to ensure they met the "sexually active" requirement for participation in the study. Any participant who answered "no" was not eligible for participation in the study. Lastly, participants were asked if they were currently involved in a relationship where they had regularly have sexual intercourse, and if they answered yes, they were further asked to indicate the length of this relationship.

Analysis

We applied both univariate and multivariable analyses in this study to examine the association between each of the outcome variables, 'use of modern contraceptive method at the first sexual contact' and 'current use of contraceptive,' and he explanatory variables sex, age, marital status, place of origin, education, ethnicity, religion, occupation, source of income, age at the first sexual intercourse, relationship type, method of participation in the first sexual intercourse, ever discussed about the importance of safe sex with partner, ever had discussed of contraceptive use with partner, and the main source of sexual and reproductive information among sexually active youths who were not planning to have a baby [21, 26–28]. A dichotomous measure indicated whether respondents had used any modern method contraception the first time they had intercourse and whether they were currently using contraceptives. We used the IBM Statistical Package for the Social Sciences (SPSS) software Version 16 (SPSS Inc., Chicago, IL, USA) complex samples procedures to account for the sampling design in the calculation of the association measures. The level of statistical significance was set at a level of $p < 0.05$.

Ethical approval

Ethical approval was granted by the University of Sydney's Human Research Ethics Committee and from the Nepal Health Research Council. Informed consent from each study participant was obtained after clear explanation about the purpose of the study. A written informed consent sheet was prepared for the parents or legal guardians of participants less than 16 years to give their signed consent on behalf of their children. The study participants and parents or legal guardians were informed that they had full right to withdraw from the study. Confidentiality of the information was assured by omitting names of study participants from the questionnaire and respondents were interviewed in a separate place to maintain their privacy.

Results

Socio-demographic characteristics

Of the total 492 sexually active young men and women, the majority of there were aged 20–24 (77% men and 79% women), had never been married (13% men and 95% women), were urban in origin (56% men and 64% women), and had ever studied at school (98% men and 92% women) women (Table 1). Most of them had the School Leaving Certificate (SLC) or above level of education (84% men and 48% women). More than half were Indo-Aryan by ethnicity (57% men and 56% women) and most were Hindu (79% men and 83% women). Men were significantly more likely than women not to be married ($p < 0.001$), ever studied at school ($p = 0.011$), have obtained a degree in higher education ($p < 0.001$), were students ($p < 0.001$), self-dependent for income ($p = 0.011$), had relationship with girlfriends ($p < 0.001$), participated willingly in a sexual activity ($p < 0.001$), had two or more sexual partners in their life time ($p < 0.001$), ever discussed of contraceptive use ($p = 0.002$) and radio was their major source of SRH information ($p = 0.002$).

Contraceptive methods used at first sex and in current relationship

Half of ever sexually active young people who were not planning a pregnancy had used a modern method of contraception at the time of their first sexual intercourse and of these, the majority (48%) had used condoms (Table 2). Condoms were also the most commonly used method amongst currently sexually active youth, with 66% of participants using a modern contraceptive method: 39% were using condoms followed by 28% injectables and 8% the oral contraceptive pill.

Determinants of contraceptive use

Use at first sexual intercourse: Seventy percent of males and 31% of females used modern contraceptive methods at their first sexual intercourse. The factors statistically associated with contraceptive use at first sexual intercourse were sex of participant, whether or not they had ever studied at school, age at first sexual intercourse and type of relationship (Table 3). The analysis suggests that compared to females, males had a 5.14 times greater odds of reporting use of contraception in their first sexual contact. Greater odds of contraceptive use were also associated with ever having studies at school, and having a relationship with a person other than a spouse. Those who had their first sexual encounter between the ages of 12–15 had significantly lower odds of having used contraception compared to women whose first sex occurred between 16 and 19 or 20 and 24 years. In the multivariable analysis only age at first sexual intercourse and relationship type with partner remained significant (Table 3).

Current use: Among young people not wanting to conceive, univariate analysis revealed greater odds of current use of contraception amongst males compared to females and amongst non-Hindus (Table 4). In the adjusted multivariate logistic we included all the

Table 1 Socio-demographic characteristics of young people aged 15–24 by sex

Background Characteristics	All (n = 492) No. (%)	Male (n = 247) No. (%)	Female (n = 245) No. (%)	*P* value
Age (in years):				
15–19	108	57 (23.0)	51 (20.7)	0.605
20–24	384	190 (77.0)	194 (79.3)	
Marital Status:				
Ever married	265	33 (13.4)	233 (95.0)	<0.001*
Never married	226	214 (86.6)	12 (5.0)	
Place of origin:				
Rural	296	139 (56.3)	157 (64.2)	0.187
Urban	196	108 (43.7)	88 (35.8)	
Ever studied at school:				
Yes	469	243 (98.3)	226 (92.2)	0.011*
No	23	4 (1.7)	19 (7.8)	
Education:				
Some secondary and below[a]	168	41 (16.4)	127 (52.0)	<0.001*
SLC and above	324	206 (83.6)	118 (48.0)	
Ethnicity:				
Tibeto-Burmese	214	106 (42.9)	108 (44.3)	0.799
Indo-Aryan	278	141 (57.1)	137 (55.7)	
Religion:				
Hindu	400	197 (79.6)	203 (83.1)	0.408
Non-Hindu[b]	92	50 (20.4)	42 (16.9)	
Occupation:				
Non-students	277	74 (29.7)	203 (83.1)	<0.001*
Students	215	173 (70.3)	42 (16.9)	
Source of income:				
Parents and others	432	205 (83.1)	227 (92.6)	0.012*
Self	60	42 (16.9)	18 (7.4)	
Age at the first sexual intercourse				
12–15	42	20 (8.0)	22 (9.1)	0.051
16–19	306	165 (67.1)	141 (57.5)	
20–24	144	62 (25.0)	82 (33.4)	
Relationship type				
Spouse	255	22 (8.8)	233 (95.0)	
Boy/girlfriend	215	205 (82.9)	10 (4.3)	<0.001*
Familiar person/ sex worker[c]	22	20 (8.3)	2 (0.7)	
Type of participation				
Willingly	457	241 (97.7)	216 (88.3)	<0.001*
Unwillingly/forcefully	35	6 (2.3)	29 (11.7)	
No. of sexual partners in life time				
One	451	107 (43.1)	244 (99.7)	<0.001*
Two and more	141	140 (56.9)	1 (0.3)	
Ever discussed of safe sex with partner				
No	120	50 (20.3)	70 (28.4)	0.100
Yes	372	197 (79.7)	175 (71.6)	
Ever discussed of contraceptive use				
No	68	20 (8.2)	48 (19.6)	0.002*
Yes	424	227 (91.8)	197 (80.4)	
Source of SRH information				
Radio	391	212 (85.9)	178 (72.9)	0.002*
Television	70	26 (10.7)	44 (17.9)	
Friends, teachers and others	31	8 (3.4)	23 (9.3)	

[a]No education: 5; Primary 22; [b]Buddhist: 69; Kirat: 12 Christian: 7; Islam: 4; [c]Familiar person: 19, Sex worker: 7; $*P < 0.05$

variables with a *p*-value less than 0.25 in the univariate analysis that comprised sex, age, place of origin, religion, source of income and ever discussed about safer sex. The only significant association that remained after multivariable logistic regression analysis was with religion

Table 2 Percentage distributions of modern contraceptive use and method mix at first sexual relationship and current use among sexually active young people in the Kathmandu valley

Contraceptive method mix	n[a]	Percent	95% Confidence Interval
Used at first sexual intercourse			
Traditional method users	38	7.7	4.7–12.4
Non-users	206	41.9	35.9–48.0
Any modern method users	248	50.4	45.0–55.8
Condom	235	47.7	42.4–53.1
Pill[b]	12	2.5	1.4–4.4
Injectables	1	0.2	0–2.5
Total	492	100.0	-
Current use of contraception			
Traditional method users	40	20.8	16.0–26.5
Non-users	26	13.0	8.6–19.4
Any modern method users	129	66.2	59.7–72.1
Condom	77	39.4	32.1–47.2
Pill	10	4.9	2.6–8.8
Injectables	36	18.7	13.6–25.2
IUCD/Implants[c]	4	2.1	0.7–6.4
Sterilisation	2	1.1	0.3–3.4
Total	195	100.0	-

[a]Weighted samples to represent population; [b]Emergency Contraceptive: 2; [c]2 each

Table 3 Factors associated with use of modern contraception at first sexual intercourse among sexually active Nepalese youth, univariate and multivariate analyses

Background Characteristics	n = 492 (%)	% of youth used modern contraceptive methods	*Univariate analyses*		*Multivariate analyses*	
			Odd ratio (95% CI)	*p*-value	Adjusted odd ratio (95% CI)	*p*-value
Sex						
Female	245 (49.8)	76 (30.9)	Ref.	<0.001*	Ref.	0.437
Male	247 (50.2)	172 (69.7)	5.14 (3.34–7.89)		1.48 (0.54–4.03)	
Place of origin						
Rural	296 (60.2)	141 (47.6)	Ref.		Ref.	0.849
Urban	196 (39.8)	107 (54.6)	1.32 (0.92–1.90)	0.128	0.96 (0.64–1.45)	
Ever studied at school						
Yes	469 (95.3)	245 (52.2)	6.51 (1.51–28.08)	0.013*	2.74 (0.74–10.21)	0.128
No	23 (4.7)	3 (14.4)	Ref.		Ref.	
Ethnicity						
Tibeto-Burmese	214 (43.6)	103 (41.6)	Ref.	0.363	Ref.	0.486
Indo-Aryan	278 (56.4)	145 (58.4)	1.18 (0.82–1.69)		1.17 (0.74–1.85)	
Religion						
Hindu	400 (81.3)	204 (82.1)	Ref.	0.671	Ref.	0.860
Non-Hindu[a]	92 (18.7)	44 (17.9)	0.91 (0.91–1.45)		0.95 (0.54–1.68)	
Age at the first sexual intercourse						
12–15	42 (8.5)	7 (2.6)	0.17 (0.07–0.41)	0.001*	0.10 (0.03–0.31)	0.001*
16–19	306 (62.3)	167 (67.5)	1.13 (0.72–1.76)		0.81 (0.50–1.33)	
20–24	144 (29.2)	74 (29.9)	Ref.		Ref.	
Relationship type with partner						
Spouse	255 (51.7)	76 (30.6)	Ref.	<0.001*	Ref.	0.003*
Boy/girlfriend	215 (43.8)	153 (61.7)	5.78 (3.88–8.61)		4.55 (1.63–12.75)	
Familiar person/sex worker[b]	22 (4.5)	19 (7.7)	15.29 (4.88–47.89)		11.85 (2.70–43.54)	
Type of participation						
Willingly	458 (93.0)	236 (95.1)	Ref.	0.064	Ref.	0.826
Unwillingly/forcefully	34 (7.0)	12 (4.9)	0.51 (0.25–1.04)		0.92 (0.44–1.95)	
Total	-	248 (50.4)				

[a]Buddhist: 69, Kirat: 12, Christian: 7, Islam: 4; [b]Familiar person: 19, Sex worker: 7; CI: Confidence Interval; Ref: Reference category; $*p < 0.05$

and current use of contraception, such that young people who belong to non-Hindu religious group had 3.24 (95% CI: 1.39-7.56; $p = 0.008$) times greater odds of using modern contraception compared to young people who stated they were Hindu.

Discussion

This study examined the timing, circumstances and use of modern contraception among sexually active youth aged 15–24 living in urban area of the Kathmandu Valley at their first and in their current sexual relationship. We found that half of young people had used a modern method of contraception at first intercourse and over two thirds in their current relationships and in both circumstances condoms were the most frequently used method followed by the oral contraceptive pill and injectables. These findings are similar to those in the 2011 National Adolescents and Youth Survey figures that revealed 46% of young people had used contraception at the time of their first sexual intercourse and of those, 91% of them used condoms, three precent the oral contraceptive pill, and one percent the injection [15]. This may relate to the fact that government of Nepal has made these methods easily available and accessible to all reproductive age men and women in Nepal. As a policy measure, findings of this study are very useful as it can inform policy and decision making in the government healthcare system to increase the contraception users among youth to

Table 4 Results of univariate and multivariate analyses for current use of contraception among sexually active Nepalese youths

Background Characteristics	n = 195 (%)	% of youth currently using modern contraceptive	*Univariate analyses*		*Multivariate analyses*	
			Odd ratio/CI	*p*-value	Adjusted odd ratio (95% CI)	*p*-value
Sex:						
Female	151 (77.3)	94 (62.4)	Ref.	0.043*	Ref.	0.232
Male	44 (22.7)	35 (79.0)	2.27 (1.03–5.03)		1.62 (0.73–3.61)	
Age (in years):						
15–19	29 (14.7)	16 (55.3)	0.58 (0.25–1.34)	0.195	0.63 (0.26–1.51)	0.287
20–24	166 (85.3)	113 (68.0)	Ref.		Ref.	
Marital Status:						
Ever married	160 (82.1)	104 (65.2)	Ref.	0.487	-	-
Never married	35 (17.9)	25 (70.7)	1.29 (0.62–2.68)			
Place of origin:						
Rural	122 (62.8)	76 (62.1)	Ref.	0.154	Ref.	0.087
Urban	73 (37.2)	53 (73.0)	1.64 (0.82–3.29)		1.87 (0.91–3.83)	
Education:						
Some secondary and below[a]	82 (41.9)	54 (65.7)	Ref.	0.927	-	-
SLC and above	113 (58.1)	75 (66.4)	1.03 (0.52–2.05)			
Ethnicity:						
Tibeto-Burmese	90 (45.9)	59 (66.0)	Ref.	0.963	-	-
Indo-Aryan	105 (54.1)	70 (66.3)	1.01 (0.60–1.69)			
Religion:						
Hindu	159 (81.6)	99 (61.9)	Ref.	0.007*	Ref.	0.008*
Non-Hindu[b]	36 (18.4)	30 (85.0)	3.49 (1.43–8.49)		3.24 (1.39–7.56)	
Occupation:						
Non-students	139 (71.4)	93 (66.9)	Ref.	0.663		
Students	56 (28.6)	36 (64.3)	0.89 (0.53–1.50)			
Source of income:						
Parents and others	179 (92.1)	116 (64.6)	Ref.	0.081	Ref.	0.209
Self	16 (7.9)	13 (84.5)	2.99 (0.97–10.34)		2.18 (0.63–7.53)	
Age at the first sexual intercourse						
12–15	19 (9.4)	11 (60.3)	0.61 (0.18–2.02)	0.582	-	-
16–19	106 (54.5)	68 (63.7)	0.70 (0.34–1.43)			
20–24	70 (36.1)	50 (71.4)	Ref.			
Relationship type						
Spouse	158 (81.3)	103 (64.8)	Ref.		-	-
Boy/girlfriend or causal partner[c]	37 (18.7)	26 (71.9)	1.39 (0.69–2.81)	0.348		
No. of sexual partners in life time						
One	170 (87.5)	113 (66.4)	Ref.	0.871	-	-
Two and more	24 (12.5)	16 (64.7)	0.93 (0.37–2.32)			
Ever discussed of safe sex with partner						
No	37 (19.1)	21 (55.6)	Ref.	0.111	Ref.	0.444
Yes	158 (80.9)	108 (68.7)	1.75 (0.87–3.50)		1.34 (0.62–2.88)	

Table 4 Results of univariate and multivariate analyses for current use of contraception among sexually active Nepalese youths *(Continued)*

Ever discussed of contraceptive use						
No	21 (10.6)	14 (69.1)	Ref.	0.720	-	-
Yes	174 (89.4)	115 (65.8)	0.86 (0.37–2.01)			
Source of SRH information						
Radio	148 (76.1)	100 (67.1)	Ref.	0.858	-	-
Television	35 (17.8)	22 (63.7)	0.86 (0.36–2.06)			
Friends, teachers and others	12 (6.1)	7 (61.7)	0.79 (0.29–2.14)			
Total	-	129 (66.2)				

[a]No education: 5; Primary 22; [b]Buddhist: 28; Christian: 5; Kirat: 2; Islam: 1; [c]Boy/girlfriend: 34, Causal partner: 3; Ref: Reference category; *$P < 0.05$

protect against unintended pregnancy and sexually transmitted infections.

The use of one of the modern contraceptive methods at first sexual encounter was, in univariate analysis, significantly associated with young people's sex, schooling, age at first sexual encounter and relationship type. However, in the multivariate analysis only age at first sexual intercourse and relationship type with a partner was statistically significantly associated with modern contraceptive use. Although it was expected that socio-cultural factors such as religion and ethnicity might influence the use of modern contraceptive use among youth, however, it did not have any significant association with use of contraception at first sexual relationship.

In contrast use of a modern method of contraception was associated with religion with significantly less odds of using a modern method of contraception if the young person identified as Hindu. Other studies have similarly reported that socio-cultural factors such as religion influence sexual attitudes and behaviour including utilisation of contraception [13, 29–32]. The possible reason for greater use of contraception by non-Hindu youths, primarily Buddhist and Christian, may relate to the more egalitarian nature of their religious and cultural beliefs and practices compared to the Hindu mores [32]. Studies have shown that there is a strong preference for childbearing immediately after marriage in Hindu societies to demonstrate that the partnership is a good one and women may not be educated about contraceptive options until after the birth of the first child [33, 34].

Although not demonstrated in our study, other research in Nepal and elsewhere has consistently shown that young people with higher education are more likely to use contraception than those who have little or no education [13, 17]. Reasons for our finding are possibly due to the sample, who were an urban population and who were likely to be aware of contraception and its benefits though exposure to mass media. This sample also excluded young women wishing to conceive who were likely to be less educated as they had chosen marriage and childbirth over tertiary studies.

Several limitations of the study should be noted. Young people provided information about their sexual relationship and contraceptive use retrospectively and there is the possibility that recall bias, social desirability and underreporting affected their responses. Another limitation of this study concerns the sample of participants. This study is limited to sexually active young people living in urban areas of the Kathmandu valley, and therefore, the generalizability of this study's findings is restricted. The responses to the question on use of contraceptives are self-reported and the validity of the respondents' claims has not been ascertained. However, the study team made a concerted effort to improve the reliability of the data by undertaking the interviews in total privacy, and using validated questions.

Conclusions

This study shows that majority of youth at their first and current sexual contact used condom to protect against unintended pregnancy and sexually transmitted infections. Age at first sexual intercourse and relationship type with a partner were associated with use of modern contraceptive first sex, whereas religion was found to be associated with current modern contraceptive use. Our results present evidence that may be useful to inform future policy direction about how to increase young people's access to contraception in Nepal. In particular sex education needs to begin early as it was the youth initiating sexual intercourse under the age of 16 who were least likely to use a modern method of contraception. Young people need better skills to be able to negotiate sexual and contraceptive decisions in their relationship and the problems of high prevalence of child marriage and early childbearing that needs to be addressed if Nepal is to reach the millennium development goal in terms of gender inequality and empowerment of women.

Abbreviations
CI: Confidence interval; HIV: Human immuno-deficiency virus; SPSS: Statistical package for the social sciences; USA: United States of America.

Acknowledgements
We are very grateful to the young men and women who participated in this study allowing us to interview them and shared information on a sensitive subject. We thank to the Center for Research on Environment Health and Population Activities for providing technical assistance in the field in carryout data collection by mobilising their interviewers and supervisors.

Authors' contributions
LT was investigator, involved in proposal writing, designing, and recruitment and training of supervisors and data collectors, analysis and write up and in all stages of the project implementation. She did most of the analysis and write up of the draft paper. CRG contributed in the designing of project proposal, reviewing and editing drafts of the manuscript, and involved in the final approval of the paper. KM provided assistance for data analysis. KB contributed in the designing of project proposal, assisted in editing and finalising the drafts of the manuscript. All authors read and approved the final manuscript.

Author details
[1]APS Prasuti Tatha Prajanan Swasthya Kendra, Link Marg 1045, Kuleshwor, Kathmandu, Nepal. [2]School of Public Health, Faculty of Medicine, The University of Sydney, Camperdown, NSW 2006, Australia. [3]Discipline of Obstetrics, Gynaecology and Neonatology, Faculty of Medicine, The University of Sydney, Camperdown, NSW 2006, Australia.

References

1. Frost JJ, Lindberg LD. Reasons for using contraception: perspectives of US women seeking care at specialized family planning clinics. Contraception. 2013;87(4):465–72.
2. Cleland J, Harbison S, Shah IH. Unmet need for contraception: issues and challenges. Stud Fam Plan. 2014;45(2):105–22.
3. Glasier A, et al. Sexual and reproductive health: a matter of life and death. Lancet. 2006;368(9547):1595–607.
4. WHO. MDG 5: Improve Maternal health 2012; Available from: http://www.who.int/topics/millennium_development_goals/maternal_health/en/. Accessed 25 May 2016.
5. Patton GC, et al. Health of the world's adolescents: a synthesis of internationally comparable data. The Lancet. 2012;379(9826):1665–75.
6. GoN and UNFPA. Health related quality of life of women suffering from pelvic organ prolapse: before and 9 to 11 months after surgical interventions. Kathmandu: Ministry of Health and Population, Department of Health Services, Family Health Division and United Nations Population Fund; 2013.
7. Puri M, Cleland J. Sexual behavior and perceived risk of HIV/AIDS among young migrant factory workers in Nepal. J Adolesc Health. 2006;38(3):237–46.
8. Puri M, Ingham R, Matthews Z. Factors affecting abortion decisions among young couples in Nepal. J Adolesc Health. 2007;40(6):535–42.
9. Bearinger L, et al. Global perspectives on the sexual and reproductive health of adolescents: patterns, prevention, and potential. Lancet. 2007;369(9568):1220–31.
10. WHO. The sexual and reproductive health of young adolescents in developing countries: reviewing the evidence, identifying research gaps, and moving the agenda. Geneva: World Health Organisation; 2011.
11. Khatiwada N, et al. Sexual and reproductive health of adolescents and youth in Nepal: trends and determinants: futher analysis of the 2011 Nepal demographic and health survey. Calverton, Maryland: Nepal Ministry of Health and Population, New ERA, and ICF International; 2013.
12. DeJong J, et al. The sexual and reproductive health of young people in the arab countries and Iran. Reprod Health Matters. 2005;13(25):49–59.
13. Dahal G, Hennink M, Hinde A. Risky sexual behaviour among young Men in Nepal, in applications and policy working paper A05/01. England: Southhampton University; 2005.
14. Puri MC, Busza J. In forests and factories: sexual behaviour among young migrant workers in Nepal. Cult Health Sex. 2004;6(2):145–58.
15. MoHP Nepal. Nepal adolescents and youth survey 2010/2011. Kathmandu: Ministry of Health and Population; 2012.
16. Adhikari R, Tamang J. Premarital sexual behavior among male college students of Kathmandu, Nepal. BMC Public Health. 2009;9(1):241.
17. MoHP Nepal, New ERA, and ICF International Inc. Nepal demographic health survey 2011. Kathmandu, Nepal: Ministry of Health and Population, New ERA and ICF International Inc, Claverton, Maryland; 2012.
18. Raj A, McDougal L, Rusch MA. Changes in prevalence of girl child marriage in south asia. JAMA. 2012;307(19):2027–9.
19. Kamal Mostafa, S.M. and C.H. Hassan. Childbearing, Unintended Pregnancy and Contraceptive Use among South Asian Married Female Adolescents. 2003; Available from: http://ghf.g2hp.net/2013/08/29/childbearing-unintended-pregnancy-and-contraceptive-use-among-south-asian-married-female-adolescents/. Accessed 25 May 2016.
20. Leone T, Matthews Z, Zuanna GD. Impact and determinants of sex preference in Nepal. Int Fam Plan Perspect. 2003;29(2):69–75.
21. Kidsley S. Contraceptive use in Nepal. University of Southampton, School of Medicine, Doctoral Thesis. 2006. p. 21. Available from: http://eprints.soton.ac.uk/210221/1.hasCoversheetVersion/00369850.pdf. Accessed 25 May 2016.
22. Cleland J, Ingham R, Stone N. Asking young people about sexual and reproductive behaviours: illustrative core instruments. Geneva: UNDP/UNFPA/WHO/World Bank Special Programme of Research, Development and Research Training in Human Reproduction; 2001.
23. MoHP Nepal, New ERA, and Macro International Inc. Nepal demographic health survey 2006. Kathmandu: Minsitry of Health and Population, New ERA and Macro International Inc; 2007.
24. Pulerwitz J, Barker G. Measuring attitudes towards gender norms among young men in brazil-development and pschometric evaluation of the GEM scale. Men Masculinities. 2008;10(3):322–38.
25. Pulerwitz J, Gortmaker S, DeJong W. Measuring sexual relationship power in HIV/STD research. Sex Roles. 2000;42(7):637–60.
26. Adhikari R. Factors affecting awareness of emergency contraception among college students in Kathmandu, Nepal. BMC Womens Health. 2009;9(1):27.
27. Frost JJ, Darroch JE. Factors associated with contraceptive choice and inconsistent method use, United States, 2004. Perspect Sex Reprod Health. 2008;40(2):94–104.
28. East L, et al. Use of the male condom by heterosexual adolescents and young people: literature review. J Adv Nurs. 2007;59(2):103–10.
29. Gaydos L, et al. An emerging field in religion and reproductive health. J Relig Health. 2010;49(4):473–84.
30. Hill NJ, Siwatu M, Robinson AK. "My religion picked My birth control": the influence of religion on contraceptive use. J Relig Health. 2014;53(3):825–33.
31. Davidson Sr JK, et al. Sexual attitudes and behavior at four universities: do region, race, and/or religion matter? Adolescence. 2008;43(170):189–220.
32. Srikanthan A, Reid RL. Religious and cultural influences on contraception. J Obstet Gynaecol Can. 2008;30(2):129–37.
33. Fisher JA, Bowman M, Thomas T. Issues for South Asian Indian patients surrounding sexuality, fertility, and childbirth in the US health care system. J Am Board Fam Pract. 2003;16(2):151–5.
34. Nath DC, Land KC, Goswami G. Effects of the status of women on the first interval in Indian urban society. J Biosoc Sci. 1999;31(01):55–69.

18

Family planning practices of women working in the Cambodian garment industry

Chisato Masuda[1], Elisa Oreglia[2], Sokhey Ly[3], Megan McLaren[4], Caroline Free[5], Camille Tijamo[3], Amra Ou[3], Michelle Helena van Velthoven[1], Amy Williamson[3] and Chris Smith[1,6*]

Abstract

Background: Women working in Cambodian garment factories have unmet needs for family planning (contraception and safe abortion) services, because of their background and living conditions. This study describes their experiences regarding abortion and contraception as part of a larger project to develop an intervention to support comprehensive post-abortion care.

Methods: We conducted semi-structured interviews with women seeking abortion services at private health facilities. In addition, we interviewed the private providers of abortion and contraception services surrounding garment factories. Interviews lasted up to 60 min and were conducted in Khmer and later translated into English. A thematic analysis was undertaken, with medical abortion experiences coded according to the Cambodia comprehensive abortion care protocol.

Results: We interviewed 16 women and 13 providers between August and November 2018. Most women reported being married and had at least one child. Among factory workers the major reported reasons for abortion were birth spacing and financial constraints. Family, friends, or co-workers were the major information resources regarding abortion and contraception, and their positive or negative experiences strongly influenced women's attitude towards both. Medical abortion pills were not always provided with adequate instructions. Half of the participants had a manual vacuum aspiration procedure performed after medical abortion. While women knew the side effects of medical abortion, many did not know the adverse warning signs and the signs of abortion completion. Only three women started post abortion family planning, as most of the women expressed fear and hesitation due to concerns about side effects of modern contraception. Fear of infertility was particularly reported among young women without children.

(Continued on next page)

* Correspondence: christopher.smith@lshtm.ac.uk
[1]School of Tropical Medicine and Global Health, Nagasaki University, Sakamoto 1-12-4, Nagasaki 852-8523, Japan
[6]Clinical Research Department, London School of Hygiene and Tropical Medicine, Keppel Street, London WC1E7HT, UK

(Continued from previous page)
Conclusion: This research shows that in this setting not all women are receiving comprehensive abortion care and contraceptive counselling. Provision of accurate and adequate information about abortion methods and modern contraception was the dominant shortfall in abortion care. Future work to address this gap could involve the development of appropriate interventions and informative tools for women in the Cambodian garment industry such as through existing client contact-centres or social media, including creation of videos or posts on topics that come from clients questions.

Keywords: Family planning services (mesh terms), Medical abortion, Contraception (mesh terms), Long-acting reversible contraception (mesh terms), Contraception, Barrier (mesh terms)

Plain English summary

Women working in Cambodian garment factories may have higher unmet need for family planning than other women in Cambodia. Most garment factory workers are living away from home and are aged under 30. Half have only primary school education. This study describes their experiences of contraception and abortion. We conducted interviews with 16 women seeking abortion services at private health facilities, and 13 private providers surrounding garment factories. Most women were married and had at least one child. Among factory workers the major reported reasons for abortion were birth spacing and financial constraints. Family, friends, or co-workers were the major information resources regarding abortion and contraception, and their positive or negative experiences strongly influenced women's attitude towards both. Medical abortion was not always provided with adequate instructions. While women knew the side effects of medical abortion, many did not know the adverse warning signs and the signs of abortion completion. Only three women started contraception after abortion, as most of the women expressed fear and hesitation of real or perceived side effects associated with modern contraception. Fear of infertility was particularly reported among young women without children. This research shows that in this setting not all women are receiving comprehensive abortion care and contraceptive counselling. Provision of accurate and adequate information about abortion methods and modern contraception was the dominant shortfall in abortion care. Future work needs to address this gap by developing appropriate and effective interventions and informative tools for women in the Cambodian garment industry.

Background

In 2017, an estimated 214 million women in low- and middle-income countries wanted to prevent pregnancy but were not using modern contraceptive methods. Of these women, 155 million used no method and 59 million used a traditional method. Estimates from global surveys indicate that yearly there could be 67 million fewer unintended pregnancies if all needs were met, thus preventing an estimated 36 million abortions and 76,000 maternal deaths [1]. In Cambodia, the use of modern contraception amongst currently married women rose from 19% in 2000 to 39% in 2014, however 18% of women were relying on traditional methods and 12% had an unmet need for family planning in 2014 [2]. More recent projection shows that about half of women using contraception choose short-acting modern methods, less than 25% of women use permanent or long-acting modern methods and slightly more than 25% rely on traditional methods [3]. Modern contraception is widely available in Cambodia, however, fear of side effects and health concerns have been identified as common reasons for non-use or discontinuation [2, 4, 5]. Perceived low risk of pregnancy, for example infrequent sexual activity due to the separation with partner, is another reason for not using contraception [4]. Thus, many Cambodian women remain at risk of unintended pregnancy.

Abortion was legalized in Cambodia in 1997 with the requirement that within the first trimester of pregnancy only qualified healthcare providers in certified health facilities can conduct abortions [6, 7]. Medical abortion, a combination of misoprostol and mifepristone, was approved in 2010 [7, 8], together with the dissemination of a national protocol for Comprehensive Abortion Care (CAC) that outlines the procedures to be followed by health providers to ensure safe abortion care [9]. Between 2010 and 2014, the proportion of medical abortions increased from 31 to 47%, while surgical abortion decreased from about 68 to 60%, and those using a traditional or unspecified method reduced from 3% to almost zero [2, 10]. Conversely, the proportion of women receiving help with abortion from a qualified health provider decreased from about 67% in 2010 to 60% in 2014 [2, 10]. These data indicate that medical abortion is increasing among Cambodian women and they are using it alone and at home. Home-based abortion is regarded as a safe method when adequate measures and support are in place [11]. However, the increasing rate of self-administration of medical abortion in Cambodia raises concerns on whether women are receiving quality comprehensive abortion services by health providers and can manage the process safely.

This study focuses on women working in a garment factory in the capital of Cambodia, Phnom Penh. Garment factories are the biggest manufacturing sector in Cambodia [12]. Roughly 800,000 people work in garment factories in Cambodia, of whom about 85% are female [13, 14]. They are potentially a vulnerable population for reproductive health issues; for example, around 70% are younger than 30 years, half of them have only a primary school education, and most have migrated from rural areas away from their family and community support [14]. According to a survey among female factory workers, they have a higher rate of abortion compared to young women in the national survey, whilst the use of contraception is comparable [2, 4, 15]. This implies that women working in garment factories have unmet needs for family planning (i.e. contraception and safe abortion) services compared with women in the general population [15, 16]. This paper aims to describe women's experiences of abortion and contraception services as part of a larger project to develop an intervention to support comprehensive post-abortion care, which follows from our previous work in Cambodia [17–19].

Methods

Study design

The study was designed as a ground-up exploratory, qualitative study to discover themes and challenges that had not been unearthed by previous research. We thus conducted semi-structured interviews with women working in garment factories to find out about their abortion and contraceptive services seeking behaviour and experience. Additionally, we interviewed private providers of abortion and contraception services to understand the availability of services at the study site and their views on practices and demands for abortion and contraception. The study was a collaboration between academics from different disciplines (medicine, information science and linguistics) and the Non-Governmental Organisation (NGO) Marie Stopes International Cambodia.

Study setting

This qualitative study was conducted from August to November 2018 in a suburb in Phnom Penh where many garment factories cluster. Table 1 provides an overview of the garment factory industry and Table 2 describes private providers of abortion and contraception in Cambodia.

Study population and recruitment process

Private providers were selected as study sites since they are the preferred option of abortion for female garment factory workers in Cambodia [4]. We recruited women seeking abortion services from three private facilities: two medical consulting cabinets and one clinic. One provider had previously worked with Marie Stopes International Cambodia on a project for contraception capacity building (not for abortion services) and the others were directly asked, and agreed, to join the research. The chief or staff of the facility asked women aged ≥18, purchasing medical abortion pills or asking for a surgical abortion, if they were interested in participation. Interested women were introduced to a local researcher working for Marie Stopes International Cambodia who then explained the reasons for the study and the procedure for an interview. When a woman agreed to participate, she was asked for consent by written signature or thumbprint and her telephone number was requested for a follow-up call. Women could end the interview at any time. To protect the privacy and confidentiality of women, we secured a closed private space for the interviews and anonymized all potentially identifying information. Women were given three to four US dollars for their travel expenses and a small towel as a gift.

Additionally, we recruited 13 providers for interviews from two clinics, five medical consulting cabinets, one pharmacy, and three factory infirmaries. Three providers were working at facilities where we recruited women seeking abortion services. Other providers were purposefully selected to involve a variety of types of facilities and providers.

Data collection methods

We developed topic guides (Appendix A and B) and modified them throughout data collection. The interviewers attended a one-day training on qualitative interviews focusing on ethics, obtaining consent from participants, and how to discuss sensitive topics. The less experienced interviewers were always accompanied by the local researcher, who also acted as an interpreter, and were shadowed by either the principle investigator and co-principle investigator for the first interviews. The interviewing teams conducted regular de-briefing after the interviews to discuss the findings as well as the interview experience. The interviews were conducted with simultaneous Khmer language translation by the local researcher who is native in Khmer and proficient in English. The interviews typically lasted 45 to 60 min. All researchers, particularly the local one, spent periods of time around the garment factories to understand the context and made notes of these observations. Interviews were recorded if women consented, transcribed in Khmer and translated into English by a Cambodian research assistant. The local researcher made follow-up calls two and 4 weeks later to women who used medical abortion to ask if the abortion was completed, if they

Table 1 The garment factory industry in Cambodia

Cambodia's garment sector employs about 85% of all Cambodian factory workers and provides 40% of the Gross Domestic Product. The minimum monthly wages of garment factory workers increased from 61 USD in 2012 to 170 USD in 2018 [13]. Workers typically work six days a week from 7 AM to 4 PM with an hour lunch break, unless there is overwork in the evening. They perform a specific task; for example, cutting fabric, stitching clothing, quality checks, or supervising other workers. Garment factory workers in Phnom Penh often share accommodation with relatives or friends within walking distance of the factory. Around the factory, there is usually a market and numerous small restaurants and shops selling commodities [15].

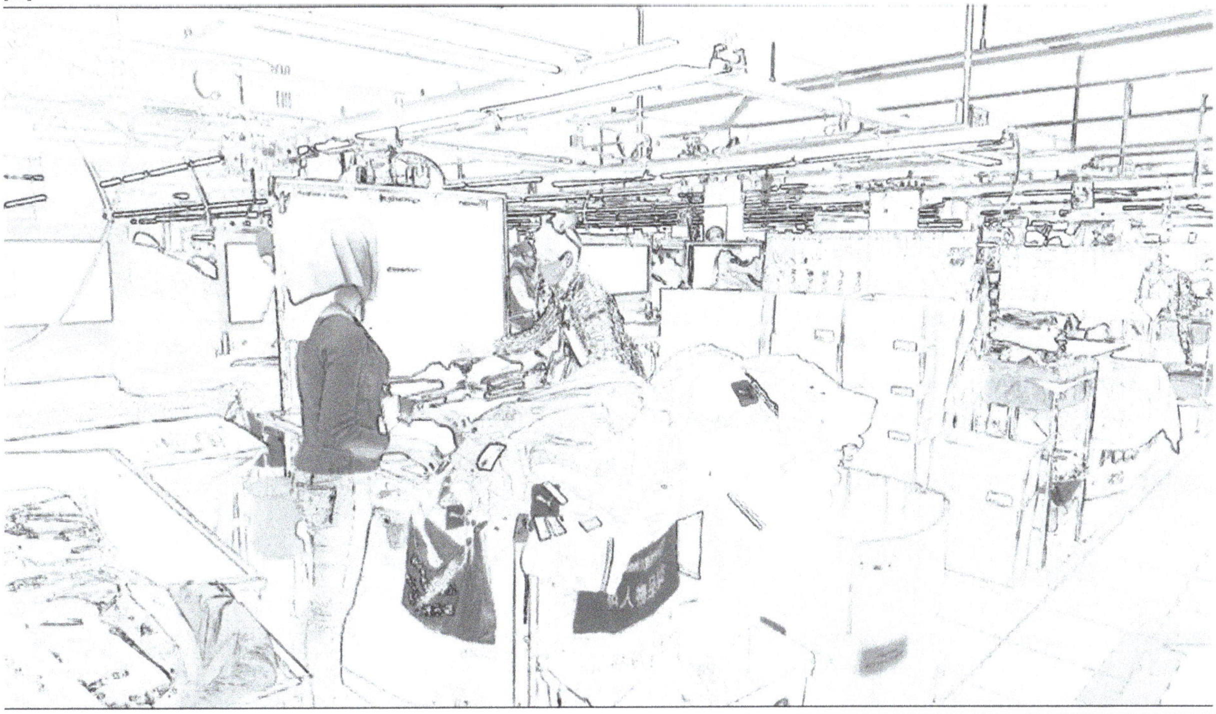

Image shows a garment factory work setting (anonymised)

Table 2 Private providers of abortion and contraception in Cambodia

The private healthcare services relevant to abortion and contraception can be roughly divided into the following types [16, 20].

1. **Medical consulting cabinet** managed by a doctor or a physician assistant. This facility provides general medical consultation and examination and maternal and child health services except for delivery. There is no inpatient space, and any type of surgery is not allowed.

2. **Prenatal consulting cabinet** managed by a secondary midwife with at least three years of professional education. This facility provides antenatal care, health education, and pre- and post-delivery vaccinations. Deliveries are not conducted here.

3. **Clinic or polyclinic** managed by a doctor with at least 5 years of experience who is either retired, has suspended their state service without pay, or has terminated their state service. Such clinics provide examination and consultation of outpatients and inpatients, conduct paramedical analysis, minor and major surgery, vaccinations, health education, maternal healthcare services including delivery and transfusion.

4. **Pharmacy** selling various medications, including medical abortion pills.

5. **Factory infirmary** managed by a doctor and one or two nurses. Factories are obliged to have the infirmary under their human resource department to provide basic medical care for general mild health problems.

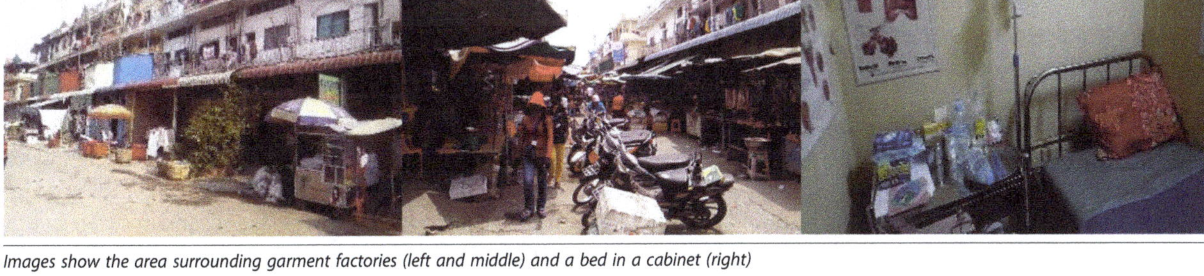

Images show the area surrounding garment factories (left and middle) and a bed in a cabinet (right)

made a follow-up visit, and to inquire about their use or plans for post-abortion contraception. Researchers also reviewed the abortion products, procedures and costs in each clinic in discussion with providers.

Data analysis

Research members individually conducted a thematic analysis of the transcribed interviews using Dedoose software [21]. Two researchers (CM, MM) used predetermined codes from the medical abortion checklist in the Cambodian national protocol for CAC [9]. Two other researchers used a ground-up coding approach (EO, AS) and applied the developed coding frame with themes and subthemes to all interviews. The predetermined and ground-up codes were combined for comprehensiveness. The findings were then organized following a number of the headings from the national protocol on CAC, in particular the example of observation checklist for medical abortion (7 P148) to show qualitative aspects of abortion care that might not surface in quantitative and survey-style research. We did not ask participants to provide feedback on the findings.

Results

Description of participants

Of 24 women seeking abortion who were interested in participation, 16 were interviewed. Eight women initially said to their provider that they wanted to participate but were later busy or had returned to their hometown. Of the 16 interviewees, we able to make follow-up calls with seven. Nine interviewees were not followed up because three had a surgical abortion after medical abortion, three did not provide a working phone number, two did not respond, and one had no time. Twelve women said that this was their first abortion, three their second, and one her fourth. Fifteen women came to Phnom Penh from rural areas of Cambodia. The ages of the women ranged from 21 to 36. Thirteen said that they were married, two divorced, and one was single in a relationship. Among the married women, two lived separately from their husbands. Fourteen women already had children, and the age of their last child ranged from eight months to three years. Twelve women had left children with family in their hometowns. All 13 private providers who we asked to participate in the interview took part: three doctors, four midwives, four nurses, one pharmacist, and one self-employed without a medical background. Nine of the providers were women.

Theme 1: factors influencing abortion-services sought and obtained by women

Theme 1 describes the findings related to abortion seeking behaviour. 'M' is used for women and 'P' for providers.

Sub-theme 1–1. Reasons and decision-making for abortion

Birth-spacing and financial constraints were the main reported reasons for abortion. All thirteen women who were married or in a relationship mentioned they made a joint decision with their husbands or partner and family.

> *M11: I wish to have one more but not now ... may be at the next two years ...*
> *M12: I think that I don't have much money and now have to pay for my daughter's milk ... I made the decision together with my husband ...*
> *M24: After tested, I discussed with my husband whether I have to keep the baby or not ... because it is not the good time for us to have the baby as our living condition is difficult and we are so young ... so we decided to have abortion.*

Sub-theme 1–2. Information sources of abortion

Women generally asked their peers, close co-workers, older family members, or relatives for information and experiences of abortion; in particular, whether to have medical or surgical abortion, and where. Hearing about other women's experiences strongly shaped the expectations, positively or negatively. Only two women said that they never sought information but went directly to the clinic. No woman said that they searched the internet for abortion information, though smartphones are widely used among factory workers.

> *M08: My friend who experienced abortion told me about abortion ... I asked her what and where she did, and she took me to here ...*

Sub-theme 1–3. Available abortion methods

Medical abortion was available at all study sites, except for factory infirmaries, which by law do not provide this service. Based on provider reports and researcher observations, pharmacies, clinics and cabinets had one or more of three pills: Medabon, Mifeso, and a 'Chinese pill' (Zizhu Pharmaceutical). Medabon and Mifeso follow the World Health Organization approved regimen which is 200 mg mifepristone and 800 μg misoprostol (4 tablets of 200 μg) [22]. The regimen of the 'Chinese pill' is two tablets of mifepristone (25 mg per tablet) for 3 days and three tablets of misoprostol (0.2 mg per tablet) on the third day. Manual Vacuum Aspiration (MVA), was available at some clinics and cabinets.

One provider reported that women typically come to have abortion on Friday or Saturday, as the process would take place during the weekend and women could return to work on Monday to avoid losing income.

Sub-theme 1–4. Cost for abortion

Women reported that Medabon or Mifeso cost between 12 and 20 US dollars (USD), sometimes with an additional charge of 5 to 30 USD for vitamin injections. MVA was provided for 60 to 200 USD. One woman reported paying 200 USD, including both medical and surgical abortion, but was satisfied with the quality of services.

> *M21: I feel ok ... not so painful ... strong enough after got service here ... I thought 200 USD is not important if I am better like this ...*

To put these amounts in context, the minimum monthly wage of a factory worker in Cambodia is USD170 [23].

Sub-theme 1–5. Selection of abortion methods

Half of the women received MVA, for the following reasons: more than 9 weeks pregnant, incomplete abortion, health care providers' advice or it was automatically included in the abortion service. Some women preferred MVA because they thought that it was cleaner and safer than medical abortion, or they did not want to come back for a follow-up or in the case of complications. Few women considered the risk of MVA as an invasive procedure and most women were afraid that medical abortion would result in an incomplete abortion.

> *M07: The provider said it is better to use vacuum aspiration...For medical abortion, I might have some difficulties when I face some problem after using it ... it will be difficult to come back again if it doesn't work well ...*

Theme 2: Women's experiences of abortion mapped against the CAC observation checklist for medical abortion

Abortion provider in Cambodia should adhere to the national protocol for CAC. Theme 2 describes women's experiences alongside the standards set by CAC.

Sub-theme 2–1. CAC task 1 – "Greets woman with respect and kindness, helps her feel comfortable and ensures privacy"

Women reported that privacy was an important factor in selecting a provider; for instance, they preferred larger providers because they afraid smaller ones may not be able to maintain confidentiality and would be less safe. Some younger and unmarried women sought a provider away from their living or working area, so that they would not encounter anyone they knew. Providers said that women never openly asked for an abortion, rather, the subject was broached indirectly.

> *P05: They just ask for a pregnancy test ... and they added that "after I did the pregnancy test, may I see you again ...".*

Sub-theme 2–2. CAC task 2 – "Assesses the woman's health: medical and reproductive history, estimates gestation based on date of last menstruation period, assess vital signs"

In this study, all women who used medical abortion were less than 9 weeks pregnant. Most women were aware of their menstrual cycle and confirmed the pregnancy immediately after they missed their period or felt morning sickness. The most common way to estimate gestational age was ultrasound, but some declined due to the cost. Four women were asked their Last Menstruation Period (LMP). No woman had a pelvic examination.

> *M13: I didn't do ultrasound ... because I missed period about 10 days ... he (provider) asked me to do ultrasound ... but I rejected as I didn't want to spend lots of money ($5 USD).*

One provider said that some clients who were over 2 months pregnant came to purchase medical abortion whilst pretending to be less than 2 months pregnant, or asked someone else to buy the drugs.

Sub-theme 2–3. CAC task 3 – "Discuss reproductive goals, including pregnancy and family planning options"

When women came to providers, most had already decided to have an abortion following discussion with their husband or family, and the decision was respected by the providers. One woman, however, told us that:

> *M24: The provider said I should have a baby now because I am young and have more energy now ... she wants me to keep the baby rather than to have abortion ...*

This was the only case of possible provider bias that we encountered.

Sub-theme 2–4. CAC task 4 – "Provide detailed information about medication-abortion side effects, warning signs, required visits and action in the event of failure of procedure"

Some women reported knowing side effects of medical abortion such as fever, exhaustion, diarrhoea, vomiting, and pain; and they received that information from providers, friends, or relatives. Most women knew that they would bleed for a few days after inserting misoprostol and needed to contact providers in case of severe bleeding. Two women experienced heavy bleeding and both visited a provider.

M19(Note): she returned to doctor on next day of inserting pills because a lot of black bleeding and much pain, used sanitary pad every hour, was very exhausted and could not eat well.

Infirmary workers encountered factory workers who came to the infirmary with serious abdominal pain, possibly caused by an incomplete abortion. Those women tried to be discreet and asked for painkillers for menstruation, although the bleeding was heavier than a normal menstruation.

Sub-theme 2–5. CAC task 5 – "Explains all aspects of the medication administration regimen, including pain management"

Most women using medical abortion were told to insert misoprostol the day after taking mifepristone. A few women took mifepristone and misoprostol on the same day, with the provider helping to insert the misoprostol. A booklet with instructions, side effects, and warning signs was available at some facilities, but some women preferred not to take any written materials for fear that other people would find out they had an abortion. Four women were provided with pain medication.

Sub-theme 2–6. CAC task 6 – "Provides emergency contact information in case the woman has questions or needs care"

Most providers gave their phone number to women and told them to call if they had a problem or needed more information. Some women returned or called providers if they were afraid of bleeding or pain.

Sub-theme 2–7. CAC task 9 – "Schedules follow-up visit to confirm completion of the medication abortion"

Most women did not return for follow-up if they did not encounter a problem. Some women who used medical abortion asked providers for a surgical abortion to ensure completion of abortion.

P04: Clients came here seeking for cleaning (surgical abortion) to make sure if it is completed since they just saw bleeding without anything.

Only a few women knew the signs of completion of medical abortion, and their knowledge was based on their previous abortion or miscarriage.

M13: I noticed it had serious bleeding and it came out along with tissue ... as remembered, when there is a miscarriage there are also coagulated blood come out and the size is about the size of a toe ...

Sub-theme 2–8. CAC task 8 – "Ensures contraceptive counselling and a method are provided if requested"

Not all women received contraceptive counselling after abortion. Some said they were informed about pills, injection, and intrauterine device (IUD), and a few women reported being advised to use traditional methods such as the calendar method. Women sought information from family members, friends, or elders in their community. Some women received contraceptive counselling at the health centre in their province after giving birth.

Of the seven women who could be followed up after abortion, three started to use modern contraception; one each of the pill, injection, and IUD. Two reasons given for not using modern contraception after abortion were still feeling weak or infrequent sex due to separation from partner.

M07: No, I have not used any contraception yet...I thought my health is still weak...we are not too often having sex...

Some women said they continued using traditional methods since they were afraid of infertility caused by using modern contraception, particularly by pills.

M24: I have learnt that one of my neighbours who used pills had uterus problem ... when she wanted to have a baby, she could not have a baby for about ten years ...

Women's' partners sometimes objected to using modern contraception because they thought that it may negatively affect their health or cause uterus problems.

M24: Actually, my husband uses the natural method (withdrawal) ... and he doesn't want me to use any other methods because we've just newly married ... he is worried that it affects my health....

Discussion

Most women seeking abortion in this study were married and had children, suggesting unmet need for contraception among female factory workers who already have children. This aligns with the data from the Cambodia demographic survey [2]. The main reasons for abortion in this study were birth spacing and financial constraints, which are same with the most common reasons for having an abortion in other countries [24]. Our findings further highlight the socio-economic context and factory work affecting the decision, such as working long hours away from their families and insufficient financial security.

Ultrasound was the most common method to determine the gestational age in our study, but some women declined it due to the cost. Gestational age can be accurately estimated based on last menstrual period and physical examination together [6, 22], therefore providers should be able to estimate the gestational age without using ultrasound. The CAC protocol rightly emphasizes the importance of clear, comprehensive, and sensitive communication with women seeking abortion services [9]. There was only one report of possible provider bias when it was recommended that the woman should continue with the pregnancy. Although we do not know how widespread this attitude is, some qualitative studies reported that provider's attitudes and values to abortion strongly affect the availability of abortion services [25, 26]. This possible provider bias in Cambodia could impede younger and women without a child from accessing safe abortion services. The National Strategy for Reproductive and Sexual Health in Cambodia 2017–2020 identifies "information" as a key area to address in order to continue making progress to strengthen safe abortion services [27]. However, it was difficult to clarify whether providers gave accurate and adequate information to women to decide on an abortion methods in our study. Half of the women underwent MVA, as it was viewed as a safer and quicker option. This preference for MVA is similar with findings in other papers [8, 28], but women in our study were not always sufficiently informed about the pros and cons of both methods. The desire to complete the abortion during weekends to minimise time off work was an important factor for factory workers in deciding the timing and methods of abortion. Reluctance to attend follow-up appointments was another reasons for choosing MVA. Similarly, detailed instruction and the process of medical abortion were not well explained. Many women did not know the signs of abortion completion and did not have enough confidence in dealing with bleeding and pain. As a result, some women returned to the provider for a surgical abortion. Only three women started post abortion family planning. Many women expressed fear and hesitation to use modern contraception as reported in previous papers [5, 29, 30], with some reporting a belief that contraceptive pills make women infertile. Most of the interviewees knew about modern contraceptive methods, which is in line with the result of a national survey among the general population and a survey among factory workers [2, 4]. However, contraception knowledge was mostly obtained from family or friends. In addition to concerns about side-effects, the infrequent sex due to separation from husbands affected the decision not to use contraception, which is consistent with a previous survey among factory workers [4].

Based on the findings from this study, we recommend two main areas for future work. The first is regarding provision of accurate and adequate information about abortion methods and modern contraception. Provision of detailed information about medical abortion procedure can be improved to empower women to manage the process by themselves. WHO's guideline recognises that women can play an essential role in the use of medical abortion, under certain conditions in which access to appropriate information and back-up health care facilities are ensured [31]. A previous study reported that effective counselling can offer women a sense of confidence by helping them prepare for possible side effects and complications [32]. A booklet with instructions was provided to woman using medical abortion. However, it was perceived to be indiscreet and few women took it, as has been reported elsewhere [32]. Therefore alternative means should be considered and future work needs to explore effective ways to deliver appropriate information privately and refer women to safe providers, such as via call-centres or social media. There is a need for reliable information on modern contraception, which can be delivered by qualified healthcare providers through in-person and alternative methods. The quality of family planning counselling should be improved to clarify the any misconceptions surrounding modern contraception and to focus on women's actual lifestyle and needs. In response to the findings of this study, we developed short videos on modern contraceptive methods and how to take medical abortion. The videos are available on the Facebook page of MSI Cambodia, and an evaluation of their impact will be reported in a separate paper. Second, there is a need to increase the opportunity to provide family planning counselling and services for married women with children. In our study most women with unmet need for family planning in Cambodia already had a child suggesting that services for married women with children should be strengthened. Women with children have several opportunities to visit health facilities for antenatal care, delivery, postnatal care, and immunizations, therefore health care providers should utilise these opportunities to provide family planning services. A study in the Philippines found that most women who wish to delay pregnancy missed the opportunity to receive family planning counselling during their public facility visits [33]. Improving the availability and quality of family planning counselling at health facilities can increase the use of contraception and reduce unintended pregnancies among women with children.

This study has some strengths and limitations. A strength of this study derives from our thorough knowledge of the Cambodian garment factory setting and the multi-disciplinary approach. The interviewers spent periods of time around the garment factories, which helped us to understand the living condition of factory workers and be sensitive to the local culture. Limitations of this study include that the sensitive nature of the research topic might have influenced the woman's decision to participate in the interview and the responses that they gave. Most of our interviewees were married. Single or unmarried women might have hesitated to participate since pregnancy outside of marriage is not socially acceptable in Cambodia [2]. In addition, characteristics of researchers such as their gender and nationality might have influenced interaction with research participants. We tried to mitigate this by alternating the foreign researchers conducting the interviews, while always having a local researcher present as translator and facilitator, and by triangulating with secondary sources and other material from our NGO partner. Some women who knew the local Marie Stopes clinic might have trusted the interviewers and may have been more inclined to participate or talk about their concerns to interviewers. We did not interview women attending public healthcare services, because garment factory workers typically seek abortions at private healthcare services which are perceived as "friendly, confidential and clean" [4, 29].

Conclusion

In conclusion, this paper described the factors influencing on seeking the abortion services and abortion experiences among women working in garment factories. While abortion and contraception services are widespread and affordable, not all women are receiving comprehensive abortion care and contraceptive counselling. Future work to address this gap could involve the development of appropriate interventions and informative tools for women in the Cambodian garment industry such as through existing client contact-centres or social media, including creation of videos or posts on topics that come from clients questions.

Interview guide for women seeking MA

Background information

What is your age?

Where are you from?

How long have you been in Phnom Penh?

Where do you work and what is your role? (Don't need specifics of factory)

How is your work?

Relationships and living situation

Are you married?

If no: do you have a relationship?

Do you have children?

How many?

How old are they?

Where do they live?

Relationships and living situation *(Continued)*

What sort of accommodation do you live in?

Who do you live with?

MA decision-making, expectations and information seeking

Have you had an abortion before?

When did you realise you were pregnant this time?

How did you realise you were pregnant?

What happened after that?FeelingsFurther confirmation soughtWho discussed it withWhy decided to have an abortion this timeDo you think this is a common reason for women to have abortion here?

How did you decide what to do?Did you talk to your family or friends?How did you make the decision?

Why did you choose this provider?

How did you learn about MA?Do you have any friends or family who have had MA?What was their experience?

Why did you choose MA instead of another way?

If have not taken MA yet:

Did you come with anyone today?

When do you think you will take the MA?

What do you expect to happen when you take the MA?

Have you been told will happen?Who has told you this?What has the provider said?

How will you manage it?

What will you do if you need more advice?

Will you need to take any time off work?

What are your feelings about taking it?

If have taken MA already:

Did you come with anyone to get the MA?

When did you take the MA?

What happened next?If any decisions made or further care sought: ask about these and why

How did you manage the bleeding?Did you use any products?How much did these cost?

Did you take any time off work?

Was the MA process what you expected?What did the provider tell you?Did anyone else tell you what to expect?

What were your feelings about taking MA?

Did anyone help you at home?

Attitudes and barriers around MA

Was it easy or hard to come to buy MA?Why was it easy/hard?What would have made it better for you?

Attitudes and barriers around MA *(Continued)*

Who would you tell and who would you not tell?Would you tell your friends?
Do people here think abortion is a bad thing?Who says this?

If have not taken MA yet:

Do you know how much the cost is?Will anyone help you pay?
Did you have to pay for transport here?

If have taken MA already:

What were the biggest challenges to taking MA?
How much did the MA (/MVA) cost?Did anyone help you pay?Did you have to pay for anything else? Transport?

Contraception

Have you used contraception before?
If yes: which methods?How long for?What was your experience of it?Why did you stop using it?
If no: why do you not use contraception?
Do you plan to use any contraception after the abortion?
If yes: do you know which method you will have?Do you know when you will get it?Do you know where?*If reported side effects:* do you know what you will do if you get the side effects?
If no: why not?How will you prevent pregnancy?Do you know which methods are available?
How do you make decisions about FP?Where would you get information about FP?Have you ever seen any videos or information online about FP?Do you and your friends ever talk about contraception?What contraception do your friends use?What do they say about it?

General life questions

What are your plans for the future with your family and your work?
Do you have a mobile phone?What type is it?What do you use it for?
How do you enjoy yourself on your day off?

Is there anything you want to ask us?

Interview guide for private providers

MA provision

How long they have been providing MA
Available types of drug for MA
Approximate number of clients per week
Information given to clients

Training

What formal training they have been given
How they keep up to date
What support they would like

Post-abortion care and support

Post-abortion issues encountered
Post-abortion care provided
Suggestions for interventions

Abbreviations

CAC: Comprehensive abortion care; MVA: Manual vacuum aspiration; IUD: Intrauterine device; LMP: Last menstruation period

Acknowledgements

We would like to appreciate many clients, factory managers and private providers who contributed to this study. We would also like to thank Marie Stopes International Cambodia for significant cooperation in the entire process of this study. Lastly, we would like to show our gratitude to Professor Tung Rathavy, Director of the National Centre for Maternal and Child Health Centre, for conceptualization and inputs on this study.

Authors' contributions

CM, EO, MM, LS, CF, CT, OA and CS contributed the conception and design of the research. CM, MM, LS, CS contributed the acquisition of data. CM, EO, MM and CS analysed and interpreted the data. CM have drafted the manuscript. EO, MV, CS substantively revised the manuscript. All authors read and approved the final manuscript.

Author's information

The local researcher who conducted interview is a local midwife working in Marie Stopes International Cambodia.

Author details

[1]School of Tropical Medicine and Global Health, Nagasaki University, Sakamoto 1-12-4, Nagasaki 852-8523, Japan. [2]Kings College London, London, UK. [3]Marie Stopes International Cambodia, Phnom Penh, Cambodia. [4]Marie Stopes International, London, UK. [5]Department of Population Health, London School of Hygiene and Tropical Medicine, Keppel Street, London WC1E7HT, UK. [6]Clinical Research Department, London School of Hygiene and Tropical Medicine, Keppel Street, London WC1E7HT, UK.

References

1. Guttmacher Institute. Adding it up: investing in contraception and maternal and newborn health. New York: Guttmacher Institute; 2017. https://www.guttmacher.org/fact-sheet/adding-it-up-contraception-mnh-2017. Accessed 25 Sep 2019.
2. National Institute of Statistics of Cambodia, Directorate General for Health of Cambodia, ICF International. Cambodia Demographic and Health Survey 2014. Phnom Penh: National Institute of Statistics of Cambodia, Directorate General for Health of Cambodia, ICF International; 2015. https://dhsprogram.com/publications/publication-FR312-DHS-Final-Reports.cfm. Accessed25 Sep 2019.
3. United Nations, United Nations Department of Economic and Social Affairs, Population Division. Contraceptive Use by Method 2019: Data booklet: United Nations; 2019. https://www.un.org/development/desa/pd/sites/www.un.org.development.desa.pd/files/files/documents/2020/Jan/un_2019_contraceptiveusebymeth/;od_databooklet.pdf. Accessed 25 Sep 2019.

4. Partnering to Save Lives, Angkor Research and Consulting Ltd. End line Survey of Reproductive, Maternal and Neonatal Health Knowledge, Attitudes and Practices among Garment Factory Workers. Phnom Penh; 2018. p. 2018. https://www.dfat.gov.au/sites/default/files/cambodia-partnering-to-save-lives-endline-survey-report-june-2018.pdf. Accessed 25 Sep 2019.
5. Hancart PP, Desclaux A. Reproductive health and HIV in Cambodia from anthropology to public health: Groupe de Recherche Culture Santé Sociétés, Sidaction, ANRS; 2010. https://hal.archives-ouvertes.fr/file/index/docid/566335/filename/Hancart_Desclaux_2010.pdf. Accessed 25 Sep 2019.
6. Cambodia passes new limits on abortion. Reproductive Free news.1997; 6(17): 7. https://www.ncbi.nlm.nih.gov/pubmed/12292784. Accessed 25 Sep 2019.
7. Hancart PP. Abortion politics in Cambodia social history, local forms and transnational issues. Global Public Health. 2018;13(6):692–701.
8. Hancart PP, Ith L, Cockroft M, Delvaux T. Towards safe abortion access: an exploratory study of medical abortion in Cambodia. Reprod Health Matters. 2015;22:47–55.
9. Ministry of Health of the Kingdom of Cambodia. National Protocol Comprehensive Abortion Care. 2010. https://abortion-policies.srhr.org/documents/countries/03-Cambodia-National-Protocol-Comprehensive-Abortion-Care-2010.pdf. Accessed25 Sep 2019.
10. National Institute of Statistics of Cambodia, Directorate General for Health, ICF Marco. Cambodia Demographic and Health Survey 2010. Phnom Penh: National Institute of Statistics of Cambodia, Directorate General for Health, and ICF Marco; 2011. https://dhsprogram.com/pubs/pdf/FR249/FR249.pdf. Accessed 25 Sep 2019.
11. Ngo TD, Park MH, Shakur H, Free C. Comparative effectiveness, safety and acceptability of medical abortion at home and in a clinic: a systematic review. Bull World Health Organ. 2011;89(5):360–70.
12. World Bank. Cambodia. https://data.worldbank.org/country/cambodia. Accessed25 Sep 2019.
13. Spies R. A sector too big to fail? Phnom Penh Post. 2018; https://www.phnompenhpost.com/business/sector-too-big-fail. Accessed 25 Sep 2019.
14. International Labour Organization, International Finance Corporation. Better Factories Cambodia. In: Towards Gender Equality Lessons from factory compliance assessments 2017–2018. Geneva: International Finance Corporation; 2018. https://betterwork.org/wp-content/uploads/2018/04/Toward-Gender-Equality-2017-18.pdf. Accessed 25 Sep 2019.
15. United Nation Population Fund. Literature review on sexual and reproductive health and rights of migrant garment factory Workers in Cambodia. 2014. https://cambodia.unfpa.org/sites/default/files/pub-pdf/SRHRofGarmentFactoryWorkerLiteratureReview_2.pdf. Accessed 25 Sep 2019.
16. Heng M, Ashish B, Chhorvann C, Bandeth R, Sopheab H, Hyunwoo JC. "Health needs, health seeking pathways, and drivers of health seeking behaviors of female garment factory Workers in Cambodia: findings from a qualitative study in Phnom Penh and Kandal provinces" policy brief. Washington DC and Phnom Penh, Cambodia: Population Council; 2017. http://evidenceproject.popcouncil.org/wp-content/uploads/2017/05/Policy-Brief-on-Health-Needs_20171.pdf. Accessed 25 Sep 2019.
17. Smith C, Scott RH, Free C, Edwards T. Characteristics and contraceptive outcomes of women seeking medical or surgical abortion in reproductive health clinics in Cambodia. Contracept Reprod Med. 2019;4:5.
18. Smith C, Ngo TD, Gold J, Edwards P, Vannak U, Sokhey L, et al. Effect of a mobile phone-based intervention on post-abortion contraception: a randomized controlled trial in Cambodia. Bull World Health Organ. 2015; 93(12):842–850A.
19. Smith C, Sokhey L, Vannak U, Warnock R, Free C. Women's views and experiences of a mobile phone-based intervention to support post-abortion contraception in Cambodia. Reprod Health. 2017;14(1):72.
20. Ministry of Health of the Kingdom of Cambodia. The Procedure and technical conditions set in the request to open or close transform or relocate private medical paramedical and medical aid services. 2001.
21. Dedoose Version 8.0.35. web application for managing, analysing, and presenting qualitative and mixed method research data. Los Angeles: Socio Cultural Research Consultants, LLC; 2018. www.dedoose.com. Accessed 25 Sep 2019.
22. World Health Organization. Medical management of abortion. Geneva: World Health Organization; 2018. https://apps.who.int/iris/bitstream/handle/10665/278968/9789241550406-eng.pdf?ua=1. Accessed 25 Sep 2019.
23. Schill A. The Footwear Sector - New Opportunities for Cambodia?. Cambodia Garment and Footwear Sector Bulletin. Int Labour Organisation. 2019;9 https://www.ilo.org/asia/publications/issue-briefs/WCMS_714915/lang%2D%2Den/index.htm. Accessed 02 May 2020.
24. Singh S, Remez L, Sedgh G, Kwok L, Onda T. Abortion Worldwide 2017: Uneven progress and unequal access. New York: Guttmacher Institute; 2018. https://wwwguttmacherorg/report/abortion-worldwide-2017 Accessed 25 Sep 2019.
25. Antieye P, Mayhew SH. Shaping legal abortion provision in Ghana: Using policy theory to understand provider-related obstacles to policy implementation. Health Res Policy Syst. 2013;11(23).
26. Harries J, Cooper D, Strebel A, Clovin CJ. Conscientious objection and its impact on abortion service provision in South Africa: a qualitative study. Reprod Health. 2014;11(16).
27. Ministry of Health of the Kingdom of Cambodia National Maternal and Child Health Centre National Reproductive Health Programme. National Reproductive Health Programme, vol. 2017. Phnom Penh: National Strategy for Reproductive and Sexual Health in Cambodia 2017-2020. https://cambodia.unfpa.org/sites/default/files/pub-pdf/Final_RSH_Strategy_2017_2020_ENG_%2830May2017%29%20pdf.pdf. Accessed 25 Sep 2019.
28. Kanstrup C, Mäkelä M, Hauskov GA. Women's reasons for choosing abortion method: a systematic literature review. Scand J Public Health. 2017;46(8): 835–45.
29. Hemmings J, Rolfe B. ABORTION IN CAMBODIA care seeking for abortion and family planning services: findings from a PEER study, conducted with women in Phnom Penh and Kandal provinces. Options Consultancy Services Ltd; 2008.
30. Sadana R, Snow R. Balancing effectiveness, side-effects and work: women's perceptions and experiences with modern contraceptive technology in Cambodia. Soc Sci Med. 1999;49(3):343–58.
31. World Health Organization. Health worker roles in providing safe abortion care and post-abortion contraception. Geneva: World Health Organization; 2015. https://www.who.int/reproductivehealth/publications/unsafe_abortion/abortion-task-shifting/en/ Accessed 6 July 2020.
32. Wainwright M, Colvin C, Swartz A, Leon N. Self-management of medical abortion: a qualitative evidence synthesis. Reprod Health Matters. 2016; 24(47):155–67.
33. Nagai M, Bellizzi S, Murray J, Kitong J, Cabral E, Sobel H. Opportunities lost: barriers to increasing the use of effective contraception in the Philippines. PLoS One. 2019;14(7):e0218187. https://doi.org/10.1371/journal.pone.0218187.

Task shifting levonorgestrel implant insertion to community midwife assistants in Malawi: Results from a non-inferiority evaluation

Dylane N. Davis[1], Clara Lemani[1], Nenani Kamtuwanje[1], Billy Phiri[1], Prisca Masepuka[1], Sally Kuchawo[1], Nivedita L. Bhushan[1,3] and Jennifer H. Tang[1,2*]

Abstract

Background: In 2013, Malawi began task shifting long acting reversible contraception (LARC) insertion from Nurse Midwife Technicians (NMTs), who undergo 3 years of training, to Community Midwife Assistants (CMAs), who undergo 18 months of training. However, there is no evidence on whether CMAs have the same competency as NMTs for LARC insertion. Therefore, we describe a non-inferiority evaluation to determine whether CMAs are non-inferior to NMTs for the insertion of levonorgestrel (LNG) contraceptive implants in Malawi.

Methods: One CMA and one matched NMT from 31 health centers across Malawi were selected for training in Malawi's 1-week LARC insertion course in October 2016, and 31 CMAs and 30 NMTs completed the training. After the course, two Family Planning Master Trainers visited the nurses' health centers over a 5-month period and used the Malawi LNG implant insertion checklist to evaluate the first five LNG implant insertions that each nurse performed during the monitoring visit. A non- inferiority margin of 10% was used to compare mean implant scores between CMAs and NMTs.

Results: We were able to fully evaluate 29 CMAs and 29 NMTs with the LNG implant insertion checklist. The CMAs and NMTs had mean scores of 90.2% and 89.7%, respectively, which were non-inferior (mean difference – 0.5%; 95% CI -3.4%, 2.4%), even when adjusted for the number of years post-graduation and the number of LNG implants inserted pre-training, during training, and since training (mean difference 1.3%; 95% CI -2.2%, 4.8%).

Conclusions: CMAs were non-inferior to NMTs with LNG implant insertion, and both cadres were generally observed to be competent with their insertions after completing their follow-up evaluations. During the evaluations, we generally saw an increase in scores with each insertion. Therefore, for both cadres, it is important to establish continued mentorship and evaluation for LARC insertion after the initial training.

Keywords: Contraception, Nurses, Assessment, Developing countries, Family planning, Health workers

* Correspondence: jennifer_tang@med.unc.edu
[1]UNC Project-Malawi, c/o Kamuzu Central Hospital, 100 Mzimba Road, Private Bag, A-104 Lilongwe, Malawi
[2]Department of Obstetrics & Gynecology, University of North Carolina at Chapel Hill, 100 Manning Drive, Chapel Hill, North Carolina, 27599-7570 CB-7570, USA

Background

Widespread shortages in healthcare providers have led to uneven distribution of healthcare access, particularly in rural settings and in countries with limited resources [1]. To circumvent this challenge, many countries have created new health cadres with fewer years of training so that more providers can be quickly trained and improve access to health services [2]. Task shifting various responsibilities and procedures to these new cadres has been proposed as a way of offloading tasks and roles from more highly trained providers so that they can focus more on the difficult and specialized cases and procedures [3]. A particular emphasis has been made on task shifting maternal and newborn health care, such as family planning (FP), to improve maternal and neonatal health access and outcomes [4].

According to the WHO, there is a current estimation of 3420 bedside midwives in Malawi, a population to midwife ratio of 5058:1, which is far higher than the recommended population to midwife ratio of 175:1 [5]. An additional 20,217 bedside midwives are needed to sufficiently address the country's health needs [5]. Malawi has thus created various auxiliary health cadres, such as Nurse Midwife Technicians (NMTs) and Health Surveillance Assistants (community health workers known as HSAs), to supplement the traditional cadres of Registered Nurses and Registered Nurse Midwives.

The newest auxiliary health cadre created in Malawi is the Community Midwife Assistant (CMA). CMAs receive 18 months of training post-secondary school and receive a certificate after completion of their studies [6]. In comparison, the NMTs receive 3 years of training and receive a diploma after completion. In Malawi, NMTs deliver the majority of FP services. They are trained to provide both short-acting and long-acting reversible contraception (LARC). However, with the growing need of personnel to deliver FP services to patients, task shifting such services from NMTs to CMAs has been considered as a potential strategy to fulfill the growing population's FP needs, and CMAs were approved to insert and provide LARC in 2013.

To help countries develop and implement task shifting programs, the WHO developed a guidance document in 2012 with "evidence-based recommendations to facilitate universal access to key, effective maternal and newborn interventions," including recommendations for FP [4]. While the WHO recommends that Registered Nurses and Diploma Nurses (such as NMTs) should be allowed to insert and remove contraceptive implants, they recommend that Auxiliary Nurse Midwives (such as CMAs) should only insert and remove implants "with targeted monitoring and evaluation" [4]. This recommendation was made because there is limited evidence about the effectiveness of allowing Auxiliary Nurse Midwives to insert and remove implants. There is currently no published evidence as to whether CMAs are competent at inserting and removing implants.

Intervention description

In light of the limited evidence for Auxiliary Nurse Midwives such as CMAs to insert contraceptive implants, we conducted a non-inferiority study to assess whether CMAs were competent at inserting the 5-year levonorgestrel (LNG) implants and whether they had similar competency as NMTs with inserting LNG implants in Malawi.

Methods

Study design

There were 200 CMAs selected by their communities, the Malawi Safe Motherhood Initiative Program, and UNC and financially sponsored for training in Malawi between 2014 and 2016 in part from the authors' institute and a foundation. Of these 200 CMAs, 31 were selected by the Malawi Ministry of Health (MoH) for deployment in October 2016 to a rural health center in the district from which they originated. For our study, we planned to train these 31 CMAs in the 1-week MoH-approved LARC insertion course in October 2016, which was provided in addition to their prior CMA training. During these trainings, we also planned to train 31 matched NMTs, one each from the same rural health center that each CMA was to be deployed.

The LARC training involved two days of didactics and then three days of practical sessions in a government health center. Each training had approximately 15 trainees and 3 trainers as per MoH guidelines. After the training, the CMAs and NMTs returned to their assigned health center. Two UNC Project-Malawi NMT Master FP Trainers then traveled to each of the health centers to evaluate the trained CMAs and NMTs in LNG implant insertion using the MoH-approved LNG Implant Insertion Checklist (Additional file 1) from November 2016 to March 2017. We were unable to evaluate nurse competency for LNG implant removal, etonorgestrel (ENG) implant insertion and removal, and intrauterine device insertion and removals due to the minimal request in the clinics for these contraceptives. The LNG Implant Insertion Checklist consists of a total of 63 assessments for a total of 63 points and includes assessment of pre-insertion counseling, screening, and preparation; insertion technique; and post-insertion tasks, including post-insertion counseling. For each CMA and NMT that could be reached during our evaluation time period, our two Master FP Trainers evaluated the first five LNG implant insertions that occurred during their monitoring visit.

Sample size calculation

The Malawi MoH deems competency in LNG implant insertion if the trainee has scored at least 85% on the LNG Implant Insertion Checklist. Therefore, for our sample size calculation, we assumed that the NMTs would have a mean LNG insertion score of 95%. We then set the non-inferiority margin at 10% so that the CMAs would still be above the 85% minimum score to meet MoH standards if they were non-inferior. To detect non-inferiority with 90% power and a one-sided alpha of 0.025, we estimated that a sample size of 200 (100 per group) would be needed. We then adjusted for clustering to account for multiple observations for the same individual. Specifically, each trained NMT and CMA would serve as their own cluster for their five scores. Using an expected intra-class correlation of 0.05, we found that we needed to have at least 115 LNG implant insertions in each group, or at least four LNG insertions per nurse if all 62 pre-selected nurses were evaluated. To account for potential loss-to-follow-up among our 62 nurses, we opted to evaluate 5 insertions per nurse to ensure that we had at least 115 insertions in each group.

Data analysis

Fisher's exact test was utilized to compare baseline characteristics between the CMAs and NMTs. We then averaged the first five evaluated scores of each CMA and each NMT to determine if each cadre was competent (mean score > 85%) for LNG implant insertion. Generalized linear models were used to evaluate if CMAs had a mean LNG implant insertion score that was within the 10% non-inferiority margin of the NMT LNG implant insertion score. Non-inferiority (NI) would be demonstrated if the lower confidence limit for the difference in mean percent of average implant insertion scores between the two cadres of nurses lay above $-\Delta$ NI = − 10. We ran both an unadjusted and adjusted models to account for the number of years since graduation and number of LNG implant insertions performed pre-training, during training, and since training by the end of their monitoring visit. The sample size and data analysis calculations were all performed using STATA, Version 11 (College Station, TX, USA).

Results

Nurse characteristics

During our LARC training in October 2016, we trained all 31 of our UNC-sponsored CMAs and 31 other health providers (29 NMTs, 1 Senior Nursing Officer, and 1 Medical Assistant) from each of their health centers. Two health centers did not have an NMT who had been previously trained in LARC insertion before, so they sent other qualified providers (a Senior Nursing Officer and a Medical Assistant, both of whom are considered qualified to place LNG implants in Malawi) instead for the training. In addition, one of the 31 pre-selected NMTs did not show up for the training.

During the 5-month evaluation period (November 2016–March 2017), we were able to evaluate at least 5 LNG implant insertions on 93.5% (29 of 31) of the CMAs and 96.7% (29 of 30) of the other trained health providers. We were unable to assess 1 CMA and 1 NMT due to travel conditions, and 1 CMA due to low clinical volume.

The CMAs and other nurse providers came from 14 of the 28 districts and from all 3 regions of Malawi (Table 1, Fig. 1). The CMAs were from a younger age

Table 1 Community Midwife Assistant and Nurse Midwife Technician characteristics

Characteristics (*N* = 58)	CMA (*N* = 29)		NMT (*N* = 29)		Fisher's Exact Test
Age					0.042
< 24	14	(48.3)	5	(17.2)	
25–30	11	(37.9)	16	(55.1)	
> 32	4	(13.8)	8	(27.6)	
District					1.000
North Rumphi, Likoma	5	(17.2)	5	(17.2)	
Central Lilongwe, Kasungu, Ntchisi	10	(34.5)	10	(34.5)	
South Blantyre, Zomba, Mulanje, Machinga, Balaka, Thyolo, Neno, Phalombe, Mangochi	14	(48.3)	14	(48.3)	
Years since graduation from school					< 0.001
< 1 year	28	(96.6)	7	(24.1)	
1–5 years	1	(3.5)	9	(31.0)	
5–10 years	0	(0.0)	9	(31.0)	
11–20 years	0	(0.0)	1	(3.5)	
21+ years	0	(0.0)	3	(10.3)	

CMA Community Midwife Assistant, *NMT* Nurse Midwife Technician, *LNG* levonorgestrel

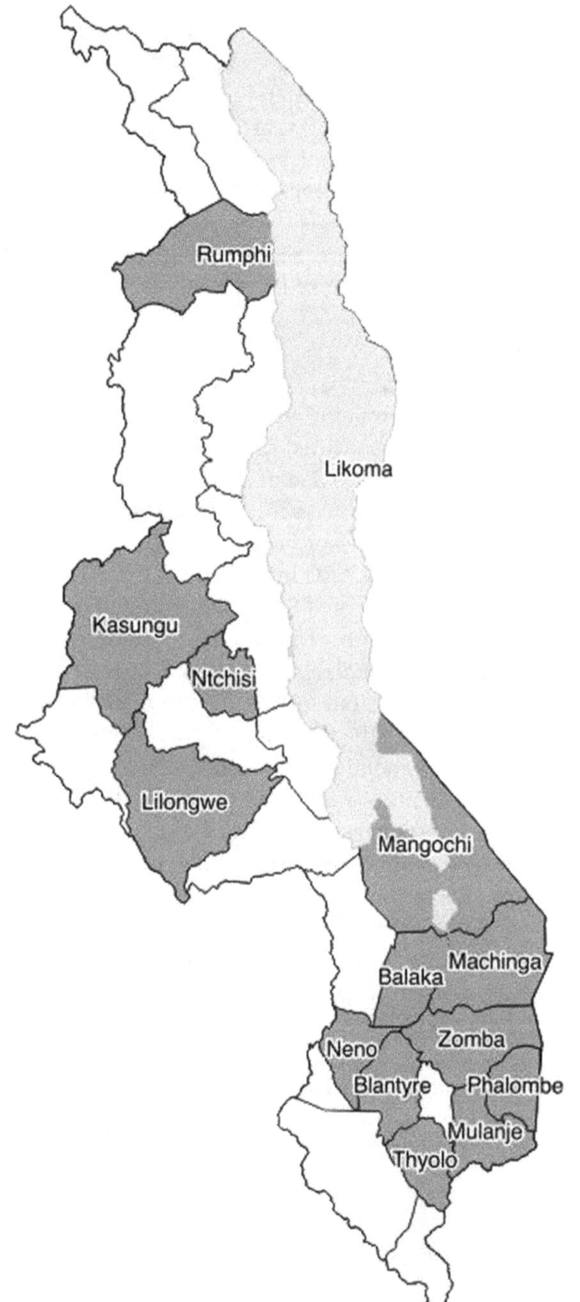

Fig. 1 Study district distribution of Malawi. One CMA and one matched NMT from 31 health centers across Malawi were selected for training in Malawi's 1-week LARC insertion course, of which 29 CMAs and 29 NMTs were used for our study analysis. After the training, the CMAs and NMTs returned to their assigned health center across Malawi. The location of these health centers are highlighted in grey, to illustrate the distribution of our study

group, with almost half below 24 years of age, whereas the NMTs were older in age, with over half between 24 and 30 years of age ($p = 0.042$). The CMAs were recent graduates, with 96.6% having graduated less than a year ago. In contrast, the NMTs had spent more time in the workforce, with only 24.1% graduating less than 1 year ago ($p < 0.001$).

Prior to the LARC training, 55% of the CMAs had never placed a LNG implant, whereas only 28% of NMTs had never placed a LNG implant ($p = 0.024$, Table 2). During the LARC training, 97% of the CMAs at least placed 1 LNG implant, but only 76% of the NMTs placed at least 1 implant ($p = 0.037$).

LNG implant insertion scores

After the LARC training, a majority of the CMAs (79.3%) and NMTs (75.8%) had placed at least 11 LNG implants at their health center ($p = 0.785$) by the end of their monitoring visit (Table 2). Overall, CMAs inserted a total of 539 LNG implants, and NMTs inserted a total of 488 LNG implants.

There was no significant difference between CMA (90%) and NMT (86%) mean LNG implant scores during the monitoring visit ($p = 0.088$). Both cadres scored above the MoH competency criterion of 85%. However, 7% of the NMTs scored below 80% (compared to 0% of CMAs) which is well below the competency level. In fact, these 2 NMTs never achieved competency as all 5 of their scores were below 85%. Thirteen (44.8%) of the CMAs and 10 (34.5%) of the NMTs had a score of < 85% on their first implant insertion during the monitoring visit, and all but the 2 NMTs were able to achieve competency within 1–3 implant insertions during the visit.

The most commonly-missed pre-insertion items on the checklist (Appendix A) were: 1) asking about allergies, 2) explaining the benefits and limitations of all contraceptive methods available, 3) asking about reproductive goals, and explanation of possible implant side effects and other health problems. The most commonly-missed items during the implant insertion were: 1) washing and drying hands (mostly due to lack of running water at the health facilities), and 2) not using sterile surgical drapes on the arm (again, due to lack of availability). Finally, the most commonly-missed post-insertion items were: 1) decontaminating the needle and syringe, 2) washing and drying hands, and 3) counselling the client about wound care.

The mean LNG implant score for the CMAs was 90.2%, versus 89.7% for the NMTs, which gave a non-inferior mean percent difference of − 0.5% (95% CI: -3.4%, 2.4%, Table 3). We also found a non-inferior mean percent difference in our adjusted model (1.3%, 95% CI: -2.2%, 4.8%).

Discussion

In our study, CMAs were non-inferior to NMTs with the insertion of LNG implants. We observed that both CMAs and NMTs were generally competent with LNG

Table 2 Community Midwife Assistant and Nurse Midwife Technician LNG implant insertion statistics

Characteristics ($N = 58$)	CMA ($N = 29$)	NMT ($N = 29$)	Fisher's Exact Test
#LNG implant placed prior to training			
0	16 (55.2)	8 (27.6)	0.024
1–10	8 (27.6)	8 (27.6)	
11–20	4 (13.8)	3 (10.3)	
21–100	0 (0.0)	6 (20.7)	
> 100	1 (3.5)	4 (13.8)	
#LNG implant placed during training			
0	1 (3.5)	7 (24.1)	0.037
1	13 (44.8)	8 (27.6)	
2	6 (20.7)	8 (27.6)	
3	6 (20.7)	1 (3.5)	
4	3 (10.3)	3 (10.3)	
5	0 (0.0)	2 (6.9)	
#LNG implant placed since training			
0–10	6 (20.7)	7 (24.1)	0.785
11–20	13 (44.8)	15 (51.7)	
> 21	10 (34.5)	7 (24.1)	
Mean LNG implant insertion score			
< 80%	0 (0.0)	2 (6.9)	0.088
81–85%	3 (10.3)	2 (6.9)	
86–90%	10 (34.5)	8 (27.6)	
91–95%	15 (51.7)	10 (34.5)	
96–100%	1 (3.5)	7 (24.1)	

There was no significant difference between CMA and NMT mean LNG implant scores during the monitoring visit ($p = 0.088$). 89.7% of CMAs had an average LNG implant insertion score above the MoH competency score of 85%, while 86.2% of NMTs had an average LNG implant insertion score above the MoH competency score of 85%

implant insertion, but it was concerning to find that 10% of CMAs and 14% of NMTs had a mean LNG implant insertion score below competency. With the increase in demand for LARC, particularly implants, in Malawi and other sub-Saharan African countries, [7–10] this study provides evidence that LNG implant insertion may be safely task shifted to Auxiliary Nurse Midwives, such as CMAs, as a way of meeting a country's FP needs.

Table 3 Difference in Mean Percentage of Observation Scores by Nurse Type

Mean % of Observational Scores	NMT $N = 29$	CMA $N = 29$	Difference* β	95% CI (Lower CI, Upper CI)
Unadjusted	90.7	89.2	−1.5	−4.4, 1.4
Adjusted**	90.5	89.4	−1.1	−5.0, 2.7

The non-inferiority margin (Δ) was set at −10 for this study. While the upper limits of the confidence interval are not interpreted for non-inferiority analyses, the lower confidence interval was interpreted and was found to be within the 10%. The mean difference between the CMAs and NMTs was also found to be within 10%

*Significant at $p < 0.05$

**Scores adjusted or number of insertions pre-training, number of insertions during training, and years since graduation

However, 40% of the nurses had initial LNG implant scores below competency, although most were able to achieve competency within a few monitored insertions. Therefore, we recommend that all nurses undergo continued mentorship and monitoring with LNG implant insertion after the initial training, particularly if they place less than 5 LNG implants during the actual training. Additionally, based on the most commonly missed pre-insertion, during insertion, and post-insertion items we recommend the improvement of reliable running water, and the availability of medical items such as sterile surgical drapes from an infrastructure standpoint.

To our knowledge, this is the first published comparative study that evaluates the competency level of Auxiliary Nurse Midwives with another cadre in LNG implant insertion. A study from Ghana also evaluated the competency level of a similar cadre of providers, called Community Health Nurses (CHNs), to insert and remove LNG implants [11]. CHNs receive 2 years of training and were previously only allowed to counsel and refer for LARC. However, in 2008, a carefully selected group of 33 CHNs across Ghana were trained to insert and remove LNG implants. They were later assessed for their skills. While more than 75% of the CHNs reported no complications with implant insertions, more than 80% of the CHNs and their managers felt that there was a need for further training in infection prevention, counseling, and management of side effects and complications. This study was similar to ours in that it specifically evaluated insertion of LNG implants among an Auxiliary health provider cadre; however, our study compared our cadre's competency level to a higher cadre to ensure that the two cadres were providing similar levels of care.

Other studies have evaluated the competency levels of Lay Health Worker cadres to insert implants. A study completed in northern Nigeria evaluated the competency of 166 Community Health Extension Workers (CHEWs) to insert both LNG and ENG implants after a 2- or 3-week training [12]. The study required that the CHEWs have at least 15 observed implant insertions before they could proceed to insert implants under supervision on actual clients. Most CHEWs reached competency after insertions on 4–5 actual clients. The authors concluded that task shifting implant insertion is a plausible option to fulfill the family planning needs in Nigeria. However, similar to our study, they also suggested that adequate training and supportive supervision was necessary to ensure high-quality implant insertion services.

Strengths and limitations

Our study had a few limitations. First, the CMAs and NMTs were evaluated over a 5-month period from November 2016 to March 2017, so the nurses who were evaluated closer towards the end of the period may have had higher scores as they may have had more implant insertions prior to evaluation. However, since the matched CMAs and NMTs for each health center were evaluated at the same visit, and we used mean average scores to compare the two groups, the potentially higher scores at the end should have been balanced out by the potentially lower scores of those CMAs and NMTs who were evaluated towards the beginning of the monitoring period. In addition, in our non-inferiority comparison, we adjusted for the number of LNG implants placed after the training.

Furthermore, our evaluations were completed by FP Master Trainers who were not blinded as to who was a CMA and who was an NMT since CMA and NMTs wear different uniforms at work. Therefore, our Master Trainers (who are both NMTs) may have been subject to bias during evaluation as they may have expected the NMTs to score higher, and the CMAs to score lower. However, we do not believe this occurred as there was a wide range of scores for both the CMAs and NMTs, and there was no difference in their mean average scores.

Despite these limitations, our study has a number of important strengths. As noted earlier, this study is the first to train and evaluate both Auxiliary Nurse Midwives and a higher cadre concurrently to assess and compare their competency levels for LNG implant insertion. In addition, we matched each CMA to another nurse working at their same health center so that we could try to control for the conditions of their health center and the population characteristics of its catchment area. We were adequately powered to analyze our primary outcome and achieved our sample size with minimal loss to follow up. Finally, we were able to evaluate CMAs and NMTs based in all 3 regions of Malawi and 14 of Malawi's 28 districts.

Conclusion

Both CMAs and NMTs generally demonstrated competency with the insertion of LNG contraceptive implants after their training, even after adjusting for the years since graduation and the number of implants place. However, almost half of the CMAs and over a third of the NMTs were not competent at the time of their first evaluated LNG implant insertion, and 2 NMTs failed to reach competency within 5 evaluated insertions. Therefore, continued mentorship and supportive supervision after training is critical to ensure that women are receiving high-quality and safe implant insertion services. Future studies could evaluate long-term client satisfaction and continuation with LNG insertion by Auxiliary Nurse Midwives or target other LARC outcomes that we were not powered to analyze. In addition, more comparative studies, such as this one, need to be done so that policymakers have the evidence they need to upgrade the family planning recommendations for various cadres of contraceptive providers.

Abbreviations

CHEW: Community Health Extension Worker; CHN: Community health nurse; CMA: Community Midwife Assistant; ENG: Etonogestrel; FP: Family planning; HEW: Health extension workers; HSA: Health Surveillance Assistants; LARC: Long-acting reversible contraception; LNG: Levonorgestrel; NMT: Nurse Midwife Technician; WHO: World Health Organization

Acknowledgements

The authors would like to thank the participating Community Midwife Assistants and Nurse Midwife Technicians and their health facilities for their support of the program. The authors would additionally like to thank Dr. Joanne Garrett and Dr. John Stanback for their statistical and study design input for this project.

Authors' contributions

DD wrote the manuscript and created Tables 1, 2 and 3. CL ran the statistical analysis for the results and assisted with the development of the project. NK and BP are the Nurse Midwife Technicians who visited each project site for data collection and contacted each NMT and CMA. SK is the statistician that performed the sample size calculation. NB and CL ran both the adjusted and unadjusted linear models that were used to evaluate the scores. Additionally, NB created Fig. 1. JT developed the methods and design of the project.

Additionally, she edited the manuscript, wrote the research protocol and proposal, and submitted to the IRB for approval. PM assisted with the mentoring and grading of the NMT and CMAs. She accompanied NK and BP for some of the follow-up visits where the checklists were performed. All authors read and approved the final manuscript.

Author details

[1]UNC Project-Malawi, c/o Kamuzu Central Hospital, 100 Mzimba Road, Private Bag, A-104 Lilongwe, Malawi. [2]Department of Obstetrics & Gynecology, University of North Carolina at Chapel Hill, 100 Manning Drive, Chapel Hill, North Carolina, 27599-7570 CB-7570, USA. [3]Department of Health Behavior, University of North Carolina at Chapel Hill, Rosenau Hall, CB #7440, Chapel Hill, North Carolina, 27599-7570 27599, USA.

References

1. Naicke S, Plange-Rhule J, Tutt R, Eastwood J. Shortage of healthcare workers in developing countries—Africa. Ethnicity & Disease. 2009;19:60–3.
2. Malawi Health Workforce Observatory. (2010). Human resources for health country profile: Malawi. Malawi health workforce observatory. [www.health.gov.mw/index.php/policies-strategies?download=12:hrh-malawi-country-profile-approved-moh]. Accessed 25 Mar 2017.
3. World Health Organization (WHO). Task Shifting: global recommendations and guidelines. 2008. [http://www.who.int/healthsystems/TTR-TaskShifting.pdf?ua=1] Accessed 25 March 2017.
4. World Health Organization (WHO). WHO recommendations: Optimizing health worker roles to improve access to key maternal and newborn health interventions through task shifting. 2012. [www.who.int/iris/bitstream/10665/77764/1/9789241504843_eng.pdf] Accessed 26 March 2017.
5. White Ribbon Alliance. Final Report on a Count of Bedside Midwives in Malawi. 2016.
6. Nurse and Midwives Council of Malawi. Syllabus for 18 months Community Midwifery Technician Programme Leading to Enrollment as a Malawi Community Midwife Technician. 2013.
7. Hubacher D, Kimani J, Steiner MJ, Solomon M, Ndugga MB. Contraceptive implants in Kenya: current status and future prospects. Contraception. 2007; 75:468–73.
8. Duvall S, Thurston S, Weinberger M, Nuccio O, Fuchs-Montgomery N. Scaling up delivery of contraceptive implants in sub-Saharan Africa: operational experiences of Marie stopes international. Glob Health Sci Pract. 2014;2:72–92.
9. National Statistical Office (NSO) [Malawi] and ICF. Malawi Demographic and Health Survey 2015–16. Zomba, Malawi, and Rockville, Maryland, USA: NSO and ICF; 2017.
10. Ghana Health Service. Family Health Division 2015 Annual Report. 2015.
11. Population Council. Increasing Access to Family Planning in Ghana through policy change: Task-sharing to enable auxilliary nurses to provide contraceptive implant services (Policy Brief). Accra, Ghana: Population Council; 2014.
12. Charyeva Z, Oguntunde O, Orobaton N, Otolorin E, Inuwa F, Alalade O, et al. Task shifting provision of contraceptive implants to community health extension workers: results of operations research in northern Nigeria. Glob Health Sci Pract. 2015.

Suboptimal child spacing practice and its associated factors among women of child bearing age in Serbo town, JIMMA zone, Southwest Ethiopia

Girma Bacha Ayane[1], Kalkidan Wondwossen Desta[2], Birhanu Wondimeneh Demissie[3*], Netsanet Abera Assefa[3] and Emebet Berhane Woldemariam[2]

Abstract

Introduction: Birth spacing is the time gaps between two consecutive life births. Optimal spacing until the next pregnancy is the resting period that allows the mother time to recover from pregnancy, and labor. Birth interval of 3 to 5 years increases maternal health and child survival and family planning programs have advocated this birth interval.

Objectives: To assess prevalence of Suboptimal Child spacing practice and its associated factors among Women of Child bearing age in Serbo town, Jimma Zone Southwest Ethiopia.

Methods: Community based cross sectional study was conducted on a total of 314 women of child bearing age from March to April 2017 who were selected by simple random sampling. A semi structured questionnaire which was pretested was used to collect the data. Data was checked for completeness and analyzed using SPSS V.20. Bi-variable logistic regression and multi- variable regression were done for predictor variables associated at p-value < 0.05 with the outcome variable.

Result: The prevalence of short birth interval in this study was 59.9%. Independent predictors like age at first marriage (AOR: 2.10, 95% CI = 1.19, 3.69), sex of index child (AOR: 1.964, 95% CI = 1.05 3.96), educational status (AOR: 3.05,95% CI = 1.68, 3.83), duration of breastfeeding (AOR: 3.09, 95% CI = 1.38, 6.96) and use of modern contraceptives (AOR: 1.94, 95% CI = 1.09, 3.45) were found to be statistically associated with short birth interval.

Conclusion and recommendation: Majority of the study respondents were practicing short birth interval. Education level, age at first marriage, having female child, short duration of breastfeeding and not using of modern contraceptives were factors associated with the outcome variable. Therefore awareness about modern contraceptive utilization, importance of breastfeeding as birth spacing mechanism and impact of early marriage are recommended.

Keywords: Suboptimal, Birth interval, Women of child bearing age, Serbo town

* Correspondence: birhanuwondimeneh@gmail.com
[3]School of Nursing, College of Health Sciences and Medicine, Wolaita Sodo University, Sodo, Ethiopia

Background

Birth spacing is the time gaps between two consecutive life births also known as the inter-pregnancy interval [1]. Optimal spacing until the next pregnancy is the resting period between pregnancies that allows the mother time to recover from pregnancy to the next pregnancy. Longer time period between births allows the next pregnancy and birth to occur more likely to be at full gestation and family planning programs have advocated three and more years intervals between births for infant and child health and survival [2].

Three to five years birth interval is safer for both the mother and child. Globally, a birth interval of less than 18 months is associated with increased risk for Neonatal mortality (AOR =3.17), Infant mortality (AOR = 3.16), and Under-five mortality AOR = 2.81). Birth interval, less than 15 month is associated with increased risk for the mother like; third trimester bleeding (AOR = 1.7), Premature rupture of membranes (AOR = 1.7), Anemia (AOR = 1.3) and Puerperal endometritis (AOR = 1.3) [3, 4].

Short birth spacing has been continued to be a problem of both developed and developing countries like; Uganda and Zimbabwe, resulting in negative infant, child, and maternal health outcomes [5]. In USA, Pregnancies that occur with birth spacing less than 18 months are associated with delayed prenatal care and adverse birth outcomes, including preterm birth, neonatal morbidity, and low birth weight [6]. In Ethiopia also there is an increased risk of maternal health problems and death at a young age among those who give birth less than two years interval between the births [7].

Beyond the health implications, closely spaced birth intervals accelerate population growth and undermining development efforts. It makes difficult for women to become productive members of society, thereby limiting their contribution to economic development [8].

Determinant for the occurrence of short birth interval includes; maternal education, maternal age, early marriage, lack of optimal breastfeeding practice and inadequate knowledge, Attitude and practice towards modern contraceptives use and different socio-demographic factors [9, 10].

Even though interventions such as promoting female education and empowerment, awareness creation and enhancing breastfeeding practice and modern contraception utilization has been done, problem of birth spacing is still evident in most parts of African countries including Ethiopia. For instance, a previous study in southern Ethiopia showed that about more than half of (57.5%) women practicing shorter birth interval with the median birth interval length of 33 months [7, 11–15]. Optimum birth spacing has an invaluable benefit for the world in building capacity to promote healthy and economic independency through balancing and managing the growth of population and budget to ensure the production of fruitful generation. Identification of factors for suboptimal child spacing practice is critical for countries like Ethiopia which is the most populated next to Nigeria in Africa with estimate population size of 102,066,540 and with current fertility rate of 4.6. It will help to design interventional program and preventive strategies. Therefore, the aim of this study was to assess suboptimal child spacing practice and its associated factors among women of child bearing age in serbo town, Southwest Ethiopia.

Methods

Study design and setting

Community based cross - sectional study was conducted from March to April 2017 in Serbo Town Jimma Zone, Oromia Regional state, South - West Ethiopia. Serbo town is located in kersa district, Jimma Zone of Oromia regional state with an attitude of 1640 km above sea level. The town is located 345 km far from Addis Ababa, Capital city of Ethiopia and about 18 km from Jimma town. The study was conducted in two kebeles (smallest administrative division in Ethiopia), namely Omaticha kebele and Wayu kebele. The town has two kebeles with total populations of 7450, of this 3650 were females. There were a total of 1649 Child bearing age mothers in the town.

Study population

The source populations were all women's of child bearing age groups (15–49) in Serbo town. And all randomly selected women of child bearing age group in Serbo town were the study population.

Eligibility criteria

Inclusion criteria

All women of child bearing age group (15–49) having at least two children were included in the study.

Sample size determination

Sample size was calculated by using the formula for single population proportion and by considering, 35.8% proportion of optimal birth interval in Lemo District, Southern Ethiopia [13] 95% level of confidence, 5% margin of error and 10% none response rate, the sample size was 388. Since the total population of reproductive age mothers in Serbo town is less than 10,000 correction formula was used to get the final sample size of 314 women's.

Sampling techniques

The sample was taken from two kebele's (smallest administrative division in Ethiopia) in Serbo town, namely

Omoticha kebele and Wayu Kebele and the study was conducted in these two kebele's. The calculated sample size was allocated proportionally to the size of populations in each kebeles. Household was selected with an interval of K for each kebele, where K was the total number of household in each kebeles divided by the total number of study subjects in each kebele's which was found to be **5** (K = 5, every 5th household) for both kebele's and the first house hold to be started from was selected by lottery method.

Method of data collection

Data was collected using a semi-structured questionnaire which was adopted and modified from different literature [13]. The questionnaire contains: socio-demographic characteristic of the study respondents, awareness of the study respondents on birth spacing, birth history of the study respondent, practice of breastfeeding and use of modern contraceptives. All eligible mothers of child bearing age were interviewed by using semi-structured questioners. The data was collected by four diploma holder nurses and two BSc. holder Environmental health professionals and the data collection was supervised by two MSc. holder nurses.

Data quality and control

The questionnaire were prepared in English version and translated into local languages (Amharic and Afan Oromo) and then back translated into English to maintain its consistency. Three days orientation training was given on the process of data collection for data collectors and supervisors. A pretest was done by 5 % of the study population three weeks before the actual data collection to evaluate the clarity of questions and validity of the instrument and reaction of respondents to the questions.

Study variables

Dependent variable

- Suboptimal birth spacing

Independent variables

Socio-demographic variables (Age, marital status, educational level, religion, occupation), fertility history, contraceptive utilization, inconsistent breastfeeding.

Operational definitions

Optimal birth interval

it denotes to 3–5 years' birth interval (including 3 and 5 years) between the birth of the child under study and the immediately preceding live and surviving birth to the mother.

Suboptimal birth interval

it refers to less than 3 years' birth interval between the birth of the child under study and the immediately preceding live and surviving birth to the mother.

Long birth interval

it refers greater than 5 years' birth interval between the birth of the child under study and the immediately preceding live and surviving birth to the mother.

Data entry and analysis

The data was cleaned manually, coded and entered into Epi data version 3.1 and exported to SPSS version 22.0 software for further analysis. Bi-variable logistic regression analysis was used to see significance of association between dependent and each independent variable. Candidate variables for the final model (multivariate binary logistic regressions) were identified at p - value < 0.20. Variables which had significant association with the outcome variable during bi-variable logistic regression analysis was introduced in to multivariable binary logistic regression and finally, predictors of suboptimal child spacing were identified at p – value < 0.05, 95% CI.

Results

Socio - demographic characteristics of mothers

A total of 314 mothers participated in the study, with response rate of 100%. From the total respondents one hundred and nine (34.7%) were in the age group of 25–29 with mean age of 30.84 (SD ± 5.956) years. Most, 292 (93.0%) of the respondents were married. Majority of the respondents 215 (68.5%) age at first marriage was 18 years and above with mean of 18.38 (SD ± 2.41) years of age. Two hundred and thirty five (74.8%) were Muslim religious followers. Almost one third of 115(36.6%) respondents were illiterate and majority of them 209 (66.6%) were housewives. More than half, 171 (54.5%) of the study participants had monthly income of less than 1000 Ethiopian birr (37 US Dollar) (Table 1).

Birth history, awareness about birth spacing and breastfeeding practice

Most of the respondents 286 (91.1%) were informed about modern contraceptives methods used by male and female to space and limit child birth. Majority 265 (84.4%) of the study respondents agreed that an optimal birth interval has health advantages both for the mother and child. Of the total respondents 47 (15.0%) did not know the health disadvantages of short birth interval for the mother and the child. Concerning with the preference of birth interval among mothers; more than half, 163 (51.9%) prefer

Table 1 Socio-demographic characteristic of mothers of child bearing age in Serbo town Jimma Zone Southwest Ethiopia, 2017 ($N = 314$)

Variables	Category	Frequency	Percent
Age of the mother	15–19	2	.6
	20–24	32	10.2
	25–29	109	34.7
	30–34	78	24.8
	35–39	59	18.8
	> = 40	34	10.8
Marital status	Married	292	93.0
	Others *	22	7.0
Age at first marriage	< 18 years	99	31.5
	> = 18 years	215	68.5
Religion	Orthodox	34	10.8
	Protestant	34	10.8
	Muslim	235	74.8
	Others**	11	3.5
Ethnicity	Oromo	266	84.7
	Amhara	18	5.7
	Gurhage	17	5.4
	Tigray	6	1.9
	Others **[a]	7	2.2
Education	Illiterate	115	36.6
	Read and write	37	11.8
	Elementary	111	35.4
	Secondary and above	51	16.2
Occupation	Employ of government or NGO	43	13.7
	House wife	209	66.6
	Merchant	41	13.1
	Others **[b]	21	6.7
Monthly income	< 1000 birr (37 US dollar)	171	54.5
	1000–1999 birr (37–74 $)	91	29.0
	2000–2999 birr (74–111$)	37	11.8
	≥ 3000 birr (≥112$)	15	4.8

*others: single, Divorced & widowed. **others: Wakefata & Catholic. **[a] Others: Wolayita, Silte & Dawuro. **[b]others: Farmer, Student and daily workers

an optimal birth interval. Almost half of the respondents 159 (50.6%) have three to four children and about thirty eight (12.1%) mothers reported child death soon after birth. Two hundred and eighty three (90.1%) of mothers have breastfed their last child, but about 31(9.9%) of them have not yet breastfed their last child due to different reasons. Among those who breastfed their last child, above three forth, 217(76.4%) breastfed their last child for 24 months and above whereas18 (6.3%) for less than 24 months (Table 2).

Distribution of birth intervals practice

More than half 188(59.9%) of the mothers were practicing short birth interval less than 36 months, followed by 112 (35.7%), and 14(4.5%) practicing optimal and long birth interval between their last two children respectively.

Table 2 Birth history, knowledge about birth spacing and breastfeeding practice among mothers of child bearing age in Serbo town Jimma Zone, Southwest Ethiopia, 2017 ($N = 314$)

Variables	Category	Frequency	Percent
Heard about modern contraceptives during two consecutive births	Yes	286	91.1%
	No	28	8.9%
Optimal birth interval has health advantage for the mother and the child	Yes	265	84.4%
	No	39	12.4%
	don't know	10	3.2%
Short birth interval has health disadvantages for the mother and the child	Yes	260	82.8%
	No	47	15.0%
	don't know	7	2.2%
Number of children born alive	2	110	35.0%
	3–4	159	50.6%
	≥5	45	14.3%
Child died soon after birth	Yes	38	12.1%
	No	276	87.9%
Mother's need to have more children after last pregnancy	Yes	191	60.8%
	No	123	39.2%
Time to become pregnant after last child	Soon after	47	24.6%
	Wait until later	144	75.4%
Mother's preference of birth interval (BI) in years	< 36 months	113	36.0%
	36–60 months	163	51.9%
	≥60 months	25	8.0%
	I don't know	13	4.1%
Sex of the last child	Male	110	35.0%
	Female	204	65.0%
Breastfeed the last child	Yes	283	90.1%
	never breastfeed	31	9.9%
Duration of breastfeeding	0–11 months	19	6.7%
	12–23 months	49	17.3%
	> = 24 months	217	76.0%
Reasons for never breastfed	new pregnancy	5	16.1%
	mother was sick	14	45.2%
	Other[a]	12	38.7%
Mother's agreement on when to stop breastfeeding	< 24 months	57	17.9%
	≥24 months	257	82.1%

[a]others include, mothers don't have breast milk b/c of unknown reason, the child refused to suck

Awareness and utilization of modern contraceptive

Two hundred and sixty six (84.7%) of the study respondents had information about modern contraceptives used to space and limit birth. Nearly two third (62.7%) of the study respondents had used those methods before the last child, 162(82.2%) for spacing purpose. One hundred fifty three (89.5%) of them were getting the service from health center and fifty one (35.7%) of those who did not use modern contraceptive mentioned religion as the main reason for not using (Table 3).

Birth spacing methods utilization

Even though more than half of the study respondents knew different modern contraceptives used to space and limit child birth, few of them used some of those contraceptives. This indicates that the awareness level about modern contraceptives of the study respondents was high while their actual utilization or practice of the methods was too low. The most frequently known contraceptive was injectable 259 (97.4%) followed by pills 233 (87.7%). Injectable was also the most frequently used 116 (58.9%) and more than half, 177 (66.5%) of the study respondents knew about condoms, but none of them utilized (Fig. 1).

Table 3 Awareness and utilization of modern contraceptive among mothers of child bear age in Serbo town Jimma Zone, Southwest Ethiopia, 2017(*N* = 314)

Variables	Category	Frequency	Percent
mothers have an awareness about modern Contraceptive	Yes	266	84.7%
	No	48	15.3%
Mother used modern contraceptives before the last child	Yes	197	62.7%
	No	117	37.3%
Purpose of using modern contraceptives	birth spacing	162	82.2%
	birth limiting	35	17.8%
Current use of modern contraceptives by mother	Yes	171	54.5%
	No	143	45.5%
The place where mother gets modern contraceptives	health post	14	8.2%
	health center	153	89.5%
	Hospital	25	14.6%
	private sector	5	2.9%
Reason of the mother not to use modern contraceptives	desire to have more children	27	18.9%
	health problem	15	10.5%
	religious reason	51	35.7%
	husband not willing	20	14.0%
	Other[a]	30	21.0%

[a]Others include, lack of service, lack of information, no husband, naturally adjusted spacing, lack of interest of modern contraceptives

Predictors of short birth interval

In bi-variable logistic regression, Educational status, age at first marriage, sex of the index child, death of child soon after birth, mother's preference of birth interval, breastfeeding of previous to last child, duration of breast feeding and use of modern contraceptives were the variables that showed statistically significant association with the outcome variable. Those variables that had association in bi variable logistic regression were introduced into multiple logistic regressions.

The likelihood of practicing short birth interval was about 2 times more likely in mothers who were married at age less than 18 years as compared to mothers who were married at age 18 years and above (AOR = 2.10, 95% CI = 1.19, 3.69). The odds of practicing short birth interval was about 3 times more likely in respondents who had no formal education as compared to those who had formal education (AOR: 3.09,95% CI = 1.68, 3.83). In the same way, the probability of having female index child was about 2 times more likely to increase the chance of getting short birth as compared to those mothers who had male index child (AOR = 1.96,95% CI = 1.046, 3.96). Study respondents who preferred birth spacing of less than 36 months were about 4 times more likely to have short birth interval as compared to those who preferred 36–60 months (AOR = 4.71,95% CI = 2.46,7.53). Mothers who had a duration of breast feeding < 24 months were 3 times more likely to have short birth interval as compared to those who breastfeed for ≥24 months (AOR = 3.09, 95% CI 1.38, 6.96). The odds of not using modern contraceptives in the mothers who practiced a short birth interval were 2 times higher than among those using modern contraceptives (AOR; 1.93, 95% CI = 1.09, 3.45) (Table 4).

Discussion

The prevalence of short birth interval in this study was found to be 59.9%. The remaining, 35.7 and 4.5% were practicing optimal and long birth interval respectively. Although, 36–60 months of interval between births is the currently recommended, still the prevalence of short birth interval outweighs the optimal one. This finding is almost consistent with a study conducted in southern Ethiopia, 57.6% of mothers were practicing short birth interval and 35.8% were practicing optimal birth interval and the remaining were long birth interval. This might be due to relative similarity in socio-economic background of the study respondents. Again, this finding was relatively similar with the study conducted in Mozambique in which 46, 35 and 19% of the women were practicing short, optimal and long birth interval respectively. However, in the current study, long birth interval was lower than study conducted in Mozambique [10, 15]. The discrepancy might be due to difference in

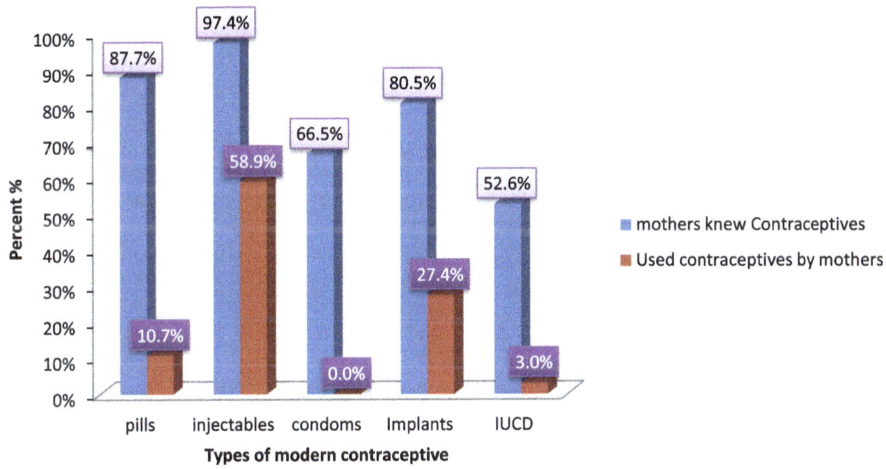

Fig. 1 Awareness and modern contraceptives utilization among mothers of child bearing age in Serbo town Jimma Zone, Southwest Ethiopia, 2017

demographic background of the study respondents of the two countries.

Those women who had married at age less than 18 years were about 2 times more likely to practice short birth interval as compared to those who had married at age 18 years or above. This finding was consistent with the study done in Uganda, Zimbabwe and Jordan [16, 17].

Sex of the index child was associated with short birth interval. According to the result of this study women's who had female index child were about 3 times more likely to have short birth interval as compared to

Table 4 Factors associated with short birth interval among mothers of child bearing age in Serbo town Jimma Zone, Southwest Ethiopia, 2017 (*N* = 314)

Variables	category	Short Birth Interval		COR(95%CI)	AOR(95%CI)
		Yes	No		
		N (%)	N (%)		
Age at first marriage	< 18 years	72 (22.9%	27 (8.6%)	2.28 (1.36,3.82)	2.09 (1.19,3.69)*
	≥18 years	116 (36.9%)	99 (31.5%)	1.00	1.00
Sex of index child	Male	33 (10.5%)	30 (9.6%)	1.00	1.00
	Female	93 (29.6%)	158 (50.6%)	1.87 (1.07,3.26)	1.96 (1.05,3.96)*
Death of child soon after birth	Yes	29 (9.2%)	9 (2.9%)	1.00	
	No	159 (50.6%)	117 (37.3%)	2.371 (1.08,5.19)	
Preference of birth interval	< 36 months	73 (23.2%)	90 (28.7%)	5.733 (3.23,10.17)	4.71 (2.46,7.53)*
	≥60 months	15 (4.8%)	10 (3.2%)	1.85 (0.70,4.36)	0.26 (0.08,0.90)
	don't know	7 (2.2%)	6 (1.9%)	1.44 (1.46,4.47)	0.27 (0.077,0.920)
	36–60 months	93 (29.6%)	20 (6.4%)	1.00	1.00
Educational status	No formal education	136 (43.3%)	92 (29.3%)	3.09 (1.68,3.71)	3.05 (1.60,3.83)*
	Formal educated	52 (16.6%)	34 (10.8%)	1.00	1.00
Breastfeeding of previous to last child	Yes	120 (38.2%)	163 (51.9%)	1.00	
	No	6 (2%)	25 (8.0%)	3.07 (1.22,7.71)	
Duration of breast feeding	< 24 months	47 (15.0%)	10 (3.2%)	3.84 (1.83,7.83)	3.09 (1.38,6.96)*
	≥24 months	141 (44.9%)	116 (36.9%)	1.00	1.00
Use of modern contraceptives	No	86 (27.4%)	31 (9.9%)	2.58 (1.57,4.25)	1.94 (1.09,3.45)*
	Yes	102 (32.5%)	95 (30.3%)	1.00	1.00

*Significant at *p*-value ≤0.05

mothers who had male index child which was consistent with studies done in Arba - minch Zuria District and Southern Ethiopia [7, 8].

Mothers who had no formal education were about 3 times more likely to have short birth interval. A similarly study conducted in Arba-Minch showed the same finding with the current study (AOR = 3.40, 95% CI: 1.80, 6.43) [7, 8]. This is also consistent with a study conducted in Illubabor zone, South West Ethiopia (AOR = 2.56, 95% CI: 1.60, 3.42) [18]. This might be due to knowledge gap about family planning methods, where to get, how to use and inability to read different advertisements about family planning.

The other predictor of short birth interval was duration of breastfeeding. Mothers who breastfeed their child for less than 24 months were about 3 times more likely to practice short birth interval as compared to those who breastfeed ≥24 months which is in line with a study conducted in Illubabor zone, South West Ethiopia (AOR = 5.36, 95% CI: 3.43, 6.34) [18]. This was lower than a study conducted in Southern Ethiopia which revealed that breastfeeding for less than 24 months was 30.8 times more likely to practice short birth interval [8]. This is due to lactation amenorrhea and this variation might be due to the difference in duration of breastfeeding practice.

The odds of not using modern contraceptive was about 2 times to have short birth interval as compared to those users of modern contraceptives (AOR = 1.94, 95% CI 1.09, 3.45). Which was similar with a study conducted in Arba-Minch district, Lemo district and rural communities of southern Ethiopia [7, 8, 15]. This is lower than a study conducted in Illubabor zone, South West Ethiopia in which those who are not using contraceptive were 4.12 times more likely to have short birth interval (AOR = 4.12, 95% CI: 2.7, 5.82) [18]. This variation might be due to the difference in health access for family planning service, unmet need due to distance and variation in awareness of women's on family planning methods.

Conclusions

The prevalence of short birth spacing among mothers of childbearing age in serbo town was high (59.9%) which shows mothers were giving birth with short birth interval.

Early marriage, sex of the index child, mother's preference of birth interval, educational status, and short duration of breast feeding and lack of modern contraceptive utilization were independent predictors of short birth interval. Therefore Minister of health and Regional Health bureau should strengthen actions to prevent early marriage and increase mothers' awareness of modern contraceptive and importance of exclusive breastfeeding for the first six month and continue breast feeding until two years old through health extension professionals, and attention should be given on actions to increase modern contraceptive utilization.

Abbreviations

AOR: Adjusted odds ratio; CI: confidence interval; SD: Standard deviation; SPSS: Statistical Package for Social Sciences.

Acknowledgements

The authors would like to thank Addis Ababa University for funding this study. Our thanks also goes to for all study participants, supervisors and data collectors for their unreserved efforts and willingness to take part in this study

Authors' contributions

GB was involved in the conception, design, analysis, interpretation, report and manuscript writing; KW and EB were participated in the design, analysis, interpretation and report writing. BW and NA were involved in the design, analysis, interpretation, report and manuscript writing; and all authors have read and approved the final manuscript.

Authors' information

1. Girma Bacha is a lecturer in department of Nursing, College of Medicine and Health Science, Jima University, Jima, Ethiopia.
2. Kalkidan Wondwossen Desta is a lecturer in school of nursing and midwifery, college of health science, Addis Ababa University, Addis Ababa, Ethiopia.
3. Birhanu Wondimeneh Demissie is a lecturer in department of Nursing, College of health Science and Medicine, Wolaita Sodo University, Wolaita Sodo, Ethiopia.
4. Netsanet Abera Assefa is a lecturer in department of Nursing, College of health Science and Medicine, Wolaita Sodo University, Wolaita Sodo, Ethiopia.
5. Emebet Berhane Woldemariam is a lecturer in school of nursing and midwifery, college of health science, Addis Ababa University, Addis Ababa, Ethiopia.

Author details

[1]Department of Nursing, College of Medicine and Health Science, Jimma University, Jimma, Ethiopia. [2]School of Nursing and Midwifery, College of Health Science, Addis Ababa University, Addis Ababa, Ethiopia. [3]School of Nursing, College of Health Sciences and Medicine, Wolaita Sodo University, Sodo, Ethiopia.

References

1. Nicole Garro at ngarro@marchofdimes.org, 2010. p. 800.
2. Saumya RJT, Ian A. Correlates of inter-birth intervals:. Population Council; . Implications of optimal birth spacing strategies in Mozambique; 2006.
3. USIAD. An activity of the catalyst consortium. In: Optimal birth spacing; 2010.
4. Hailu D, Gulte T. Determinants of short inter birth interval among reproductive age mothers in Arba Minch District, Ethiopia. International journal of reproductive medicine. 2016;2016.
5. Mcguire C, Stephenson R. Community factors influencing birth spacing among married women in Uganda and Zimbabwe. Afr J Reprod Health. 2015;19(1):14–24.
6. DeFranco EASL, Greenberg JM, Muglia LJ. Influence of inter pregnancy interval on neonatal morbidity. Am J Obstet Gynecol. 2015;12(3):386.
7. Begna, et al. Determinants of inter birth interval among married women living in rural pastoral communities of southern Ethiopia: a case control study. BMC Pregnancy and Childbirth. 2013;13(116).
8. Hailu D, Gultie T, Workineh Y. Barriers to adherence of optimal birth spacing: a qualitative study among mothers and their husbands in Arba Minch Zuria district, Ethiopia. American Journal of Health Research. 2014; 2(4):188–95.
9. RamaRao S, Townsend J, Askew I. Correlates of inter-birth intervals: implications of optimal birth spacing strategies in Mozambique: Frontiers in reproductive health. Population Council. 2006.

10. Christina A. Nti CG, Sarah N.A. Dodoo, Bernice Ofosu EAaMA-D.Knowledge, attitude and practice of birth spacing among Ghanaian mothers; implications for maternal and child nutritional status. World Appl Sci J 2014; 31 (11):1971–1978.
11. Rasheed P. BKA-D. birth interval: perceptions and practices among urban-based Sausi Arabians women. Eastern Mediteranean health. Journal. 2007; 13(4):884–6.
12. Hossein Fallahzadeh ZF, Emam Z. Duration and determinants of birth interval in Yazd, Iran: a population study. Iran J Reprod Med. 2013;11(5):379–84.
13. WHO U. UNFPA, World Bank. Maternal mortality in 2005: estimates developed by WHO, UNICEF. UNFPA and the World Bank. Geneva: World Health Organization; 2007.
14. Tarekegn SM, Lieberman LS, Giedraitis V. Determinants of maternal health service utilization in Ethiopia: analysis of the 2011 Ethiopian demographic and health survey. BMC pregnancy and childbirth. 2014;14(1):1.
15. Yohannes et al. Duration and determinants of birth interval among women of child bearing age in southern Ethiopia. BMC Pregnancy and Child birth. 2011;11:38.
16. Youssef RM. Duration and determinants of inter birth interval: community-based survey of women in southern Jordan eastern Mediterranean health journal, . 2005; 11, No. (4):559.
17. Exavery A, SM, AS, KB, DM, G, et al. Non-adherence of WHO recommended inter-birth interval in Rufiji, Tanzania 2010.
18. Dereje T, Muluneh S, Kebebe B. Practice of child spacing and its associated factors among women of child bearing age (15 to 49 years) in Illubabor zone, south West Ethiopia. International Journal of Nursing and Midwifery. 9(7):102–8.

21

Process evaluation of a mobile phone-based intervention to support post-abortion contraception in Cambodia

Chris Smith[1,4*], Sokhey Ly[2], Vannak Uk[2], Ruby Warnock[3], Phil Edwards[1] and Caroline Free[1]

Abstract

Background: The MObile Technology for Improved Family Planning (MOTIF) trial assessed a mobile phone-based intervention comprising voice messages and counsellor support to increase post-abortion contraception at four Marie Stopes International clinics in Cambodia. The aim of this process evaluation was to assess participants' interaction with the intervention from a service provider perspective.

Methods: (1) We conducted a descriptive analysis to assess participants' interaction with the intervention. (2) In order to explore how the intervention might work, we assessed associations between interaction with the intervention and contraception use using logistic regression analysis. (3) We undertook a logistic regression analysis to assess associations between baseline socio-demographic factors and *ever* requesting to speak to a counsellor (pressing '1'), a variable found to be associated with contraception use.

Results: Amongst 249 women that received six interactive voice messages +/− counsellor support for contraception, around half actively requested to speak to a counsellor (pressed '1') and over 90% spoke to a counsellor at some stage. Women who spoke to the counsellor having requested to (by pressing '1') were more than four times as likely to be using effective contraception at four months compared to women who didn't request or speak to the counsellor (Odds Ratio 4.39; 95% CI: 1.15-16.71). There was a small, non-statistically significant increase in contraception use amongst women that spoke to the counsellor without requesting a call. Increased parity, a history of >2 previous induced abortions, lower socio-economic status, and medical abortion (after adjusting for age, socio-economic status and residence) were associated with requesting to speak to a counsellor.

Conclusions: The interactive message can identify a subgroup of women in whom counselling will be more effective and appears to be equitable in terms of engaging those most in-need. The intervention could be adapted based on the findings of this study.

Plain English summary

Our MObile Technology for Improved Family Planning (MOTIF) trial assessed a mobile phone-based intervention comprising six interactive voice messages +/− counsellor support to increase post-abortion contraception at four Marie Stopes International clinics in Cambodia. The aim of this process evaluation was to assess participants' interaction with the intervention from a service provider perspective to further understand what worked or didn't work and to inform future implementation. We analysed data collected during the delivery of the intervention. This included women's response to the messages and number of contacts with the counsellor. We assessed associations between women's response to the intervention and subsequent contraception use, and associations between women's background factors and engagement with the intervention.

We found that amongst 249 women that received the intervention, around half actively requested to speak to a counsellor and over 90% spoke to a counsellor at some stage. Women who requested to speak to a counsellor were more likely to be using effective contraception at

* Correspondence: christopher.smith@lshtm.ac.uk

[1]Department of Population Health, London School of Hygiene and Tropical Medicine, Keppel Street, London WC1E 7HT, UK

[4]Room 150, Department of Population Health, London School of Hygiene and Tropical Medicine, Keppel Street, London WC1E 7HT, UK

four months compared to women who didn't request to speak to a counsellor. Women with living children, a history of >2 previous abortions, of lower socio-economic status, and those who had a medical rather than surgical abortion were more likely to request to speak to a counsellor.

In conclusion, the interactive voice message can identify a subgroup of women in whom counselling will be more effective and appears to be equitable in terms of engaging those most in-need. The intervention could be adapted based on the findings of this study.

Background

The past decade has seen rapid expansion in delivery of health-care interventions by mobile phone ('mHealth') [1]. In the field of contraception, mobile phone-based interventions have been developed to support uptake of methods or reduce discontinuation, for example by providing reminders, or support for clients experiencing side-effects [2]. However, the effects of interventions delivered by mobile phone for improving contraception use have not been reliably established [2].

Our trial, MObile Technology for Improved Family Planning (MOTIF), randomised 500 women seeking elective induced abortion services aged 18 years or older to a personalised mobile phone-based behaviour change intervention or to a control group. The trial results and a detailed description of the intervention and its development are reported elsewhere [3, 4]. In brief, the intervention comprised a series of automated interactive 'real-time' voice messages over the three-month post-abortion period in addition to standard care. Women would receive the first message within one week of attending the clinic, and then every two weeks, with a total of six messages. The message was designed to remind women about contraception methods available to them and provide a conduit for additional support [5]. Women could press '1' to request to speak to a counsellor, press '2' if they did not require a call back, or press '3' to opt-out of receiving further messages. Women who pressed '1', or who did not respond, received a phone call from a counsellor. The phone calls provided individualised counselling intending to encourage contraception use by reminding women about available methods and providing support for side-effects. Counsellors could make appointments for implant or intra-uterine device insertions or women could opt to receive additional oral contraceptive pill or injectable reminder messages. The counsellor could discuss contraception with the husband or partner, if the woman requested or women could call in to the service to request to speak with a counsellor.

The intervention increased self-reported use of an effective contraception method at four months post-abortion (135/211 (64·0%) vs. 101/220 (45·9%) risk ratio (RR) 1·39, 95% CI 1·17-1·66; $p < 0 \cdot 001$), but not after 12 months (84/ (49.7%) vs. 68/ (42.8%) RR 1.16, 95% CI 0.92-1.47; $p = 0.208$). However, self-reported long-acting contraception use was increased at four and 12 months [3].

As a complex intervention delivered by automated voice messages and phone counselling, it is not clear what components of the intervention resulted in behaviour change. Our intervention was based on literature on the determinants of contraceptive use and a similar approach to Lester (2010) who hypothesized that regular structured mobile phone-based support could improve HIV medication adherence [4, 6]. However, for research conducted in 'real-life' settings, it cannot be assumed that the delivery of a complex intervention will be exactly as planned in the design stage of a trial. Process evaluation of randomised controlled trials can lead to a greater understanding of what works, and provide meaningful interpretation of the effects on an intervention to inform future implementation [7, 8]. In a subsequent paper we will report findings from interviews conducted with participants that received the intervention. The aim of this study was to assess participants' interaction with the intervention from a service provider perspective and to consider how the intervention could be improved. Specific objectives were to:

1. Describe the response to voice messages and number of counsellor contacts over the intervention duration
2. Examine associations between interaction with the intervention and subsequent contraception use
3. Assess associations between baseline socio-demographic factors and interaction with the intervention

Methods

This quantitative study used data collected during the intervention and trial. First, we undertook a descriptive analysis to assess how participants interacted with the intervention. Counsellors delivering the intervention made a record of all mobile phone communications with participants. We report the response to voice messages, the number and type of counsellor contacts and number of women that opted out of the intervention or that the counsellor was unable to contact using descriptive statistics.

Second, in order to explore how the intervention might work, we assessed associations between interaction with the intervention and effective and long-acting contraception use using logistic regression analysis. Using data collected by counsellors delivering the intervention we created variables based on response to the voice messages and whether women spoke to the counsellor or received pill or injection reminder messages. We conducted a pre-specified per-protocol analysis to assess the impact of the intervention among participants who responded to at least one voice message [5]. We estimated odds ratios (OR) with 95% confidence intervals (CI).

Third, we undertook a logistic regression analysis to assess associations between baseline socio-demographic factors and *ever* requesting to speak to a counsellor (pressing '1'), a variable that was found to be associated with contraception use in the previous analysis. As the voice message stated *"Press 1 if you would like me to call you back to discuss contraception"* we considered plausible, 'a priori' confounders that might be associated with contraception use in Cambodia. Age, socio-economic status, residence, education and number of living children are associated with contraception use in Cambodia and were included in the adjusted analysis [9, 10]. As almost all the women in the trial (>99%) were able to recognise numbers on a phone and spoke Khmer as their mother tongue, we did not consider confounders that might be associated with the ability to understand or respond to a voice message. For categorical variables in the adjusted analysis, we assessed the statistical significance of the crude association, controlled for the effect of the confounding variables using the Likelihood ratio test. Ethical approval for the MOTIF study was obtained from ethics committees at the London School of Hygiene and Tropical Medicine and Marie Stopes International and the Cambodia Human Research ethics committee.

Results

Interaction with the intervention

Figure 1 shows the response to voice messages over time. The proportion of '1' responses (requesting a call) decreased from 27% at voice message one to 8% by message six. Overall, 49% of clients ever pressed '1' (to request to speak to the counsellor). The proportion of '2' responses (not requiring a call back) increased from 26–38%. The proportion of 'call failed' (no response to the voice message) increased from 35–53% at voice message six. The proportion of clients that spoke to a counsellor decreased from 64% at voice message one to 26% at voice message six. In total, there were 210 (15%) '1' responses, 452 (32%) '2' responses, 109 (8%) '3' responses, 657 (46%) 'no responses', 613 calls from the counsellor to client (outgoing) and approximately 100 calls from the client to the counsellor (data not systematically recorded). The mean number of outgoing phone calls per client was 2·46 (standard deviation 1·48). Overall, 92% of participants ever spoke to a counsellor. It is not clear how often the counsellor discussed contraception with the women's husband or partner, as this information was not systematically recorded.

Twenty per cent (49/249) of participants receiving the intervention opted to receive oral contraceptive or injection reminders at some stage. Of the 24 women that received a reminder message three months after receiving the injectable, 83% (20/24) reported continued use at four-month follow up. Of the 25 women that received monthly oral contraceptive reminders, 68% (17/25) reported continued pill use at four-months.

By voice message six, 15 (6%) clients had opted out. Reported reasons according to the counsellors notes were that they were 'too busy' and had 'no time', or the 'phone was answered by someone else'. Six participants (2%) randomised to the intervention did not receive any

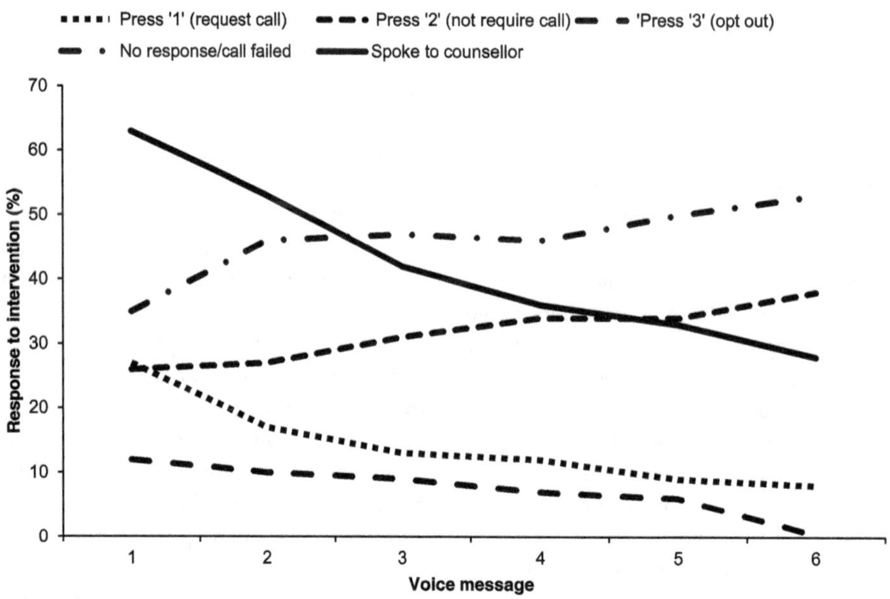

Fig. 1 Interaction with intervention over time

messages; five due to non-functioning phone number and in one case someone not known to the participant answered the phone.

Association between interaction with the intervention and contraception use

Table 1 shows associations between interaction with the intervention and effective and long-acting contraception use at four months. The following factors were associated with effective contraception use at four months: Requesting to speak to a counsellor (pressing '1') compared to not pressing '1' after the first voice message (OR 3.37; 95% CI: 1.62-6.98); *ever* requesting to speak to a counsellor (pressing '1') compared to *never* requesting to speak to a counsellor (OR 2.51; 95% CI: 1.41-4.47); speaking to the counsellor having requested to (pressed '1') compared to *never* speaking and requesting to speak to the counsellor (OR 4.39; 95% CI: 1.15-16.71) or speaking to the counsellor having not requested to (OR 1.79; 95% CI 0.47-6.79); received pill or injection reminder compared to not received a pill or injection reminder (OR 4.63; 95% CI: 2.11-10.16). The following factors were associated with long-acting contraception use at four months: Requesting to speak to a counsellor (pressing '1') compared to not pressing '1' after the first voice message (OR 2.05; 95% CI: 1.09-3.88); *ever* compared to *never* requesting to speak to a counsellor (OR 2.88; 95% CI: 1.52-5.45); speaking to the counsellor and *ever* pressing '1' compared to speaking to the counsellor and *never* pressing '1' (OR 2.76; 95% CI: 1.44-5.29).

Association between baseline variables and response to the intervention

Table 2 shows the association between socio-demographic baseline variables and response to the intervention. The following socio-demographic factors were associated with ever requesting to speak to the counsellor (pressing '1'): Age greater than 25 compared to less than 25 (unadjusted OR 1.78; 95% CI: 1.05-3.02) but not after adjusting for confounding variables; lower compared to higher socio-economic status (unadjusted OR 2.92; 95% CI: 1.23-6.90) which remained statistically significant; being married or living together compared to never married or living together (unadjusted OR 4.25; 95% CI: 1.17-15.46) but not in the unadjusted analysis; having one or more compared to no children (unadjusted OR 2.25; 95% CI: 1.30-3.91) which remained statistically significant; having two or more previous abortions as opposed to none (unadjusted OR 3.34; 95% CI: 1.50-7.44) which remained statistically significant; planning to use (unadjusted OR 3.58; 95% CI: 1.09-11.70) or being undecided about PAFP (unadjusted OR 3.71; 95% CI: 1.16-11.82) as opposed to not planning to use PAFP at the time of randomisation but not in the adjusted analysis. Medical compared to surgical abortion became associated with requesting to speak to the counsellor (adjusted OR 1.77; 95% CI: 1.03-3.07) after adjusting for the confounding variables.

Discussion

Summary of main results

In summary, amongst 249 women that received six interactive voice messages +/− counsellor support for PAFP, around half actively requested to speak to a counsellor (pressed '1') and over 90% spoke to a counsellor at some stage. Women who spoke to the counsellor having requested to (by pressing '1') were more than four times as likely to be using effective contraception at four months compared to women who didn't request or speak to the counsellor. There was a small, non-statistically significant increase in contraception use amongst women that spoke to the counsellor *without* requesting a call. Increased parity, a history of >2 previous induced abortions, lower socio-economic status, and medical abortion were associated with requesting to speak to a counsellor (pressing '1') after adjusting for age, socio-economic status and residence, education and number of living children.

Strengths & limitations

A strength of this study is the use of prospectively collected quantitative data on participant characteristics and response to the intervention which provides some insight into the active components of the intervention. The main limitation of this study is that it only considers a provider perspective and does not consider the views and experiences of users; this will be assessed in a subsequent paper. The main limitation affecting the logistic regression analysis was the relatively small sample size, particularly in some of the subgroups, resulting in lack of statistical power to detect differences. Hence, whilst odds ratios may appear to vary greatly between subgroups, the confidence intervals are wide, and so these trends should be interpreted with caution. It was not possible to adequately evaluate the effect of the pill or injection reminders as they were sent to a relatively small number of women, without a control group, and part of a complex intervention. A further limitation concerns the generalisability of this study and the findings might not be applicable to other settings.

Interpretation & comparison with existing literature

To our knowledge, this is the first process evaluation of an interactive mobile phone-based intervention for contraception that includes a detailed assessment of provider-participant communication. Other trials of mobile phone-based interventions to improve contraception use have involved unidirectional text messages, and thus provide limited opportunity for comparison [11–14]. However, some comparisons can be made with other

Table 1 Association between interaction with intervention and effective and long-acting contraception use at four months

	Using effective contraception No/total no. of respondents (%)	OR	*p* value	Using long-acting contraception No/total no. of respondents (%)	OR	*p* value
Per-protocol analysis						
Responded to 1–2 voice messages (r)	33/55 (60%)	1.00		18/55 (33%)	1.00	
Responded to >2 voice messages	89/124 (72%)	1.70 (0.87-3.30)	0.121	40/124 (32%)	0.98 (0.50-1.93)	0.951
Response to voice message 1						
Call failed (r)	40/69 (58%)	1.00		16/69 (23%)	1.00	
1	49/60 (82%)	3.23 (1.44-7.26)	0.005	24/60 (40%)	2.21 (1.03-4.73)	0.041
2	36/58 (62%)	1.19 (0.58-2.42)	0.639	18/58 (31%)	1.49 (0.68-3.28)	0.321
3	10/24 (42%)	0.52 (0.20-1.33)	0.171	3/24 (12%)	0.47 (0.12-1.79)	0.271
Response to voice message 1						
Didn't press '1' (r)	86/151 (57%)	1.00		37/151 (25%)	1.00	
Pressed '1'	49/60 (82%)	3.37 (1.62-6.98)	0.001	24/60 (40%)	2.05 (1.09-3.88)	0.026
Whether participant ever pressed '1'						
Never (r)	53/100 (53%)	1.00		18/100 (18%)	1.00	
1 or more	82/111 (74%)	2.51 (1.41-4.47)	0.002	43/111 (39%)	2.88 (1.52-5.45)	0.001
Spoke to counsellor after voice message '1'						
No (r)	44/74 (59%)	1.00		20/74 (27%)	1.00	
Yes	91/137 (66%)	1.35 (0.75-2.42)	0.315	41/137 (30%)	1.15 (0.61-2.17)	0.658
Whether participant ever spoke to counsellor						
Never (r)	4/11 (36%)	1.00		1/11 (9%)	1.00	
1 or more	131/200 (66%)	3.32 (0.94-11.74)	0.062	60/200 (30%)	4.29 (0.54-34.23)	0.170
Whether pressed '1' if spoke to counsellor						
Spoke to counsellor & never pressed '1' (r)	49/90 (54%)	1.00		17/90 (19%)	1.00	
Spoke to counsellor & ever pressed '1'	82/110 (75%)	2.45 (1.35-4.45)	0.003	43/110 (39%)	2.76 (1.44-5.29)	0.002
Combinations of pressing '1' and speaking to counsellor						
Never pressed '1' & never spoke to counsellor (r)	4/10 (40%)	1.00		1/10 (10%)	1.00	
Never pressed '1' & spoke to counsellor	49/90 (54%)	1.79 (0.47-6.79)	0.390	17/90 (19%)	2.10 (0.25-17.68)	0.496
Pressed '1' & spoke to counsellor	82/110 (75%)	4.39 (1.15-16.71)	0.030	43/110 (39%)	5.78 (0.71-47.22)	0.102
Pressed '1' & never spoke to counsellor	0/1 (0%)	1.00 (.-.)	.	0/1 (0%)	1.00 (.-.)	.
Whether received pill or injection reminders						
Didn't receive pill or injection reminder (r)	96 (59%)	1.00		60 (37%)	1.00	
Received pill or injection reminder	39 (83%)	4.63 (2.11-10.16)	<0.001	1 (2%)	0.08 (0.01-0.62)	0.015
All participants	135/211 (64%)			61/211 (29%)		

The per-protocol analysis included 179 participants. Participants were categorised as 'highly protocol adherent' if they responded (i.e. pressed number '1' or '2') to more than three messages and 'less protocol adherent' if they responded to three or fewer messages

studies, in particular the process evaluation of the text message component of Lester's intervention for anti-retroviral medication adherence [15].

Response to the intervention

Despite sending the messages at the clients preferred time (e.g. morning or evening), the proportion of participants not responding to voice messages (i.e. pressing '1' or '2') was greater than non-responses to interactive text messages reported in trials in Kenya and the USA [6, 14]. The most likely explanation for this is that our 'real-time' voice message required an immediate response (there was no voice-mail), whereas clients can respond to a text message at their convenience. The proportion of women actively responding to voice messages decreased over time, similar to decrease in responses observed in

Table 2 Association between baseline variables and interaction with intervention

	Never pressed '1' N = 127	Ever pressed '1' N = 122	Crude OR	*p* value	Adjusted OR[a]	*P* value
Age group						
Age <25 (r)	53 (60%)	35 (40%)	1.00			
Age >25	74 (46%)	87 (54%)	1.78 (1.05-3.02)	0.032	1.06 (0.52-2.19)	0.864
Residence (urban/rural)						
Urban (r)	48 (56%)	37 (44%)	1.00			
Rural	79 (48%)	85 (52%)	1.40 (0.82-2.36)	0.215	1.49 (0.86-2.59)	0.153
Socio-economic status						
Access to motorised transport (r)	119 (54%)	102 (46%)	1.00			
No access to motorised transport	8 (29%)	20 (71%)	2.92 (1.23-6.90)	0.015	3.36 (1.35-8.40)	0.009
Education						
Secondary or above (r)	85 (54%)	71 (46%)	1.00			
None or primary	42 (45%)	51 (55%)	1.45 (0.87-2.44)	0.155	1.02 (0.58-1.80)	0.936
Marital status						
Never married or living together (r)	12 (80%)	3 (20%)	1.00			
Married/living together	112 (48%)	119 (52%)	4.25 (1.17-15.46)	0.028	3.13 (0.76-12.91)	0.091
Divorced/separated	3 (100%)	0 (0%)	1.00 (.-.)	.	1.00 (.-.)	
# living children						
0 (r)	51 (65%)	28 (35%)	1.00			
1 or more	76 (45%)	94 (55%)	2.25 (1.30-3.91)	0.004	2.24 (1.07-4.72)	0.033
# previous abortions						
0 (r)	81 (56%)	63 (44%)	1.00			
1 or more	46 (44%)	59 (56%)	1.65 (0.99-2.74)	0.053	1.68 (0.96-2.94)	0.067
# previous abortions						
0	81 (56%)	63 (44%)	1.00			
1	36 (52%)	33 (48%)	1.18 (0.66-2.10)	0.576	1.26 (0.68-2.33)	0.014
2 or more	10 (28%)	26 (72%)	3.34 (1.50-7.44)	0.003	3.49 (1.45-8.40)	
Previous contraception use						
No (r)	57 (54%)	49 (46%)	1.00			
Yes	70 (49%)	73 (51%)	1.21 (0.73-2.01)	0.452	1.00 (0.57-1.74)	0.997
Contraception decision-making						
Joint decision (r)	70 (51%)	68 (49%)	1.00			
Mainly participant	26 (47%)	29 (53%)	1.15 (0.61-2.15)	0.665	0.89 (0.45-1.76)	0.931
Mainly husband/partner	17 (45%)	21 (55%)	1.27 (0.62-2.62)	0.514	1.06 (0.48-2.35)	
Mobile phone access						
Never shares (r)	65 (52%)	61 (48%)	1.00			
Shares	62 (50%)	61 (50%)	1.05 (0.64-1.72)	0.852	0.99 (0.59-1.68)	0.979
Disclosure of abortion to others						
No (r)	10 (59%)	7 (41%)	1.00			
Yes	52 (49%)	54 (51%)	1.48 (0.53-4.19)	0.457	1.14 (0.36-3.56)	0.825
PAFP intentions						
No (r)	14 (78%)	4 (22%)	1.00			
Undecided	68 (49%)	72 (51%)	3.71 (1.16-11.82)	0.027	2.69 (0.80-9.12)	0.248
Yes	45 (49%)	46 (51%)	3.58 (1.09-11.70)	0.035	2.46 (0.71-8.55)	

Table 2 Association between baseline variables and interaction with intervention *(Continued)*

Fertility plans						
Have a/another child (r)	82 (53%)	73 (47%)	1.00			
No more/none	34 (50%)	34 (50%)	1.12 (0.63-1.99)	0.690	0.67 (0.34-1.31)	0.388
Undecided	11 (42%)	15 (58%)	1.53 (0.66-3.55)	0.319	1.15 (0.46-2.86)	
Abortion method						
Surgical (r)	80 (54%)	67 (46%)	1.00			
Medical	47 (46%)	55 (54%)	1.40 (0.84-2.32)	0.196	1.85 (1.06-3.22)	0.030
Phone credit						
Always (r)	53 (55%)	44 (45%)	1.00			
Usually	38 (58%)	27 (42%)	0.86 (0.45-1.61)	0.631	0.91 (0.47-1.77)	0.480
Sometimes	36 (41%)	51 (59%)	1.71 (0.95-3.06)	0.073	1.35 (0.73-2.52)	

[a]Adjusted for age, socio-economic status, residence, education and number of living children

previous trials of interactive text message or pager interventions [15–17].

More women requested to speak to a counsellor at voice message one than at message six and the proportion of women not requesting a call back increased over time, which might be expected as issues were resolved. By message six, 15 (6%) clients had opted out mainly because they reported being too busy or shared their phone with someone else, which is common in Cambodia [18]. Six participants (2%) randomised to the intervention did not receive any messages mainly due to non-functioning phone number. A text message trial in the USA reported similar intervention discontinuation (42/480; 9%) and number of participants that never received messages (4/480; 0.9%) [11].

Previous studies have reported greater than 40% discontinuation of short-acting methods by 12 months [19]. In our study, 17% of women that received an injectable reminder message and 32% of women that received a pill reminder message had discontinued at four-months. It is not possible to determine the added value of these additional messages within the whole intervention, as we did not have a comparison group of women using pill or injectable not receiving reminder messages. However, pooled analysis suggests that text message reminders for medication adherence have at best small effects [20]. Elsewhere, a trial in the USA reported that participants receiving text message reminders had a lower mean number of days between scheduled appointment and actual attendance for contraceptive injection for the first, but not subsequent appointments [14].

Assessing associations between interaction with the intervention and contraception use provided further insights regarding possible active components of the intervention. Compared to women that never requested a call (pressed '1') or spoke to the counsellor, women who pressed '1' and spoke to the counsellor were over four times more likely to be using effective contraception at four months. In contrast, there was a lesser, non-statistically significant increase in contraception use amongst women that spoke to the counsellor *without* requesting a call. We did not find evidence that contraception or fertility intentions at the time of seeking abortion services were associated with requesting to speak to a counsellor, after adjusting for the confounding variables. The finding that phoning women who requested a call is associated with subsequent use of effective contraception suggests that the interactive message can identify a subgroup of women in whom counselling will be more effective.

Public health implications

Our finding that women were more likely to request a call back from a counsellor (pressing '1') if they were of lower socio-economic status or increased parity suggests that the intervention is equitable in terms of engaging those most in-need and could have public health benefits at scale. Older women and those with increased parity are at greater than average obstetric risk from subsequent unintended pregnancies [21]. Poor women are most likely to experience complications related to unsafe abortion from subsequent unintended pregnancies [22].

Age was associated with pressing '1' in the unadjusted analysis was because older women were poorer, less educated, had more children or previous abortions and more likely to live in rural areas. In contrast to other studies, we didn't find that residence was associated with response to the voice message [15]. However, it is possible that lack of access to motorised transport (proxy for socio-economic status) was a barrier to accessing face-to-face health services.

Women with one or more child might have requested to speak to a counsellor due to increased motivation to prevent another unintended pregnancy. Engagement by women who have had several abortions could reflect problems with contraception in the past or post-abortion health concerns. Women opting for medical abortion might be more likely to request to speak to a counsellor for support regarding managing their symptoms at home [23]. Although it is safe to use a full-range of contraceptive methods apart from intra-uterine device on the day of medical (misoprostol) treatment, [24] some women might want to postpone decisions about contraception use until the abortion is complete.

Implications for practice/research

First, given that women were more likely to subsequently use contraception if they requested to speak to a counsellor (i.e. pressed '1'), the intervention could be further refined so that counsellors only phone women that request to speak to a counsellor. As the cost of counselling is likely to be the main limitation to scaling up the intervention, this change would reduce costs but any effect of the intervention amongst women that speak to the counsellor *without* requesting a call would be lost. Second, in settings where smartphones use is high, the intervention could be adapted whereby the voice message is sent via an instant messaging application and listened to at the woman's convenience, and can be listened to several times. This might increase the response rate to the messages. Use of such applications provides additional opportunities to add other low-literacy content such as stickers/cartoons and future research could evaluate such interventions.

Conclusions

The interactive message can identify a subgroup of women in whom counselling will be more effective and appears to be equitable in terms of engaging those most in-need. The intervention could be adapted based on the findings of this study.

Acknowledgments

We thank all clients and clinic staff who participated in the study; Channe Suy at the InSTEDD iLab South East Asia; Sieklot Chinn, Melissa Cockcroft, Sarah Cooper, Nicky Jurgens, Michelle Phillips, Sras Thorng and Stefanie Wallach at Marie Stopes International; Clara Calvert, Tim Collier at the London School of Hygiene & Tropical Medicine. CS is supported by a Medical Research Council (MRC) Population Scientist Fellowship.

Authors' contributions

CS undertook the data analysis and drafted the manuscript. LS, RW and UV collected data and assisted with the descriptive analysis. PE advised on statistical analysis. CS and CF designed the intervention and the trial. RW, LS, UV, PE and CF commented on the manuscript. All authors read and approved the final manuscript.

Author details

[1]Department of Population Health, London School of Hygiene and Tropical Medicine, Keppel Street, London WC1E 7HT, UK. [2]Marie Stopes International, Phnom Penh, Cambodia. [3]Department of Obstetrics, Gynecology and Reproductive Sciences, University of California, San Francisco, USA. [4]Room 150, Department of Population Health, London School of Hygiene and Tropical Medicine, Keppel Street, London WC1E 7HT, UK.

References

1. Mechael P, Batavia H, Kaonga N, Searle S, Kwan A, Goldberger A, et al. Barriers and Gaps Affecting mHealth in Low and Middle Income Countries: Policy White Paper. Centre for Global Health and Economic Development. USA: Earth Institute, Columbia University; 2010.
2. Smith C, Gold J, Ngo T, Sumpter C, Free C. Mobile phone-based interventions for improving contraception use (Review). Cochrane Database Syst Rev [Internet]. 2015;(6). Available from: http://onlinelibrary.wiley.com/doi/10.1002/14651858.CD011159.pub2/full
3. Smith C, Ngo T, Gold J, Edwards P, Vannak U, Sokhey L, et al. Effect of a mobile phone-based intervention on post-abortion contraception: a randomized controlled trial in Cambodia. Bull World Health Organ. 2015;93(12):842–50.
4. Smith C, Vannak U, Sokhey L, Ngo T, Gold J, Free C. Mobile Technology for Improved Family Planning (MOTIF): the development of a mobile phone-based (mHealth) intervention to support post-abortion family planning (PAFP) in Cambodia. Reprod Health. 2016;13(1):1–8. Reproductive Health.
5. Smith C, Vannak U, Sokhey L, Ngo TD, Gold J, Khut K, et al. MObile Technology for Improved Family Planning services (MOTIF): study protocol for a randomised controlled trial. Trials. 2013;14(427):1–9. Available from: http://www.trialsjournal.com/content/14/1/427.
6. Lester R, Ritvo P, Mills E, Kariri A, Karanja S, Chung M, et al. Effects of a mobile phone short message service on antiretroviral treatment adherence in Kenya (WelTel Kenya1): a randomised trial. Lancet. 2010;376(9755):1838–45.
7. Reynolds J, DiLiberto D, Mangham-Jefferies L, Ansah EK, Lal S, Mbakilwa H, et al. The practice of "doing" evaluation: lessons learned from nine complex intervention trials in action. Implement Sci. 2014;9(1):75. Available from: http://www.pubmedcentral.nih.gov/articlerender.fcgi?artid=4079170&tool=pmcentrez&rendertype=abstract.
8. Craig P, Dieppe P, Macintyre S, Michie S, Nazareth I, Petticrew M. Developing and evaluating complex interventions: new guidance [Internet]. Sciences-New York. 2008. Available from: www.mrc.ac.uk/complexinterventionsguidance
9. National Institute of Statistics, Directorate General for Health and IM. Cambodia Demographic and Health Survey 2010 [Internet]. Health (San Francisco). 2010. Available from: http://www.measuredhs.com/pubs/pdf/FR249/FR249.pdf
10. Westoff C. Unmet Need for Modern Contraceptive Methods: DHS Analytical Studies No. 28. Calverton, Maryland, USA: ICF International; 2012.
11. Castano P, Bynum J, Andres R, Lara M, Westhoff C. Effect of Daily Text Messages on Oral Contraceptive Continuation; A randomised controlled trial. Obstet Gynecol. 2012;119(1):14–20.
12. Hou M, Hurwitz S, Kavanagh E, Fortin J, Goldberg A. Using daily text-message reminders to improve adherence with oral contraceptives: a randomized controlled trial. Obstet Gynecol. 2010;116(3):633–40.
13. Tsur L, Kozer E, Berkovitch M. The effect of drug consultation center guidance on contraceptive use among women using isotretinoin: a randomized, controlled study. J Women's Heal. 2008;17(4):579–84.
14. Trent M, Thompson C, Tomaszewski K. Text messaging support for urban adolescents and young adults using injectable contraception: Outcomes of the DepoText pilot trial. J Adolesc Heal [Internet]. Elsevier Inc.; 2015;57(1):100–6. Available from: http://dx.doi.org/10.1016/j.jadohealth.2015.03.008
15. van der Kop M, Karanja S, Thabane L, Marra C, Chung M, Gelmon L, et al. In-Depth Analysis of Patient-Clinician Cell Phone Communication during the WelTel Kenya1 Antiretroviral Adherence Trial. Coyne J, editor. PLoS One [Internet]. 2012 Sep 25 [cited 2012 Sep 27];7(9):e46033. Available from: http://dx.plos.org/10.1371/journal.pone.0046033
16. Simoni J, Huh D, Frick P, Pearson C, Andrasik M, Dunbar P, et al. An RCT of Peer Support and Pager Messaging to Promote Antiretroviral Therapy Adherence and Clinical Outcomes among Adults Initiating or Modifying Therapy in Seattle, WA. USA J Acquir Immune Defic Syndr. 2009;52(4):465–73.
17. Hardy H, Kumar V, Doros G, Farmer E, Drainoni M, Rybin D, et al. Randomized Controlled Trial of a Personalized Cellular Phone Reminder System to Enhance Adherence to Antiretroviral Therapy. Behav Psychosoc Res. 2011;25(3):153–61.
18. Bullen P. Operational Challenges in the Cambodian mHealth revolvution. J Mob Technol Med. 2013;2(2):20–3. Available from: http://www.journalmtm.com/2013/operational-challenges-in-the-cambodian-mhealth-revolution/.
19. Ali M, Cleland J, Shah I. Causes and consequences of contraceptive discontinuation: evidence from 60 demographic and health surveys. 2012. Available from: http://apps.who.int//iris/handle/10665/75429.

20. Free C, Phillips G, Galli L, Watson L, Felix L, Edwards P, et al. The effectiveness of mobile-health technology-based health behaviour change or disease management interventions for health care consumers: a systematic review. PLoS Med. 2013;10(1), e1001362.
21. Cleland J, Conde-Agudelo A, Peterson H, Ross J, Tsui A. Contraception and health. Lancet. 2012;380(9837):149–56.
22. Guttmacher Institute. Facts on Induced Abortion Worldwide [Internet]. Most. 2012. Available from: http://www.guttmacher.org/pubs/fb_IAW.pdf
23. Constant D, de Tolly K, Harries J, Myer L. Mobile phone messages to provide support to women during the home phase of medical abortion in South Africa: a randomised controlled trial. Contraception. 2014;90(3):226–33. Elsevier Inc.
24. USAID. High Impact Practices in Family Planning (HIP). Postabortion family planning: strengthening the family planning component of postabortion care. Washington DC: USAID; 2012. Available from: http://www.fphighimpactpractices.org/resources/postabortion-family-planning-strengthening-family-planning-component-postabortion-care.

Maternal and community factors associated with unmet contraceptive need among childbearing women in Northern Nigeria

Bola Lukman Solanke[1*], Funmilola Folasade Oyinlola[1], Olaoye James Oyeleye[1,2] and Benjamin Bukky Ilesanmi[1]

Abstract

Background: Unmet need for modern contraceptive remains a critical reproductive health challenge in Nigeria. Numerous studies in Nigeria and other countries have investigated the patterns, prevalence and associated factors of unmet contraceptive need. In spite of these, the associated factors of unmet contraceptive need in Northern Nigeria have remained insufficiently explored. The few studies that focused on Northern Nigeria have mainly examined maternal individual factors leaving out higher level factors such as community-level factors that may be associated with unmet contraceptive need. This study examines the extent to which maternal and community factors are associated with unmet contraceptive need in Northern Nigeria.

Method: Data was pooled from 2008 to 2013 Nigeria Demographic and Health Surveys. A weighted sample size of 26, 730 women was analysed. The outcome variable was unmet contraceptive need, dichotomised into no unmet need and unmet need. The explanatory variables were individual maternal characteristics such as age, education, number of living children, age at marriage, pregnancy termination experience, and death of a child, and selected community characteristics such as community socioeconomic status, community literacy level, community knowledge of modern contraceptive and geo-political zone. The Multilevel Logistic Regression Model (MLRM) was applied.

Result: Results showed a prevalence of 18% unmet contraceptive need among Northern women in Nigeria. Maternal age of 35 years or older (AOR = 0.873; $p < 0.05$, CI: 0.780–0.976), having five or more living children (AOR = 1.813; $p < 0.001$, CI: 1.663–1.977), higher maternal education (AOR = 0.787; $p < 0.05$, CI: 0.625–0.993), and never experience death of a child (AOR = 0.866; $p < 0.001$, CI: 0.805–0.933) are the maternal factors significantly associated with unmet contraceptive need, while high community literacy level (AOR = 1.230; $p < 0.05$, CI: 1.041–1.454), moderate (AOR = 0.862; $p < 0.05$, CI: 0.767–0.968) or high (AOR = 0.821; $p < 0.05$, CI: 0.726–0.929) community knowledge of modern contraceptive, and geo-political zone of residence are the community-level characteristics significantly associated with unmet contraceptive need among women in Northern Nigeria.

Conclusion: Maternal and community factors are significantly associated with unmet contraceptive need, but based on the ICC maternal factors have more significance in Northern Nigeria. The expansion of existing family planning delivery points to cover all communities including rural and remote areas in the region is imperative.

Keywords: Unmet need, Contraceptive, Reproductive health, Women, Maternal health, Northern Nigeria

* Correspondence: modebolasolanke@gmail.com; bsolanke@oauife.edu.ng
[1]Department of Demography and Social Statistics, Obafemi Awolowo University, Ile-Ife, Nigeria

Background

Unmet contraceptive need exists when women desire to limit childbearing or delay next pregnancy, but are not using any form of contraception to actualise such reproductive desire [1–3]. Unmet contraceptive need remains a public health concern in developing countries particularly in sub-Saharan Africa, where it is currently high but expected to reduce if the countries increase public expenditure on family planning and improve access to modern contraceptives [4, 5]. It is important to address the current high unmet contraceptive need in developing countries because it elevates the exposure of childbearing women to unintended pregnancies, high-risk births, and unsafe abortion, in addition to preventing women from engaging in optimal economic productivity, and thus, may undermine the attainment of the post-2015 development agenda [6–9].

Numerous studies in Nigeria [10–12] and in other countries [13–19] have investigated the patterns, prevalence and associated factors of unmet contraceptive need. These studies not only provided information on the various reasons for unmet contraceptive need among women, but also raise public awareness on the consequences of unmet contraceptive need. In spite of these numerous studies, the associated factors of unmet contraceptive need in Northern Nigeria have remained insufficiently explored. The few studies that focused on Northern Nigeria [20–22] have mainly examined maternal individual factors associated with unmet contraceptive need. The studies provided evidence of low use of modern contraceptive among women in Northern Nigeria. A particular study found 10.3% unmet need for family planning among rural women in the region [21], which was much higher than the 2% reported in a more recent study in the region [22]. The studies also provided evidence of male control over women's utilisation of modern contraceptives in the region [21, 22]. Higher levels of influence on unmet contraceptive need such as community-level characteristics were largely ignored in the existing Northern Nigerian studies.

As observed in an earlier study [23], the determinants of low use of modern contraceptives, and high unmet need among women in low and middle-income countries are similar and operate at multiple levels of the social and physical environment such as the individual level, household level, community level, and health service level. Each level of influence has both joint and independent effects on the level of contraceptive use as well as level of unmet contraceptive need in specific context. For instance, two women with similar or the same socio-demographic characteristics may have different likelihood of contraceptive use due to living in different communities with different proportions of women who had economic empowerment in the community. By examining factors beyond the maternal level, the research prospect of identifying more relevant factors to be targeted in family planning interventions is enhanced across developing countries. It is against this backdrop that the current study focused on maternal and community factors associated with unmet contraceptive need in Northern Nigeria. The study is guided by the research question: to what extent are maternal and community factors associated with unmet contraceptive need in Northern Nigeria?

Methods

Study context

The Federal Republic of Nigeria, an Anglo-phone West African country is the current seventh most populous country in the world, and Africa's most populous country [24]. Population within the country is unevenly distributed between the Southern and Northern regions of the country, with the Northern region being the most populous region in the country. However, in terms of socio-economic development, the Northern region is the poorest in the country with several parts of the region currently undergoing armed insurgency that have gone a long way in reducing availability and utilisation of reproductive health services including family planning services [25–27]. The Northern region of Nigeria is predominantly Islamic with well-entrenched patriarchal social order that thrives on polygynous marriages which has been associated with lower contraceptive use in the country [28]. The region is a high fertility zone [29] with persistence of high parity [30, 31] which has been associated with adverse maternal and child health outcomes in Northern Nigeria [32, 33], as well as in other countries [34–36], and low contraceptive use among high parous women [37]. The region also had the least percentage of family planning demand satisfied by modern methods in the country [38]. Nevertheless, many women in the region still face fertility challenges [39]. Most other indicators of demographic and health situation in the country such as contraceptive prevalence, infant and child health, maternal mortality, and female genital mutilation/cutting reveal that the Northern region is not only worst off in the country, but also deserves more reproductive health attention, which is been promoted through series of health initiatives [40] in addition to ongoing implementation of national population and health policies [41–43].

Data source and sample size

Data analysed in the study was pooled from 2008 and 2013 Nigeria Demographic and Health Surveys (NDHSs) which was part of the Demographic and Health Survey (DHS) being implemented across developing countries to provide national estimates of basic demographic and health information such as fertility, family planning, maternal and child health, female genital mutilation/cutting, and domestic violence. The DHS are nationally representative surveys based on similar methodology and design across the developing countries [44]. In each country where the surveys are conducted, the national population or statistical agency is usually the agency to implement the survey with technical and financial support from the USAID through MEASURE DHS. The 2008 and 2013 NDHSs are the fourth and fifth rounds of the survey in Nigeria. Samples in the surveys were selected in a three-staged stratified cluster designs. In both surveys, information was obtained from respondents using DHS model questionnaires. Interviews were conducted sequel to obtaining informed consent from respondents. The design of the surveys has been widely published [38, 45]. In the current study, the 2008–2013 data were pooled to form a large mass of data that enhance statistical precision and inference. The study used the survey weights provided by the DHS to weight the sample. Hence, a weighted sample size of 26,730 women was analysed. Women included in the sample were: women who want to postpone their next pregnancy or birth but not using a contraceptive method; women who want no more children but not using a contraceptive method; and women who either had a current mistimed or unwanted pregnancy. Those excluded from the study were women from the Southern region and other women that are not relevant to the study such as women who are not currently married, and those not sexually active.

Research variables

The outcome variable was unmet contraceptive need, which was categorised into unmet need and no unmet need. The category of interest in the study was the unmet need category. This group represents the proportion of women who desire to either delay the next pregnancy or limit child birth, but not using any method of contraception [1–3]. The explanatory variables were individual maternal characteristics such as age, age at marriage, number of living children, pregnancy termination experience, education, female autonomy on household decision, and experience of death of a child, and community-level characteristics such as community socioeconomic status, community literacy level, community knowledge of modern contraceptive, proportion of women ever used modern contraceptive in community, place of residence, and geo-political zone. These variables were selected based on their significance in previous studies [11, 12, 14, 15, 23]. Four community-level characteristics, namely, community education level, community socioeconomic status, proportion ever used modern contraceptive method, and community knowledge of modern contraceptive were divided into three categories of 'low, medium, and high' based on the percentiles. Two health service factors, namely, visitation by family planning worker and barriers to healthcare, and two male-partner factors, namely partner education and couple fertility desire were selected for statistical control in the study. Table 1 provides further information on variable definition and measurement.

Data analysis

Data were analysed at the univariate, bivariate and multivariate levels. Prevalence of unmet contraceptive need was described using the pie chart, while the respondents' characteristics were described using percentages and frequency distribution at the univariate level. At the bivariate level, Unadjusted Odds Ratio (UOR) of binary logistic regression was used to examine the likelihood of unmet contraceptive need due to change in each specific explanatory variable. Variables that show statistical significance at this level were selected for inclusion in Multilevel Logistic Regression Model (MLRM). The MLRM was used based on the hierarchy of influence on unmet contraceptive need, namely, individual maternal level and community level, and to show effects that vary by community. The MLRM consists of fixed effects (regression coefficients that vary but not being modelled), and random effects (the regression coefficients being modelled) [46, 47].

The MLRM fitted in the study was specified as:

$$logit\left(P_r\left(Y_{ij}=1\right)\right)=\alpha_0+\alpha_{oj}+\alpha_1 x_{1ij}+\ldots+\alpha_k x_{kij}+\beta_1 z_{1j}+\ldots\beta_m z_{mj}$$

Where:

$x_{ij}-x_{kij}$ are the maternal characteristics

$z_{1j}-z_{mj}$ are the community-level characteristics

The fixed effects of MLRM were assessed using the binary logistic Adjusted Odds Ratio (AOR), while the random effects of the MLRM were measured using Intra-Cluster Correlation (ICC) and Median Odds Ratio (MOR). The ICC calculated as: $\frac{\sigma_{ui}^2}{\sigma_{ui}^2+\left[\frac{\pi^2}{3}\right]}$ where σ_{ui}^2 is the variance at the community level [48] shows the variation in unmet contraceptive need due to the community-level characteristics, and ranges from 0 to 1 but may be expressed in percentage. The higher the values of the ICC, the more important are the community-level characteristics. The MOR calculated as: $\exp(0.95)\sqrt{\sigma_{ui}^2}$ [49] is the median increased odds of reporting unmet contraceptive need if a woman moves to another community with higher likelihood of unmet contraceptive need. The higher the MOR, the more are the importance of the community-level characteristics in predicting variations in unmet contraceptive need. In the absence of community-level characteristics, the value of MOR will be equal to 1 [48]. Model adequacy was checked using the LR test.

Table 1 Variable definition and measurement

S/No.	Name of variable	Measurement	Category/code
Outcome variable			
1.	Unmet contraceptive need	Women who desire to delay next pregnancy or limit child birth, but not using any form of contraception	1. Unmet contraceptive need 0. No unmet need
Individual maternal characteristics			
2.	Age	Current age of respondent	0. 15–24 years 1. 25–34 years 2. 35 years or older
3.	Education	Maternal level of educational attainment	1. None 2. Primary 3. Secondary 4. Higher
4.	Age at first marriage	Age of respondent at the first marriage	1. 17 years or less 2. 18–24 years 3. 25 years or older
5.	Female autonomy	The sole, joint or non-participation of women in three household decision of own healthcare, purchase of large items, and visit to friends and family	1. Full autonomy 2. Joint autonomy 3. No autonomy
6.	Pregnancy termination	Respondents' experience of pregnancy termination	1. Never experienced 2. Ever experienced
7.	Child mortality experience	Whether respondent has experience or never experienced death of a child	1. Never experienced 2. Ever experienced
8.	Number of living children	Respondent number of children ever born that are alive	1. Four or less 2. Five or more
Partner and health service factors (Control variables)			
9.	Partner education	Educational attainment of respondent male partner	1. None 2. Primary 3. Secondary 4. Higher
10.	Couple fertility desire	The fertility preference of respondent and the male partner on family size	1. Both want same 2. Husband want more 3. Husband want fewer 4. Don't know
11.	Visitation by family planning worker	Whether respondent was visited by a family planning worker in the last 12 months preceding the survey	1. Not visited 2. Visited
12.	Barriers to healthcare	Whether respondent perceived that getting partner permission to access healthcare, getting money for treatment, or distance to health facility constitute a barrier to accessing healthcare	1. No barrier 2. At least one barrier
Community characteristics (Higher level of influence)			
13.	Community education level	The proportion of women who had at least secondary education in the community. Not directly available in data but generated from maternal education through method of aggregation at the cluster level	1. Low 2. Medium 3. High
14.	Community socioeconomic status	The proportion of women in richest household wealth quintile in the community. Not directly available in data but generated from household wealth quintile through method of aggregation at the cluster level	1. Low 2. Medium 3. High
15.	Proportion ever used modern contraceptive in community	The extent to which women in the community had ever used modern contraceptive method. Not available directly in data but generated from women's ever use of modern contraceptive method through method of aggregation at the cluster level	1. Low 2. Medium 3. High
16.	Community knowledge of modern contraceptive	The proportion of women in the community who have knowledge of at least one modern contraceptive. Not directly available in data but generated through method of aggregation at the cluster level	1. Low 2. Medium 3. High
17.	Place of residence	Whether respondent place of residence is rural or urban type community	1. Urban 2. Rural
18.	Geo-political zone	The geographic/administrative residence of sampled women	1. North-central 2. North-east 3. North-west

Statistical significance is accepted at $p < 0.05$. All analyses were performed using Stata version 14 [50].

Results

Figure 1 presents the prevalence of unmet contraceptive need among the respondents. As shown in the figure, nearly one-fifth of the respondents had unmet contraceptive need, while the majority of the respondents had no unmet contraceptive need. Table 2 presents the socio-demographic characteristics of the respondents. Slightly more than a quarter of the respondents were less than 25 years, while the rest were 25 years or older. The majority of respondents were 17 years or younger at the time of marriage, while slightly more than one-fifth of the respondents were in the age range of 18 to 24 years at the time of their marriage. The majority of the respondents had four or fewer number of living children, while less than one-third of the respondents had five or more living children. The majority of the respondents had no formal education, but the dominant educational attainment among the educated was primary education. The majority of respondents had no autonomy on household decisions. Slightly more than one-tenth of the respondents had experienced at least one pregnancy termination, while more than half of the women had never experienced the death of a child.

The distribution of the respondents by community literacy level was nearly equal among the respondents. However, slightly higher proportion of the respondents lives in communities with low proportion of women who had secondary education compared to other community educational categories. Nearly half of the respondents live in communities with low socioeconomic status, while one-third of the respondents live in communities with high socioeconomic status. The distribution of respondents by community knowledge of modern contraceptive was nearly equal among the women. But higher proportions of the respondents live in communities with low proportion of women who had ever used contraceptive. The majority of respondents are rural dwellers. Respondents from the North-west geo-political zone were dominant in the sample. Virtually all the respondents were not visited by a family planning worker in the last 12 months preceding the survey. The majority of respondents had no barrier to accessing healthcare. More than half of respondents' partners had no formal education, but secondary education was the dominant level among educated partners. More than two-fifths of respondents' partners desired more children compared to the respondents.

Table 3 presents the bivariate results of the analyses. As maternal age increases, the likelihood of unmet contraceptive need increased significantly among the women particularly among women in the advanced reproductive age of 35 years or older (UOR = 1.335; $p < 0.001$). Likewise, as number of living children increased from four or less to five or more, the likelihood of unmet contraceptive need increased significantly among the women (UOR = 1.672; $p < 0.001$). On the contrary, as age at marriage increases, the likelihood of unmet contraceptive need reduced among the respondent, but this was without statistical significance. Maternal education had mixed relationship with unmet contraceptive need. At the primary and secondary educational levels, the likelihood of unmet need increased, but at higher educational level, the likelihood of unmet contraceptive need reduced significantly (UOR = 0.817; $p < 0.05$). Female autonomy and pregnancy termination were not significantly related to unmet contraceptive need among the women. Women who had never experienced death of a child were less likely to have unmet contraceptive need compared with women who had experienced death of a child (UOR = 0.832; $p < 0.001$).

As community literacy improves from low to medium and high, the likelihood of unmet contraceptive need increased among the women indicating a positive relationship between community literacy level and unmet contraceptive need. Though, the relationship between community socioeconomic status was also positive, but the relationship was without statistical significance. In contrast, as community knowledge of modern contraceptive improved from low to medium and to high, the likelihood of unmet contraceptive need reduced significantly among the respondent. Women who live in communities with high proportion of women who had ever used contraceptive were significantly more likely to have unmet contraceptive need (UOR = 1.086; $p < 0.05$). Place of residence and geo-political zones of the respondents were significantly associated with unmet contraceptive need. Visitation by family planning worker was the only control variable not significantly related to unmet contraceptive need among the women. The variables

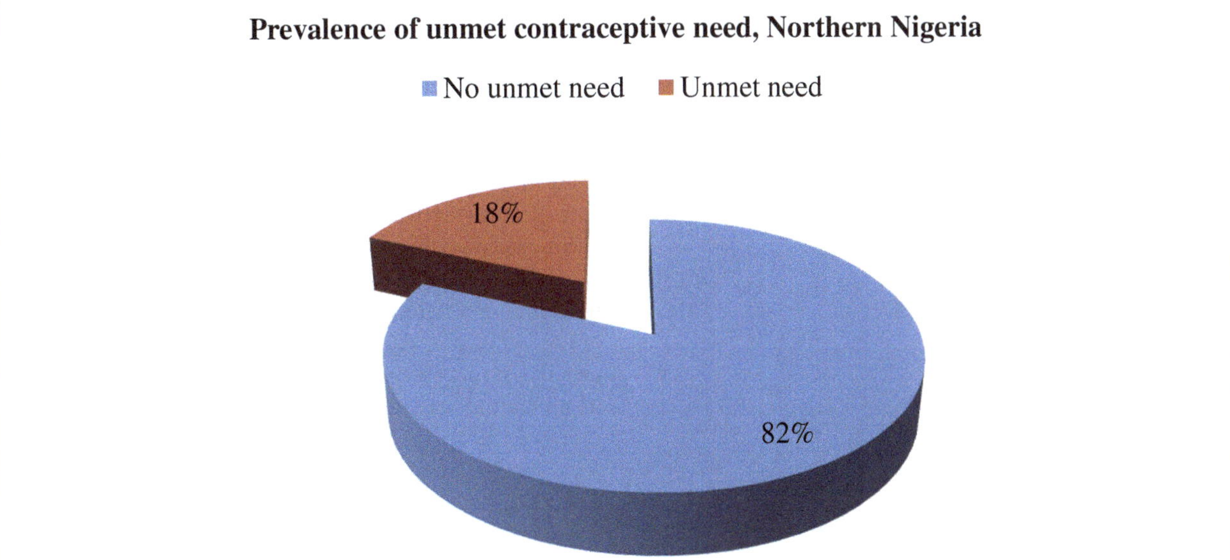

Fig. 1 Prevalence of unmet contraceptive need in Northern Nigeria

Table 2 Respondents' Socio-demographic characteristics

Characteristic	Number of Women (*n* = 26,730)	Percentage
Maternal age		
15–24 years	7870	29.4
25–34 years	9785	36.6
35 years or older	9075	34.0
Age at first marriage		
17 years or younger	20,192	75.5
18–24 years	5619	21.0
25 years or older	919	3.5
Number of living children		
Four or less	18,775	70.2
Five or more	7955	29.8
Education		
None	18,851	70.5
Primary	3990	14.9
Secondary	3076	11.5
Higher	813	3.1
Female autonomy		
Sole	220	0.8
Joint	4631	17.3
No autonomy	21,879	81.9
Pregnancy termination		
Never experienced	23,432	87.7
Ever experienced	3298	12.3
Death of a child		
Ever experienced	10,818	40.5
Never experienced	15,912	59.5
Partner education		
None	15,864	59.4
Primary	3840	14.4
Secondary	4422	16.5
Higher	2604	9.7
Barriers to healthcare		
At least one barrier	3220	12.1
No barrier	23,510	87.9
Visitation by family planning worker		
Not visited	25,813	96.6
Visited	917	3.4
Couple fertility desire		
Both want same	6526	24.4
Husband want more	11,874	44.4
Husband want fewer	859	3.2
Don't know	7471	28.0
Place of residence		
Urban	6104	22.8
Rural	20,626	77.2
Community literacy level		
Low	9476	35.4
Medium	8916	33.4
High	8338	31.2
Community socioeconomic status		
Low	12,174	45.5
Medium	5642	21.1
High	8914	33.4
Community knowledge of modern contraceptive		
Low	8741	32.7
Medium	8840	33.1
High	9149	34.2
Proportion ever used contraceptive in community		
Low	9648	36.1
Medium	9058	33.9
High	8023	30.0
Geo-political zone		
North-central	4680	17.5
North-east	6898	25.8
North-west	15,152	56.7

Source: Author analysis based on 2008–2013 NDHSs

that showed no statistical significance at the bivariate level, namely, age at first marriage, female autonomy, pregnancy termination, community socioeconomic status, and visitation by family planning worker were excluded from the multivariate analyses.

Table 4 presents the fixed effects of the MLRM. The Wald chi-square tests confirm that the models are adequately fitted. In Model 1, the four maternal characteristics included in the model, namely, maternal age, number of living children, education, and experience of death of a child revealed statistically significant associations with unmet contraceptive need. The inclusion of the community-level characteristics in Model 2 did not cause any change in the statistical significance of the maternal characteristics. In the model, community literacy level, community knowledge of modern contraceptive, and geo-political zones were the community-level characteristics significantly associated with unmet contraceptive need.

In Model 3, four maternal characteristics (maternal age, number of living children, experience of death of a child, and maternal education), and three community characteristics (community literacy level, community knowledge of modern contraceptive, and geo-political

Table 3 Unadjusted odds ratio of binary logistic regression showing association between specific explanatory variable and unmet contraceptive need

Variable	UOR	*p*-value	95% CI
Maternal age			
15–24 years [a]	–	–	–
25–34 years	1.162*	$p < 0.001$	1.074–1.258
35 years or older	1.335*	$p < 0.001$	1.234–1.444
Age at first marriage			
17 years or younger[a]	–	–	–
18–24 years	0.997	0.933	0.925–1.074
25 years or older	0.915	0.278	0.779–1.075
Number of living children			
Four or less [a]	–	–	–
Five or more	1.672*	$p < 0.001$	1.568–1.782
Maternal education			
None [a]	–	–	–
Primary	1.102**	$p < 0.05$	1.013–1.199
Secondary	1.072	0.152	0.975–1.179
Higher	0.817	$p < 0.05$	0.686–0.972
Female autonomy			
Sole	–	–	–
Joint	0.991	0.955	0.715–1.373
No autonomy	0.913	0.579	0.663–1.258
Pregnancy termination			
Never experienced [a]	–	–	–
Ever experienced	1.089	0.065	0.995–1.192
Death of a child			
Ever experienced [a]	–	–	–
Never experienced	0.832*	$p < 0.001$	0.782–0.885
Partner education			
None [a]	–	–	–
Primary	1.038	0.419	0.949–1.135
Secondary	1.109**	$p < 0.05$	1.019–1.206
Higher	1.038	0.468	0.938–1.149
Barriers to healthcare			
At least one barrier [a]	–	–	–
No barrier	1.191**	0.001	1.077–1.318
Visitation by family planning worker			
Not visited [a]	–	–	–
Visited	0.888	0.171	0.750–1.052
Couple fertility desire			
Both want same [a]	–	–	–
Husband want more	1.004	0.911	0.929–1.085
Husband want fewer	1.025	0.790	0.855–1.229
Don't know	1.180*	$p < 0.001$	1.085–1.283

Table 3 Unadjusted odds ratio of binary logistic regression showing association between specific explanatory variable and unmet contraceptive need *(Continued)*

Variable	UOR	*p*-value	95% CI
Place of residence			
Urban [a]	–	–	–
Rural	0.901**	0.005	0.838–0.969
Community literacy level			
Low [a]	–	–	–
Medium	1.091**	0.024	1.012–1.177
High	1.130**	0.001	1.048–1.219
Community socioeconomic status			
Low [a]	–	–	–
Medium	1.001	0.979	0.923–1.085
High	1.025	0.484	0.956–1.099
Community knowledge of modern method			
Low [a]	–	–	–
Medium	0.927**	0.048	0.861–0.999
High	0.911**	0.014	0.845–0.982
Proportion ever used contraceptive in community			
Low [a]	–	–	–
Medium	1.021	0.592	0.947–1.101
High	1.086**	0.031	1.007–1.171
Geo-political zone			
North-central [a]	–	–	–
North-east	0.996	0.929	0.915–1.085
North-west	0.865*	$p < 0.001$	0.798–0.937

[a]RC: *Reference category*, *$p < 0.001$, **$p < 0.05$

zone) were the variables significantly associated with unmet contraceptive need. Women who were 35 years or older were 12.7% less likely to have unmet contraceptive compared to women in the 15–24 years age range (AOR = 0.873; $p < 0.05$, CI: 0.780–0.976). However, women who had five or more living children were 81.3% more likely to have unmet contraceptive need compared to women who had four or fewer number of living children (AOR = 1.813; $p < 0.001$, CI: 1.663–1.977). Women who attained higher education were 21.2% less likely to have unmet contraceptive need compared to uneducated women (AOR = 0.787; $p < 0.05$, CI: 0.625–0.993). Also, women who had never experienced death of a child were 13.4% less likely to have unmet contraceptive need compared to women who had experienced death of a child (AOR = 0.866; $p < 0.001$, CI: 0.805–0.933).

The model further reveals that women who live in communities with high literacy level were 23% more likely to have unmet contraceptive need compared to women in the reference category (AOR = 1.230; $p < 0.05$, CI: 1.041–1.454). On the contrary, women who live in communities with high knowledge of modern contraceptive were 17.9% less likely to have unmet contraceptive need compared to women in communities with low knowledge of modern contraceptive need (AOR = 0.821; $p < 0.05$, CI: 0.726–0.929). Likewise, women in the North-west geo-political zone were 16.8% less likely to have unmet contraceptive need compared to women in the North-central geo-political zone (AOR = 0.832; $p =$ 0.001, CI: 0.748–0.926). Barrier to healthcare was the only control variable that reveals significant association with unmet contraceptive need. Table 5 presents random effects of the MLRM. Diagnosis of the model adequacy using the LR test reveals that the empty model as well as the three fitted models were adequate for examining the significance of contextual influence on unmet contraceptive need ($p < 0.001$). However, the results of the ICC only reveal marginal importance of the community level characteristics compared with the maternal characteristics. Across the fitted models, the ICC showed that community factors accounted for less than 5 % of the variation in unmet contraceptive need among the women, which was buttressed by the median odds ratios that indicate a low context effect in the three models.

Discussion

This study examined the extent to which maternal and community factors were associated with unmet contraceptive need in Northern Nigeria. The study not only provided additional information on the prevalence and associated factors of unmet contraceptive need, but has also made two key significant contributions to the literature on unmet need for family planning. Firstly, the study focused on Northern Nigeria which is the region with the poorest contraceptive prevalence in the country, and has only been covered in few studies on unmet contraceptive need in the region [20–22]. The situation of unmet need for family planning in Northern Nigeria has therefore been brought further to the fore of national family planning awareness, which may draw the attention of family planning programming officers in the country. Secondly, the study extended search for significant correlates of unmet contraceptive need in Nigeria by examining the likely community characteristics that may shape the level of unmet need for family planning in Northern Nigeria. This addressed the limitation of previous studies in the region [20–22], and provides information on wider range of variables to be targeted by family planning policy makers in the region. Based on the findings five key issues emerged from the study.

One, the prevalence of unmet contraceptive need in Northern Nigeria is 18%. This prevalence is higher than the 10.3% reported in an earlier study in the region [21] and much higher than the 2% reported in a recent study in the region [22]. This variation may be explained by the fact that the previous studies in the region [20–22] were small scale surveys compared to the NDHSs which were nationally representative and covered more women in the region. The result is however similar to the 17.1% reported in a study in Indonesia [15], the 17.4% reported by a study in Ethiopia [16], and the 17.4% reported in a study conducted in Iran [14]. However, the level of unmet contraceptive need found in this study is much lower than the 31.1% reported by a study in North-west region of Cameroon [18], the 44% found in a study in Dessie Town of Ethiopia [17], as well as the 32.4% reported in a study conducted in Burundi [19]. The level of unmet contraceptive need found in this study is thus comparable to findings elsewhere, and suggests need for fresh initiatives in Northern Nigeria to reduce unmet need for family planning among childbearing women in the region.

This is particularly important because high unmet contraceptive need further expose women to unintended pregnancies, unsafe abortion, and hinder women from effective economic participation, which also have implications for family health [6–9]. Bearing in mind, that Northern Nigeria is a high fertility zone in the country [29], there is need for urgent steps to be taken to reduce unmet need for family planning in Northern Nigeria. This may include expansion of existing family planning delivery points to cover all communities including rural and remote areas in the region. Such initiative should take advantage of the existing negative relationship between community knowledge of modern contraceptive and unmet contraceptive need as found in the study. In communities with high knowledge of modern contraceptive, the odds of unmet need were lower to indicate that expansion in knowledge of modern contraceptive may further reduce unmet need among women. It is therefore important that expansion in service delivery points should be accompanied with expansion in women's education which is currently poor as found in this study, as this may boost awareness and utilisation of modern contraceptives among women in the region.

Two, the study found that women who had five or more living children had higher likelihood of unmet contraceptive need in Northern Nigeria. This situation is detrimental to maternal and child health in the region due to widespread evidence that high parity among women elevates the risk of adverse maternal and child health outcomes [32–36]. It is therefore important for additional contraceptive information, education and communication programme in the country to specifically target women with high parity in Northern Nigeria. Such programme could be designed and implemented by Primary Health Care agencies which are the nearest health facility to most women in the region.

Three, the study reveal that women with higher education had the least likelihood of unmet contraceptive

Table 4 Fixed effects on the likelihood of unmet contraceptive need, Northern Nigeria

Characteristic	Model 1 (Wald chi-sq = 266.1; $p < 0.001$)			Model 2 (Wald chi-sq = 298.1; $p < 0.001$)			Model 3 (Wald chi-sq = 325.2; $p < 0.001$)		
	AOR	*p*-value	95% CI	AOR	*p*-value	95% CI	AOR	*p*-value	95% CI
Maternal age (years)									
15–24 years[a]	–	–	–	–	–	–	–	–	–
25–34 years	0.977	0.622	0.893–1.070	0.964	0.429	0.880–1.056	0.969	0.500	0.885–1.062
35 years or older	0.885	$p < 0.05$	0.792–0.988	0.867	$p < 0.05$	0.776–0.969	0.873	$p < 0.05$	0.780–0.976
Number of living children									
Four or fewer[a]	–	–	–	–	–	–	–	–	–
Five or more	1.801	$p < 0.01$	1.652–1.963	1.808	$p < 0.01$	1.658–1.971	1.813	$p < 0.01$	1.663–1.977
Maternal education									
None[a]	–	–	–	–	–	–	–	–	–
Primary	1.081	0.105	0.984–1.188	1.030	0.548	0.935–1.136	1.013	0.809	0.913–1.123
Secondary	1.124	$p < 0.05$	1.005–1.257	1.044	0.476	0.927–1.175	1.022	0.747	0.896–1.165
Higher	0.869	0.176	0.710–1.065	0.778	$p < 0.05$	0.630–0.960	0.788	$p < 0.05$	0.625–0.993
Death of a child									
Ever experienced[a]	–	–	–	–	–	–	–	–	–
Never experienced	0.882	0.001	0.819–0.949	0.867	$p < 0.01$	0.805–0.934	0.866	$p < 0.01$	0.805–0.933
Community literacy level									
Low[a]				–	–	–	–	–	–
Medium				1.138	0.052	0.999–1.296	1.128	0.069	0.991–1.285
High				1.247	$p < 0.05$	1.054–1.474	1.230	$p < 0.05$	1.041–1.454
Community Knowledge of modern contraceptive									
Low[a]				–	–	–	–	–	–
Medium				0.861	$p < 0.05$	0.766–0.968	0.862	$p < 0.05$	0.767–0.968
High				0.815	0.001	0.721–0.923	0.821	$p < 0.05$	0.726–0.929
Proportion ever used modern contraceptive in community									
Low[a]				–	–	–	–	–	–
Medium				0.989	0.849	0.881–1.110	0.988	0.835	0.880–1.108
High				1.030	0.654	0.906–1.170	1.025	0.700	0.903–1.164
Place of residence									
Urban[a]				–	–	–	–	–	–
Rural				0.909	0.060	0.822–1.004	0.916	0.088	0.829–1.013
Geographic region									
North-central[a]				–	–	–	–	–	–
North-east				0.881	$p < 0.05$	0.788–0.985	0.887	$p < 0.05$	0.793–0.994
North-west				0.827	$p < 0.01$	0.745–0.917	0.832	0.001	0.748–0.926
Barriers to healthcare									
At least one barrier[a]							–	–	–
No barrier							1.162	$p < 0.05$	1.040–1.299
Partner education									
None[a]							–	–	–
Primary							1.016	0.761	0.915–1.128
Secondary							1.100	0.088	0.986–1.228
Higher							1.048	0.514	0.911–1.205
Couple fertility desire									

Table 4 Fixed effects on the likelihood of unmet contraceptive need, Northern Nigeria *(Continued)*

Characteristic	Model 1 (Wald chi-sq = 266.1; $p < 0.001$)			Model 2 (Wald chi-sq = 298.1; $p < 0.001$)			Model 3 (Wald chi-sq = 325.2; $p < 0.001$)		
	AOR	*p*-value	95% CI	AOR	*p*-value	95% CI	AOR	*p*-value	95% CI
Both want same[a]							–	–	–
Husband want more							1.057	0.215	0.968–1.153
Husband want fewer							1.011	0.911	0.832–1.229
Don't know							1.193	$p < 0.01$	1.087–1.309

[a]RC: *Reference Category*, $p < 0.01$ or $p < 0.05$ is statistically significant

need in Northern Nigeria which was consistent with findings in previous Nigerian studies [11, 12]. This implies that initiatives to improve women's access to formal education in the region should not be limited to primary and secondary educational levels but should seeks to make higher education more accessible to women in the region. Higher education for women not only provides them with economic empowerment, it also enhances their ability to take reproductive decisions with little male involvement. Though, higher education among women may also create some problems such as the problems associated with delayed marriage and childbearing, but such problem can be properly handled through adequate family life education curriculum. In spite of the significance of maternal education, it was revealed in the study that high community literacy level was associated with higher odds of unmet contraceptive need. This seems counter-productive but may be explained by the fact that when there is high proportion of women who had secondary or higher education in the community, there is also higher likelihood of postponement of marriage or childbearing among women in the community. In such community, women will most likely use contraceptive for spacing and not limiting. This may create unmet contraceptive need among women particularly when family planning delivery is poor in the community.

Four, the study reveals that women who had never experienced death of a child had less likelihood of unmet contraceptive need. This finding has two implications. Firstly, it may suggest that women who had lost a child in the region tend to desire replacement of the dead child irrespective of current number of living children. For women still at the lower echelons of the reproductive life span, such fertility desire may not be injurious to their reproductive health, but for women already in advanced reproductive age who may no longer have fertility desire such attempt to replace a dead child may lead to serious health complications. Secondly, it tends to draw attention to boosting child survival in the region. Presently, child health is poorest in Northern Nigeria compared to Southern Nigeria [38] and needs to be improved upon to discourage some women from continuing to have deliveries with the mind-set that some of the new-borns may not survive to adulthood, hence another pregnancy is desired as possible replacement.

Five, the study revealed that the odds of unmet contraceptive need was higher among women who had no barrier to accessing healthcare. Ordinarily, women who had no barrier to accessing healthcare should have reduced unmet contraceptive need since such women will have more likelihood of receiving facility-based counselling and education on family planning. The results however may also indicate that in some situations, having access to healthcare services may not necessarily translate to utilisation of the services. This is possible in many Islamic settings such as Northern Nigeria where women may not utilise available services due to preference for female healthcare providers or personnel who may not be readily available in some health facility, particularly in rural and remote areas. Thus, repositioning family planning services in Northern Nigeria may require the development and implementation of more religion or culture specific strategies. This may be particularly more relevant in the North-east and North-west geopolitical zones of the region because the two zones have the poorest levels of contraceptive prevalence in the country.

The analysis performed in the study suffers from two drawbacks. One, the study pooled data from surveys

Table 5 Multilevel logistic regression model showing random-effects on unmet contraceptive need, Northern Nigeria

Parameter	Empty Model	Model 1	Model 2	Model 3
Community-level variance (S.E.)	0.139 (0.019)	0.137 (0.019)	0.127 (0.018)	0.123 (0.018)
ICC	4.1%	4.0%	3.7%	3.6%
Log-likelihood	−12,910.7	−12,773.9	−12,756.3	−12,740.8
LR test	$\chi^2 = 166.0$; $p < 0.001$	$\chi^2 = 159.4$; $p < 0.001$	$\chi^2 = 139.4$; $p < 0.001$	$\chi^2 = 133.7$; $p < 0.001$
Median Odds Ratio (MOR)	0.96	0.96	0.92	0.91

Notes: $p < 0.001$ is statistically significant

conducted in 2008 and 2013. This will treat the sample analysed as sampling done with replacement, and will not allow the findings to be specifically linked to either to 2008 or 2013 but jointly as a single period of 2008–2013. It is therefore important to understand the inference made in the study with caution despite the precision attributable to pooled data. Also, the cross-sectional nature of the data did not allow the investigation of causality. Hence, the analyses were limited to investigating associations between the research variables.

Conclusion

This study analysed maternal and community factors associated with unmet contraceptive need in Northern Nigeria. Data were extracted from the 2008–2013 Nigeria Demographic and Health Surveys. Findings revealed that some maternal and community factors were significantly associated with unmet contraceptive need in Northern Nigeria. However, based on the results of the ICC, individual maternal characteristics showed more significance than community characteristics. The expansion of existing family planning delivery points to cover all communities including rural and remote areas in the region is imperative.

Abbreviations

DHS: Demographic and Health Survey; MLRM: Multilevel Logistic Regression Model; NDHS: Nigeria Demographic and Health Survey

Acknowledgements

The authors expresses gratitude to the National Population Commission (NPC) [Nigeria], ICF International and MEASURE DHS Project for granting authorisation to analyse the datasets.

Authors' contributions

FFO developed the original concept. BLS modified the concept and reviewed literature. BLS, OJO and BBI analysed the data. All authors discussed the findings. All authors read through the manuscript for intellectual content. All authors read and approved the final manuscript.

Author information

BLS is a Senior Lecturer in Demography and Social Statistics, Obafemi Awolowo University, Ile-Ife, Nigeria. His research interests are fertility, contraception, and women's health issues. FFO and BBI are doctoral students while OJO is a graduate student in the Department of Demography and Social Statistics, Obafemi Awolowo University, Ile-Ife, Nigeria.

Author details

[1]Department of Demography and Social Statistics, Obafemi Awolowo University, Ile-Ife, Nigeria. [2]Action Against Hunger, ACF-International, Damaturu, Yobe State, Nigeria.

References

1. Bradley SEK, Casterline JB. Understanding unmet need: history, theory, and measurement. Stud Fam Plan. 2014;45(2):123–50. https://doi.org/10.1111/j.1728-4465.2014.00381.x.
2. Cleland J, Harbison S, Shah IH. Unmet need for contraception: issues and challenges. Stud Fam Plan. 2014;45(2):105–22.
3. Sedgh G, Ashford LS, Hussain R. Unmet need for contraception in developing countries: examining Women's reasons for not using a method. New York: Guttmacher Institute; 2016.
4. Darroch JE, Singh S. Trends in contraceptive need and use in developing countries in 2003, 2008, and 2012: an analysis of national surveys. Lancet. 2013;381:1756–62.
5. Alkema L, Kantorova V, Menozzi C, Biddlecom A. National, regional, and global rates and trends in contraceptive prevalence and unmet need for family planning between 1990 and 2015: a systematic and comprehensive analysis. Lancet. 2013;381:1642–52. https://doi.org/10.1016/S0140-6736(12)62204-1.
6. Yamey G, Cohen CR, Bukusi EA. Meeting an unmet need for family planning. BMJ. 2012;344:e4160. https://doi.org/10.1136/bmj.e4160.
7. Cleland J, Conde-Agudelo A, Peterson H, Ross J, Tsui A. Contraception and health. Lancet. 2012;380:149–56. https://doi.org/10.1016/S0140-6736(12)60609-6.
8. Canning D, Schultz TP. The economic consequences of reproductive health and family planning. Lancet. 2012;380:165–71. https://doi.org/10.1016/S0140-6736(12)60827-7.
9. Bishwajit G, Tang S, Yaya S, Feng Z. Unmet need for contraception and its association with unintended pregnancy in Bangladesh. BMC Pregnancy Childbirth. 2017;17:186. https://doi.org/10.1186/s12884-017-1379-4.
10. Ogunjuyigbe PO, Akinlo A, Oni GO. Violence against women as a factor in unmet need for contraception in Southwest Nigeria. J Fam Violence. 2010;25:123–30. https://doi.org/10.1007/s10896-009-9275-y.
11. Austin A. Unmet contraceptive need among married Nigerian women: an examination of trends and drivers. Contraception. 2015;91:31–8. https://doi.org/10.1016/j.contraception.2014.10.002.
12. Alaba OO, Olaomi JO, Olubusoye OE. Spatial pattern and determinants of unmet need of family planning in Nigeria. S Afr Fam Pract. 2015;57(5):306–12. https://doi.org/10.1080/20786190.2015.1071536.
13. Withers M, Kano M, Pinatih GDE. Desire for more children, contraceptive use and unmet need for family planning in a remote area of Bali, Indonesia. J Biosoc Sci. 2010;42:549–62. https://doi.org/10.1017/S0021932010000052.
14. Motlaq ME, Eslami M, Yazdanpanah M, Nakhaee N. Contraceptive use and unmet need for family planning in Iran. Int J Gynecol Obstet. 2013;121:157–61. https://doi.org/10.1016/j.ijgo.2012.11.024.
15. Ayuningtyas D, Oktaviana W. Misnaniarti. Factors contributing to unmet need for contraception in Nusa Tenggara Barat, Indonesia. J Reprod Contracept. 2015;26(4):239–48. https://doi.org/10.7669/j.issn.1001-7844.2015.04.0239.
16. Genet E, Abeje G, Ejigu T. Determinants of unmet need for family planning among currently married women in Dangila town administration, Awi zone, Amhara regional state; a cross sectional study. Reprod. 2015;12:42. https://doi.org/10.1186/s12978-015-0038-3.
17. Tegegn M, Arefaynie M, Tiruye TY. Unmet need for modern contraceptives and associated factors among women in the extended postpartum period in Dessie town, Ethiopia. Contracept Reprod Med. 2017;2:21. https://doi.org/10.1186/s40834-017-0048-3.
18. Edietah EE, Njotang PN, Ajong AB, Essi MJ, Yakum MN, Mbu ER. Contraceptive use and determinants of unmet need for family planning; a cross sectional survey in the north west region, Cameroon. BMC Womens Health. 2018;18:171. https://doi.org/10.1186/s12905-018-0660-7.
19. Nzokirishaka A, Itua I. Determinants of unmet need for family planning among married women of reproductive age in Burundi: a cross-sectional study. Contracept Reprod Med. 2018;3:11. https://doi.org/10.1186/s40834-018-0062-0.
20. Duze MC, Mohammed IZ. Male knowledge, attitudes, and family planning practices in northern Nigeria. Afr J Reprod Health. 2006;10(3):53–65.
21. Doctor HV, Findley SE, Afenyadu GY, Uzondu C, Ashir GM. Awareness, use, and unmet need for family planning in rural northern Nigeria. Afr J Reprod Health. 2013;17(4):107–17.
22. Sinai I, Nyenwa J, Oguntunde O. Programmatic implications of unmet need for contraception among men and young married women in northern Nigeria. Open Access J Contracept. 2018;9:81–90. https://doi.org/10.2147/OAJC.S172330.
23. Wulifan JK, Brenner S, Jahn A, De Allegri M. A scoping review on determinants of unmet need for family planning among women of reproductive age in low and middle income countries. BMC Womens Health. 2016;16:2. https://doi.org/10.1186/s12905-015-0281-3.
24. Population Reference Bureau. 2018 World population data sheet with focus on changing age structures. Washington DC: PRB; 2018.
25. Ager AK, Lembani M, Mohammed A, Ashir GM, Abdulwahab A, de Pinho H, Delobelle P, Zarowsky C. Health service resilience in Yobe state, Nigeria in the context of the Boko Haram insurgency: a systems dynamics analysis using group model building. Confl Health. 2015;9:30. https://doi.org/10.1186/s13031-015-0056-3.

26. Solanke BL. Factors associated with use of maternal healthcare services during the Boko Haram insurgency in North-East Nigeria. Med Confl Surviv. 2018;34(3):158–84. https://doi.org/10.1080/13623699.2018.1511358.
27. Chukwuma A, Ekhator-Mobayode UE. Armed conflict and maternal health care utilization: evidence from the Boko Haram insurgency in Nigeria. Soc Sci Med. 2019;226:104–12. https://doi.org/10.1016/j.socscimed.2019.02.055.
28. Audu B, Yahya S, Geidam A, Abdussalam H, Takai I, Kyari O. Polygamy and the use of contraceptives. Int J Gynecol Obstet. 2008;101:88–92. https://doi.org/10.1016/j.ijgo.2007.09.036.
29. Izugbara CO, Ezeh AC. Women and high fertility in Islamic northern Nigeria. Stud Fam Plan. 2010;41(3):193–204.
30. Akinyemi A, Adedini S, Hounton S, Akinlo A, Adedeji O, Adonri O, et al. Contraceptive use and distribution of high-risk births in Nigeria: a sub-national analysis. Glob Health Action. 2015;8:29745. https://doi.org/10.3402/gha.v8.29745.
31. Rabiu A, Abubakar IS, Garba I, Haruna IU. Contraceptive choices among grand multiparous women at Murtala Mohammed Specialist Hospital, Kano. Ann Afr Med. 2016;15:58–62. https://doi.org/10.4103/1596-3519.176203.
32. Geidam AD, Audu BM, Oummate Z. Pregnancy outcome among grand multiparous women at the University of Maiduguri Teaching Hospital: a case control study. J Obstet Gynaecol. 2011;31(5):404–8. https://doi.org/10.3109/01443615.2011.561383.
33. Omole-Ohonsi A, Ashimi AO. Grand multiparity: obstetric performance at Aminu Kano teaching hospital, Kano, Nigeria. Niger J Clin Pract. 2011;14(1):6–9. https://doi.org/10.4103/1119-3077.79231.
34. Teguete I, Maiga AW, Leppert PC. Maternal and neonatal outcomes of grand multiparas over two decades in Mali. Acta Obstet Gynecol Scand. 2012;91:580–6. https://doi.org/10.1111/j.1600-0412.2012.01372.x.
35. Lahti M, Eriksson JG, Heinonen K, Kajantie E, Lahti J, et al. Maternal grand multiparity and the risk of severe mental disorders in adult offspring. PLoS One. 2014;9(12):e114679. https://doi.org/10.1371/journal.pone.0114679.
36. Al-Shaikh GK, Ibrahim GH, Fayed AA, Al-Mandeel H. Grand multiparity and the possible risk of adverse maternal and neonatal outcomes: a dilemma to be deciphered. BMC Pregnancy Childbirth. 2017;17:310. https://doi.org/10.1186/s12884-017-1508-0.
37. Ibrahim G, Rabiu A, Abubakar IS. Knowledge, attitude and practice of contraceptives among grand multiparous women attending antenatal clinic in a specialist hospital, Kano, Nigeria. Niger J Basic Clin Sci. 2015;12:90–4. https://doi.org/10.4103/0331-8540.169277.
38. National Population Commission (NPC) [Nigeria], ICF International. Nigeria Demographic and Health Survey 2013. Abuja and Rockville: NPC and ICF International; 2014.
39. Iliyasu Z, Galadanci HS, Abubakar S, Auwal MS, Odoh C, Salihu HM. Et. Phenotypes of intimate partner violence among women experiencing infertility in Kano, Northwest Nigeria. Int J Gynaecol Obstet. 2016;133:32–6. https://doi.org/10.1016/j.ijgo.2015.08.010.
40. Doctor HV, Findley SE, Ager A, Cometto G, Afenyadu GY, Adamu F, Green C. Using community-based research to shape the design and delivery of maternal health services in northern Nigeria. Reprod Health Matters. 2012; 20(39):104–12. https://doi.org/10.1016/S0968-8080(12)39615-8.
41. National Population Commission. National Policy on population for sustainable development. Abuja: NPC; 2004.
42. Federal Ministry of Health. Revised National Health Policy. Abuja: FMoH; 2004.
43. Federal Ministry of Health. Saving newborn lives in nigeria: newborn health in the context of the integrated maternal, newborn and child health strategy. 2nd ed. Abuja: FMoH, Save the Children, Jhpiego; 2011.
44. ICF International. Survey Organization Manual for Demographic and Health Surveys, MEASURE DHS. Calverton: ICF International; 2012.
45. National Population Commission (NPC) [Nigeria], ICF Macro. Nigeria Demographic and Health Survey 2008. Abuja: NPC and ICF Macro; 2009.
46. Gelman A, Hill J. Data analysis using regression and multilevel/hierarchical models. New York: Cambridge University Press; 2007.
47. Austin PC, Merlo J. Intermediate and advanced topics in multilevel logistic regression analysis. Stat Med. 2017. https://doi.org/10.1002/sim.7336.
48. Merlo J, Wagner P, Ghith N, Leckie G. An original stepwise multilevel logistic regression analysis of discriminatory accuracy: the case of Neighbourhoods and health. PLoS One. 2016;11(4):e0153778. https://doi.org/10.1371/journal.pone.0153778.
49. Goicolea I, San Sebastian M. Unintended pregnancy in the amazon basin of Ecuador: a multilevel analysis. Int J Equity Health. 2010;(14):9. https://doi.org/10.1186/1475-9276-9-14.
50. StataCorp. Stata: Release 14. Statistical Software. College Station: StataCorp LP; 2015.

23

Return of fertility after discontinuation of contraception

Tadele Girum* and Abebaw Wasie

Abstract

Introduction: Along with increasing availability and utilization of contraception, It is also important to confirm that the effects of contraception use on resumption of fertility after discontinuation However currently evidences on resumption of fertility after contraception use are inconclusive and practically fertility after termination of contraception remains a big concern for women who are using contraception. This fear poses a negative impact on utilization and continuation of contraception. Therefore, Estimating the rate of pregnancy resumption after contraceptive use from the available reports and identifying the associating factors are important for designing a strategy to overcome the problem.

Methods: The review was conducted through a systematic literature search of articles published between 1985 and 2017. Five bibliographic databases and libraries: PubMed/Medline, Global Health Database, Embase, the Cochrane Library, and African Index Medicus were used. After cleaning and sorting, analysis was performed using STATA version 11. The pooled rate of conception was estimated with a random-effects model. Heterogeneity was assessed by the I^2 and publication bias through funnel plot.

Results: Twenty two studies that enrolled a total of 14,884 women who discontinued contraception were retained for final analysis. The pooled rate of pregnancy was 83.1% (95% CI = 78.2-88%) within the first 12 months of contraceptive discontinuation. It was not significantly different for hormonal methods and IUD users. Similarly the type of progesterone in specific contraception option and duration of oral-contraceptive use do not significantly influence the return of fertility following cessation of contraception. However the effect of parity in the resumption of pregnancy following cessation of contraception was inconclusive.

Conclusion and recommendation: Contraceptive use regardless of its duration and type does not have a negative effect on the ability of women to conceive following termination of use and it doesn't significantly delay fertility. Therefore, appropriate counseling is important to assure the women to use the methods as to their interest.

Keywords: Return of fertility, Contraceptives, Intrauterine device, Implants, Pills

Background

Wide ranges of effective and safe reversible modern contraceptives are available in the contemporary world. Despite the advancement in contraceptive technologies and organized international effort over the last few decades; the concern of women who use reversible contraception related to time to return of fertility still remained unanswered [1–3]. Most contraceptives have been modified to improve their safety and tolerability without compromising efficacy. It is also important to know the effect of contraception use on the subsequent fertility [1, 3].

However, currently evidences regarding resumption of pregnancy after contraceptive discontinuation are inconclusive. Delay of fertility after termination of contraception remains a big concern for women who are using contraception. Particularly women who ever experienced post pill amenorrhea or fail to become pregnant within expected date of fertility after termination of contraception have speculated contraceptive options cause delayed return of fertility.

* Correspondence: girumtadele@yahoo.com
Department of Public Health, College of Medicine and Health Sciences, Wolkite University, Wolkite City, Ethiopia

Controlling unwanted fertility with highly effective reversible contraception allowed couples to have the number of children they want at the time they want to have. On the other hand fertility delay or impairment as a result of prior contraception use may lead to dissatisfaction and lower contraception use irrespective of actual desire [3–7].

Approximately 15% of couples experience infertility (fail to get pregnant within 1 year) [6], women who use hormonal contraception have considerable concern of delayed or impaired fertility upon discontinuation. Delayed return of fertility or infertility among previous contraceptive users is commonly linked to their contraceptive use. Therefore, this premise that leads to misconception among family planning users need to be synthesized and tested using the available evidences across the globe.

These concerns were also raised by scholars from early reports that Oral Contraceptive use may cause secondary amenorrhea, which is associated with anovulation and reduced reproductive fecundity. IUD may also cause infertility secondary to pelvic inflammatory disease (PID) [7]. It was believed that exogenous hormonal therapy causes delayed return of normal function of hypothalamic/pituitary/ovarian axis [8–11] and temporary infertility [12]. However these concerns were disproved from more recent studies partly from development of low dose hormonal contraception, prevention of PID and implementation of scientific technique [13–16].

There are a number of studies and few specific reviews conducted to assess the effect of different forms of contraceptives on subsequent pregnancies. The findings were inconclusive, in some studies contraception shown to have only an initial (temporary) delay in conception for the first few months after discontinuation [13–16]. While in recent studies no association was observed between contraceptive use and secondary amenorrhea [17–19] except with higher doses of oestrogen [20]. On the other hand many studies have reported that, the type of intrauterine device as well as duration of use has not been found to be related to fertility return [21].

Therefore, we aimed to conduct a comprehensive systematic review and meta-analysis through reviewing globally published observational studies on the effect of fertility return after discontinuation of different contraception among married and in union. Return of fertility is measured in terms of pooled rate of fertility return within 1 year in order to bring conclusive evidence. So that policy makers and other stakeholder could have synthesized evidence to rely on in decision making on prospect of the problem.

Methods and material

Literature search strategy

This systematic review and meta analyses is conducted according to PRISMA (Preferred Reporting Items for Systematic Reviews and Meta-Analyses) guideline [22]. Systematic literature search of articles was made. Articles published between 1985 and 2017 containing information on rate of pregnancy following cessation of reversible contraception were retained for systematic review and meta-analysis. Electronic bibliographic databases and libraries including PubMed/Medline, Global Health Database, Embase, the Cochrane Library, and African Index Medicus were used to retrieve published articles. Combination of search terms were used with (AND, OR, NOT) Boolean (Search) Operators. (1: contraception discontinuation; 2: IUD discontinuation; 3: Implant discontinuation; 4: Hormonal contraception discontinuation; 5: 1 or 2 or 3 or 4; 6: return to fertility; 7: rate of fertility; 8: time to pregnancy; 9: planned pregnancy; 10: fecundity; 11: delay in conception; 12: time to conception; 13: pregnancy delay; 14: time to ovulation, 15: 6 or 7 or 8 or 9 or 10 or 11 or 12 or 13 or 14; 16: 5 and 15). In addition the reference lists of primary and pertinent review articles were also uploaded into an EndNote XI library (EndNote, Carlsbad, CA, USA) to identify cited studies not captured by the electronic search and after all checked for duplications.

Study selection process and eligibility criteria

Studies published in English language anywhere in the world that reported a 12 month pregnancy rates following discontinuation of a reversible contraceptive method with the intention to get pregnant, with sample size of 100 women and above, and prospective clinical/observational study designs were the inclusion criteria for this systematic review and meta-analysis. One-year pregnancy rate was used to exclude women who developed secondary infertility. Unable to conceive despite of unprotected sexual intercourse with optimum frequency for 1 year and above is called infertility, but the scope of this review is delayed return of fertility after cessation of contraceptive use. Therefore, 1 year rate of pregnancy is more informative to assess delayed resumption to fertility than other time scales. The outcome of interest was the rate of pregnancy among modern reversible ex-contraception users. However studies reporting rate of delivery as the only outcome, Studies published before 1985, studies assessing fertility after abortion or post abortion contraception were excluded. Also Studies conducted in the same location during the same time period were considered as potential duplicates and therefore excluded from the analysis. Three experts reviewed each article and decided based on the inclusion and exclusion criteria.

Data extraction and abstraction

Titles and abstracts derived through primary electronic search were thoroughly assessed for possibility of reporting pregnancy rates within 1 year period and filtered for potential eligibility. If needed, and whenever possible, the authors were contacted for clarifications. From each eligible research, the following information was extracted based on the preformed database (Excel, Microsoft, 2010) format: about author, study participants, studies (study design, sample size, study setting), Type of contraception, length of use, year of publication, year of study start and end, eligibility criteria, rate of pregnancy, etc. All data were extracted independently and in duplicate using a standardized extraction form. Returned abstracts were reviewed and full texts retrieved if they contained relevant information. At the same time, each selected research was assessed for methodological quality and possibility of bias. The outcome variable (rate of pregnancy) was defined as the proportion of women who were pregnant within 1 year of contraception discontinuation. The effect size is measured in rates/ proportion.

Assessment of risk of bias in individual studies and across studies

Risk of bias in individual studies and across studies was assessed through evaluating reliability and validity of data for each important outcome variables. Methods used to assess the outcome variable in each study were also used to assess risk of bias. For all studies; the study design, study participants, the outcome, presence of loss to follow up were assessed based on the eligibility criteria and quality assessment check list. Moreover all studies were prospective studies which employed the same participants and outcome was measured in the same standard. The risk of publication bias and heterogeneity was assessed through the standard statistical approaches. However there are still uncontrolled biases at the selection of study participants, analysis of the result and presentation/publication of the report.

Data analysis

After cleaning and sorting the final database was exported into STATA 11.0 for analysis (STATA, College Station, TX, USA). An outcome of interest was rate of pregnancy after discontinuation of contraception before or at 12th month. Estimate of pregnancy rate was assessed for each study and standardized mean with 95% confidence interval was used. These were calculated with a random effects model according to the DerSimonian and Laird method [23]. Heterogeneity was assessed by the I^2 and values greater than 50% considered representing significant heterogeneity. When heterogeneity between studies was found to be significant, pooled estimates were based on random-effect models and the Hedges method of pooling. Results were displayed visually in forest plots. Bias was investigated by construction of funnel plots and Analysis was performed using the 'metan' and related functions in STATA version 11 (College Station, TX).

Results

Studies included

From 114 studies initially identified, 22 [24–44] were retained for final analysis based on the inclusion and exclusion criteria and quality assessment. From the initial search, literatures were identified as abstract, bibliography and full text research from the selected electronic data bases. After reviewing the abstracts, 62 possible researches were transferred to preformed format of endnote, searched for full text research and cleaned for duplications and 32 abstracts of articles were identified for full text review. Of these reviewed in full text, 30 were removed prior to analysis for different reasons: 5 studies overlapped with larger studies, 3 studies were out of time boundary and for 2 studies the design was ambidirectional (retrospective & prospective) cohort study (Fig. 1).

Description of findings

The studies enrolled a total of 14,884 women who discontinued contraception for the sake of pregnancy. Of them 735 discontinued implants, 139 discontinued injectable contraception, 2374 women discontinued IUD and 11,636 discontinued oral contraception. The primary outcome of the studies was rate of pregnancy after discontinuation of contraception at 12 month. Some studies also assessed the possible reasons for delay in resumption of pregnancy. With duplicates, 5 studied implants [24–29], 2 injectables [30, 31], 5 oral contraception [32–36] and the rest 12 assessed return of fertility after discontinuation of IUD [37–43]. All included studies were prospective cohort and prospective observational designs conducted in different parts of the world and published between 1985 and 2017 with English language.

The mean exposure time (duration of use) of implant users extend from 29.1-55.8 months, injectable users have exposure time of 21.3-35.7 months, while oral contraception users were exposed for 24-84 months and IUD users retained for 19-28 months. Survey characteristics are described in (Table 1).

The 12 month pregnancy rate following discontinuation of different forms of implant with the intension to have pregnancy was measured in 8 studies (with duplicates). Based on this estimates, 74.7% of ex-implant users get pregnant within 12 months. Moreover a study reporting exceptionally lower rate of pregnancy (48.8% among Implanon and 37.5% among Implant II-VI) [24]

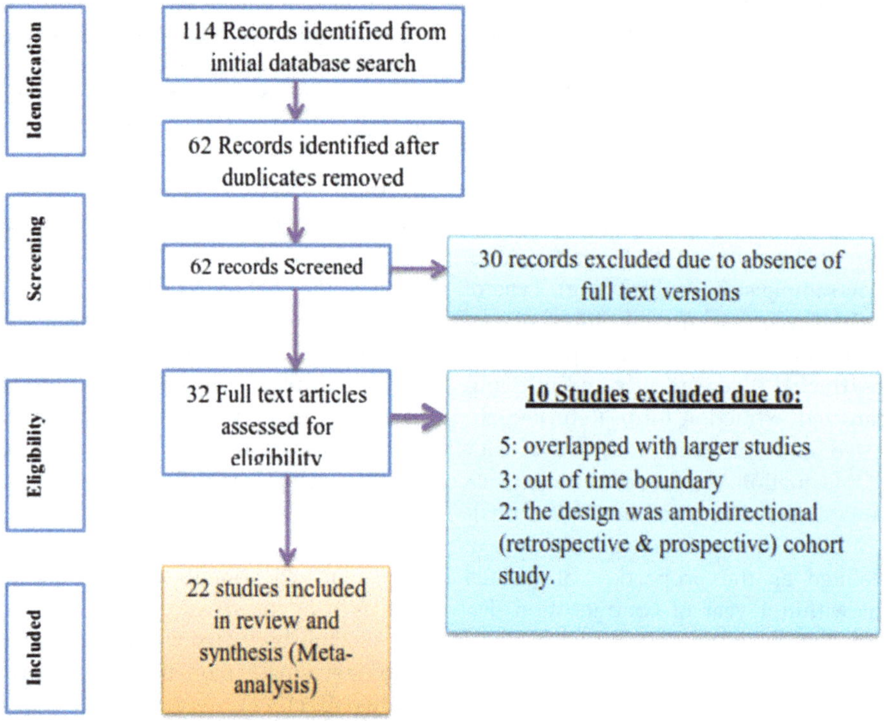

Fig. 1 Flow chart for study search, selection and screening for the review

is removed, the mean weighted pregnancy rate increases to 83.45%. With the same hormonal composition ex-injectable contraception users have a pregnancy rate of 77.74% which is estimated only with two studies and ex-oral contraception users have a pregnancy rate of 87.04.

One year pregnancy rate following cessation of different types of Intrauterine device (IUD) was 84.75%, which is weighted among 13 studies (with duplicates). The studies also noted that there is no significant difference between different types of IUD in terms or fertility resumption. Also in this case pregnancy was resumed with in a brief period of time following cessation of use or removal of the device.

The highest rate of pregnancy among implant users of 90% was reported by Singh et al. [27] in Singapore, while the highest resumption rate of 95% following cessation of oral contraception was reported by Zimmermann et al. [36] among German women and as high as 96.4% of ex-IUD users in Belhadji et al. [42] report were conceived within 1 year. There is a wide overlap in the reported 1-year pregnancy rates after discontinuation of different forms of contraception. The rate of pregnancy was unexpectedly higher among ex-oral contraception users, followed by IUD users. However this difference was not statistically significant.

Pooled estimates and tests

Heterogeneity tests showed significant variations between studies ($Q = 611.5$, $P = 0.000$), where Q-value, the weighed sum of squares on a standardized scale was significantly different compared with expected weighed sum of squares and I-squared showed that 95.3% of the observed dispersions are attributed to real rather than spurious variations. Also the funnel plot showed evidence of bias with some of the studies missing at the bottom rather than around the main effect. Accordingly, the Duval and Tweedie's trim and fill test was applied to adjust for the publication bias.

The presence of heterogeneity and publication bias resulted in adjustment of the point estimate of the rate of pregnancy following cessation of different types of contraception under a random effect model from 84.36 to 83.1%. In a fixed effect model the pooled estimate of pregnancy rate was 84.36% (95% CI = 83.3-85.4%) and in a random effect model the pooled estimate of pregnancy rate became 83.1% (95% CI = 78.2-88%), while estimates of each study are unchanged. In all cases pooled estimate from random effect model was used for report and discussion (Fig. 2).

The effect of some demographic characteristics, like age at contraceptive discontinuation and parity on resumption of pregnancy were inconclusive from these findings. Some studies reported a decrease in resumption of pregnancy rates with increasing age [25, 26, 33, 37, 38, 41, 43] and others showing no such decrease with increased age [30, 34, 40, 42]. In addition, the effect of parity on pregnancy rates was inconsistent, with some

Table 1 Characteristics of studies included in the review

Authors & FP method	Publication year	Type of contraception	Sample size	Duration of use	Pregnancy rate	Design of the study	Setting
Implants							
[24] Affandi et al.	1999	Implanon	80	mean 35.3 month	48.80	Prospective	Indonesia
[24] Affandi et al.	1999	Norplant	80	mean 55.8 month	37.50	Prospective	Indonesia
[25] Buckshee et al.	1995	Norplant II	159	30.0 ± 11.5 months	80.30	Prospective	India
[26] Sivin et al.	1992	Norplant II	116	Mean 29.1 month	84.00	Prospective obs.	Not specified
[26] Sivin et al.	1992	Norplant VI	62	Mean 33.6 ± 1.9	83.00	Prospective obs.	Not specified
[27] Singh et al	1989	Norplant	100		90.00	prospective	Singapore
[28] Affandi et al	1987	Norplant VI	51	32.4 ± 8.8 months	76.50	Prospective	Indonesia
[29] Diaz et al	1987	Norplant VI	87	1–8 years	85.6	Prospective	Chile
waited mean (12 month Return rate of pregnancy among ex-users of implants)					74.70		
Injectable							
[30] Bahamondes et al.	1997	Cyclofem-monthly	70	7.1 ± 4.6 cycle	82.90	Prospective	4 countries[a]
[31] ICMR task Force	1986	Norethisterone	69	11.9 ± 4.9 months	72.50	Prospective	India
Waited mean (12 month Return rate of pregnancy among ex-users of injectable)					77.74		
Oral contraceptives							
[32] Barnhart et al.	2009	Oralcontraceptives	21		81.00	Prospective	multicenter
[33] Cronin et al.	2009	Oralcontraceptives	2064	7.2 yrs	79.40	Prospective obs.	7 countries[b]
[34] Wiegratz et al.	2006	30 mcg EE/2 mgDNG	706	21.5 ± 16.8 cycle	94.00	Prospective obs.	Germany
[35] Farrow et al	2002	Oralcontraceptives	8497		88.00	Prospective	England
[36] Zimmermann	1999	31 mcg EE/2 mgDNG	348	med. 4-6 cycle	95.00	Prospective obs.	Germany
Waited mean (12 month Return rate of pregnancy among OC ex-users)					87.04		
Intra uterine device (IUD)							
[37] Delbarge et al	2002	GyneFix	128	mean104.6 ± 93wk	88.00	Prospective	Belgium
[38] Tadesse et al	1996	Copper T-200	780	med. 3.5 years	86.00	Prospective obs.	Ethiopia
[39] Anderson et al	1992	Nova-T	71	Median 21 month	71.20	Prospective	5 countries[c]
[39] Andersson et al	1992	LNG-20 IUS	138	Median 19 months	79.10	Prospective	5 countries
[26] Sivin et al.	1992	TCu380Ag	103	mean 38.9 months	77.00	Prospective obs.	Not specified
[26] Sivin et al.	1992	LNG-20 IUS	91	mean 30.2 months	84.00	Prospective obs.	Not specified
[40] Gupta et al.	1989	Copper plus Prog.	91	56% b2 years	92.30	prospective	Not specified
[28] Affandi et al	1987	Lippes C IUDs	75	31.8 ± 8.6 month	74.70	Prospective	Indonesia
[41] Skjeldestad et al	1987	Copper IUDs	101	56% b24 months	81.00	Prospective obs.	Norway
[42] Belhadji et al.	1986	TCu380Ag	50	23.96 months	91.10	Prospective	Not specified

Table 1 Characteristics of studies included in the review *(Continued)*

Authors & FP method	Publication year	Type of contraception	Sample size	Duration of use	Pregnancy rate	Design of the study	Setting
[31] *ICMR Task Force*	1986	Copper T-200	110	28.2 ± 14.7 months	83.60	Prospective	India
[42] Belhadji et al.	1986	LNG-20 IUS	60	22.72 months	96.40	Prospective	Not specified
[43] Randic et al	1985	all forms of IUD	576	59% b3 years	86.10	Prospective	Yugoslavia
Waited mean (12 month Return rate of pregnancy among IUD ex-users)					84.75		

obs **observational,** ***FP*** **Family planning,** ***OC*** **oral contraception**
[a]Brazil, Chile, Columbia, Peru
[b]Austria, Belgium, Denmark, France, Germany, Netherlands, UK
[c]Denmark, Finland, Hungary, Norway, Sweden

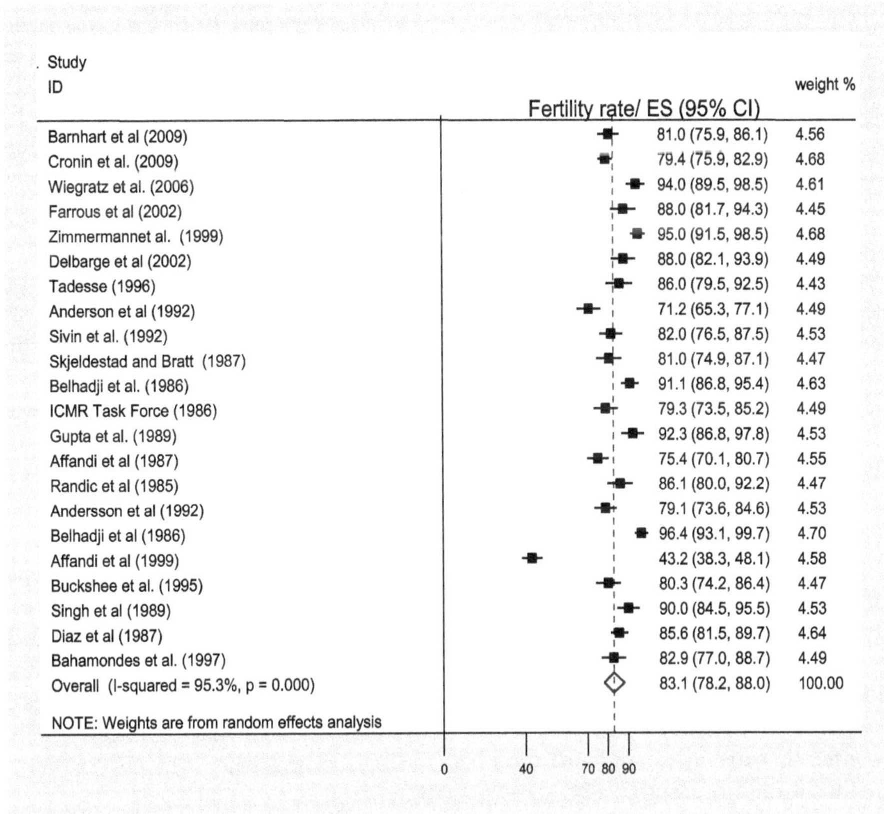

Fig. 2 Forest plot showing the rate of one year pregnancy following discontinuation of contraception, weighted according to random-effects model

studies suggesting that age-adjusted pregnancy rates were significantly higher in multiparous women [33], while in another study it was lower among nulliparous women [41], unaffected by parity [26] and significantly lower among multiparous women in Delbarge et al. [37] report. The possible effect of hormonal contraception and prolonged use of oral contraception on impaired fertility was not supported in these findings [25–31]. Higher level of fertility was observed among non-hormonal contraception users in many studies [37–43] however the difference was not statistically significant.

Discussion

According to this review 83.1% (95% CI = 78.2-88%) of women who discontinued contraception became pregnant within the first 12 months. Return of fertility at the first year was not significantly different for hormonal methods and IUD users. Similarly type of progesterone in contraception and duration of oral-contraceptive use do not significantly influence return of fertility following cessation of contraception. However effect of parity in resumption of pregnancy following cessation of contraception was inconclusive.

The rate of fertility return in this review was comparable to other reports of reviews and articles which assessed specific types of contraception [45–48]. The rate of pregnancy for oral contraceptives, copper IUDs and the LNG-IUS ex-users was also overlap with each other and comparable to previous findings. However the finding was slightly lower than reports of women who discontinued barrier methods or using no contraceptive method of 85.2– 94% [49, 50]. This difference may be due to the fact that hormonal contraceptives commonly take months to clear from the body which results in temporary delay in resumption of pregnancy for months [44, 47, 48].

One year pregnancy rate of (37.5-90%) following cessation of Implant also overlaps across different studies [45, 46]. There are studies which report exceptionally low rate of pregnancy within 1 year after cessation of contraception as evidenced by Affandi et al. [24] which reports (37.5 and 48.8% for Norplant and Implanon ex-users respectively). However when the study with low rate of pregnancy after cessation of contraception is removed the rate of fertility return is comparable to other methods. Moreover, no significant difference was reported between different forms of Implants. This may be explained by the fact that implants are impregnated with similar hormone which doesn't create a difference.

Return of fertility following termination of IUD was not compromised at all and resumption ranges between (71-96%) with a mean of 84.75%. Moreover, type of IUD and duration of use as well as addition of hormones to the device do not compromise pregnancy [37–43]. In line with this finding Mansour et al. [45] reported pregnancy rate of 86.1 to 92.3% following termination of IUD which is comparable to natural method users and non-users. This finding also witnesses that prompt resumption of fertility after termination of IUD. As explained by other findings type and duration of IUD use doesn't matter the rate of pregnancy after cessation [46, 47].

It is commonly believed that oral contraception may compromise conception, however, this review reported higher rate of conception (87%). In line with this finding other researchers reported comparable return of fertility after cessation of oral contraception [47–50] However, this review and meta-analysis appreciate presence of brief delay in return of fertility after cessation of hormonal contraception use until the bioavailability of the hormone in blood is completely cleared. It is also noted that the 3 months hormonal contraception use hinders pregnancy, but the effect is extremely low for12 month users and no effect for 24 month users [32–36, 47–49]. The Concern of impaired fertility which was reported with high-dose of oral contraceptive pills in early years is not a problem currently. This is due to presence of low dose contraception regimen for use [33, 34, 48].

Our review also shows that the duration of contraception use was not significantly affected with return of fertility. It is in line to many studies included in the review [24–44] and the report of some other researches [45–49]. On the other hand there are evidences which narrate women who used oral contraceptives for a longer duration may had a slightly lower rate of pregnancy than did women using oral contraceptives for a shorter period of time [44] which could be the effect of age, in which fertility decreases as age advances.

However, since none of the studies were randomized control trials and most of the studies had small sample sizes, the possible relationship between extended use of hormonal contraception and the rate of resumption of pregnancy may not come across through appropriate and reliable conclusion.

Similarly our review showed that the progestin type had no major effect on the rate of pregnancy over the short term and long-term. This is because rather than duration, dose matters. However currently only low dose preparations are in use. Therefore, delay in fertility may not be common following termination of contraception use. In addition, return of fertility among women discontinuing extended or continuous OC regimens is similar to that observed with cyclic OCs [32–36]. This result was also reported from previous reviews assessing the return of fertility following cessation of oral contraception [45–50].

The effect of parity on the rate of fertility was inconclusive. The finding of this review shows that parity may or may not enhance fertility. Studies included in the review particularly compared nulliparous and multiparous women which ignored the rate of infertility [44]. Therefore, higher rate of pregnancy among multiparous women who are proved to be fertile are expected. In all cases baseline prevalence of infertility may influence fertility rates of women seeking pregnancy following discontinuation of a contraceptive method.

Conclusion and recommendation

Resumption of fertility following cessation of contraception was not affected by use of contraception, type of contraception, duration of use and type of progesterone. However the effect of parity in the resumption of pregnancy following cessation of contraception was inconclusive. Therefore, it is important to counsel women that prior contraceptive use regardless of its duration and type does not have a negative effect on subsequent fertility, so that they can choose and use the duration they want.

Abbreviations

FP: Family planning; IUD: Intrauterine device; LARC: Long acting reversible contraception; MeSHs: Medical subject headings; PRISMA: Preferred reporting items for systematic reviews and meta-analyses

Acknowledgments

For all authors who provided us information whenever we contacted them.

Authors' contributions

TG: Conceived the project, took the primary role in data acquisition, analysis, interpretation writing the manuscript, and publication of the project. AW: revised the project, involved in interpretation and manuscript preparation. Both authors revised the final draft of the manuscript.

Authors' information

TG: is Bsc/public health, MPH in Epidemiology and Biostatistics, Lecturer at Department of Public health, College of Medicine and Health Sciences, Wolkite University, Wolkite, Ethiopia.
AW: is Bsc/public health, MPH in Reproductive health, Lecturer at Department of Public health, College of Medicine and Health Sciences, Wolkite University, Wolkite, Ethiopia.

References

1. Jacobstein R. Long acting and permanent contraception: an international development, service delivery perspective. J Midwifery Womens Health. 2007;52(4):361–7.
2. Family Health International. Addressing Unmet Need for Family Planning in Africa. 2007. [Accessed 15 Sept 2017]; Available from: http://www.k4health.org/ system/files/ unmetneed for FP_Africa. pdf
3. Kulier R, O'Brien PA, Helmerhorst FM, Usher-Patel M, D'Arcangues C. Copper containing, framed intra-uterine devices for contraception. Cochrane Database Syst Rev. 2007;4:CD005347.

4. Fotherby K, Yong-En S, Howard G, Elder MG, Muggeridge J. Return of ovulation and fertility in women using norethisteroneoenanthate. Contraception. 1984;29:447–54.
5. Pardhaisong T, Gray RH, McDaniel EB. Return of fertility after discontinuation of depot medroxyprogesterone acetate and intra-uterine devices in northern Thailand. Lancet. 1980;I:509–12.
6. Kaplan B, Nahum R, Yairi Y, Hirsch M, Pardo J, Yogev Y, et al. Use of various contraceptive methods and time of conception in a communitybased population. Eur J Obstet Gynecol Reprod Biol. 2005;123:72–6.
7. McIver B, Romanski SA, Nippoldt TB. Evaluation and management of amenorrhea. Mayo Clin Proc. 1997;72:1161–9.
8. Shearman RP. Amenorrhea after treatment with oral contraceptives. Lancet. 1966;2:1110–1.
9. Horowitz BJ, Solomkin M, Edelstein SW. The oversuppression syndrome. Obstet Gynecol. 1968;31:387–9.
10. Halbert DR, Christian CD. Amenorrhea following oral contraceptives. Obstet Gynecol. 1969;34:161–7.
11. MacLeod SC, Parker AS, Perlin IA. The oversuppression syndrome. Am J Obstet Gynecol. 1970;106:359–64.
12. Bracken MB, Hellenbrand KG, Holford TR. Conception delay after contraceptive use: the effect of estrogen dose. Fertil Steril. 1990;53:21–7.
13. Harlap S, Baras M. Conception-waits in fertile women after stopping oral contraceptives. Int J Fertil. 1984;29:73–80.
14. Archer DF, Jensen JT, Johnson JV, Borisute H, Grubb GS, Constantine GD. Evaluation of a continuous regimen of levonorgestrel/ethinyl estradiol: phase 3 study results. Contraception. 2006;74:439–45.
15. Hassan MA, Killick SR. Is previous use of hormonal contraception associated with a detrimental effect on subsequent fecundity? Hum Reprod. 2004;19: 344–51.
16. Davis AR, Kroll R, Soltes B, Zhang N, Grubb GS, Constantine GD. Occurrence of menses or pregnancy after cessation of a continuous oral contraceptive. Fertil Steril. 2008;89:1059–63.
17. Archer DF, Thomas RL. The fallacy of the postpill amenorrhea syndrome. Clin Obstet Gynecol. 1981;24:943–50.
18. Speroff L, Fritz M. Clinical gynecologic endocrinology and infertility.7th ed. Baltimore, MD: Lippincott Williams and Wilkins; 2004.
19. Tolis G, Ruggere D, Popkin DR, Chow J, Boyd ME, De Leon A, et al. Prolonged amenorrhea and oral contraceptives. Fertil Steril. 1979;32:265–8.
20. Vessey MP, Wright NH, McPherson K, Wiggins P. Fertility after stopping different methods of contraception. BMJ. 1978;1:265–7.
21. Silverberg SG, Haukkamaa M, Arko H, Nilsson CG, Luukkainen T. Endometrial morphology during long term use of levonorgestrelreleasing intrauterine devices. Int J Gynecol Pathol. 1986;5:235–41.
22. Moher D, Liberati A, Tetzlaff J, Altman DG, The PRISMA Group. Preferred reporting items for systematic reviews and metaanalyses: the PRISMA statement. PLoS Med. 2009;6:e1000097.
23. DerSimonian R, Laird N. Meta-analysis in clinical trials. Control Clin Trials. 1986;7:177–88.
24. Affandi B. Pregnancy after removal of etonogestrel implant contraceptive (Implanon). Med J Indones. 1999;8:62–4.
25. Buckshee K, Chatterjee P, Dhall GI, et al. Return of fertility following discontinuation of Norplant(R)-II subdermal implants. ICMR task force on hormonal contraception. Contraception. 1995;51:237–42.
26. Sivin I, Stern J, Diaz S, et al. Rates and outcomes of planned pregnancy after use of Norplant capsules, Norplant II rods, or levonorgestrelreleasing or copper TCu 380Ag intrauterine contraceptive devices. Am J Obstet Gynecol. 1992;166:1208–13.
27. Singh K, Viegas OA, Singh P, Ratnam SS. Norplant contraceptive subdermal implants: two-year experience in Singapore. Adv Contracept. 1989;5:13–21.
28. Affandi B, Santoso SS, Djajadilaga, Hadisaputra W, Moeloek FA, Prihartono J, et al. Pregnancy after removal of Norplant implants contraceptive. Contraception. 1987;36:203–9.
29. Diaz S, Pavez M, Cardenas H, Croxatto HB. Recovery of fertility and outcome of planned pregnancies after the removal of Norplant subdermal implants or copper-T IUDs. Contraception. 1987;35:569–79.
30. Bahamondes L, Lavin P, Ojeda G, et al. Return of fertility after discontinuation of the once-a-month injectable contraceptive Cyclo-fem. Contraception. 1997;55:307–10.
31. Anonymous. ICMR (Indian Council of Medical Research) task force on hormonal contraception. Return of fertility following discontinuation of an injectable contraceptive-norethisterone enanthate (NETEN) 200mg dose. Contraception. 1986;34:573–82.
32. Barnhart KT, Schreiber CA. Return to fertility following discontinuation of oral contraceptives. Fertil Steril. 2009;91:659–63.
33. Cronin M, Schellschmidt I, Dinger J. Rate of pregnancy after using drospirenone and other progestin-containing oral contraceptives. Obstet Gynecol. 2009;114:616–22.
34. Wiegratz I, Mittmann K, Dietrich H, Zimmermann T, Kuhl H. Fertility after discontinuation of treatment with an oral contraceptive containing 30 mcg of ethinyl estradiol and 2 mg of dienogest. Fertil Steril. 2006;85:1812–9.
35. Farrow A, Hull MGR, Northstone K, Taylor H, Ford WCL, Golding J. Prolonged use of oral contraception before a planned pregnancy is associated with a decreased risk of delayed conception. Hum Reprod. 2002;10:2754–61.
36. Zimmermann T, Dietrich H, Wisser KH, Munch C. Fertility after discontinuation of the dienogest-containing oral contraceptive Valette. First data of an ongoing study. Drugs Today. 1999;35:89–95.
37. Delbarge W, Batar I, Bafort M, et al. Return to fertility in nulliparous and parous women after removal of the GyneFix intrauterine contraceptive system. Eur J Contracept Reprod Health Care. 2002;7:24–30.
38. Tadesse E. Return of fertility after an IUD removal for planned pregnancy: a six-year prospective study. East Afr Med J. 1996;73:169–71.
39. Andersson K, Batar I, Rybo G. Return to fertility after removal of a levonorgestrel-releasing intrauterine device and Nova-T. Contraception. 1992;46:575–84.
40. Gupta BK, Gupta AN, Lyall S. Return of fertility in various types of IUD users. Int J Fertil. 1989;34:123–5.
41. Skjeldestad FE, Bratt H. Return of fertility after use of IUDs (Nova-T,MLCu250 and MLCu375). Adv Contracept. 1987;3:139–45.
42. Belhadj H, Sivin I, Diaz S, et al. Recovery of fertility after use of the levonorgestrel 20 mcg/d or copper T 380 ag intrauterine device. Contraception. 1986;34:261–7.
43. Randic L, Vlasic S, Matrljan I, Waszak CS. Return to fertility after IUD removal for planned pregnancy. Contraception. 1985;32:253–9.
44. Doll H, Vessey M, Painter R. Return of fertility in nulliparous women after discontinuation of the intrauterine device: comparison with women discontinuing other methods of contraception. Br J Obstet Gynaecol. 2001; 108:304–14. [26] Cronin
45. Mansour D, Kristina GD, Inki P, Jeffrey TJ. Fertility after discontinuation of contraception: a comprehensive review of the literature. Contraception. 2011;84:465–77.
46. French R, Sorhaindo AM, Van Vliet HAAM, Mansour DD, Robinson AA, Logan S, et al. Progestogen-releasing intrauterine systems versus other forms of reversible contraceptives for contraception. Cochrane Database Syst Rev 2004, Issue 3. Art. No.: CD001776.
47. Barnhart KT, Schreiber CA. Return to fertility following discontinuation of oral contraceptives. Fertil Steril. 2009;91:3.
48. Inka W, Katrin M, Horst D, Thomas Z, Herbert K. Fertility after discontinuation of treatment with an oral contraceptive containing 30microgram of ethinyl estradiol and 2 mg of dienogest. Fertil Steril. 2006;85:6.
49. Hassan J, Kulenthran A, Thum YS. The return of fertility after discontinuation of oral contraception in Malaysian women. Med J Malaysia. 1994;49:348–50.
50. Hassan MA, Killick SR. Is previous aberrant reproductive outcome predictive of subsequently reduced fecundity? Hum Reprod. 2005;20:657–64.

24

Effect of performance based financing home visiting on the use of modern methods of contraception in the kumbo east health district, Cameroon

Thomas Obinchemti Egbe[1*], Julius Atashili[2], Emmanuella Talla[3] and Mary Bih Suh Atanga[4]

Abstract

Background: The use of modern methods of contraception (MMC) as defined by the World Health Organization still remains a challenge in most of Sub-Saharan Africa. Performance Based Financing (PBF) home visit was introduced in 2012 to increase the use of those modern methods in the Kumbo East Health District (KEHD), Cameroon.
We determined the utilization rates of MMC in areas in the KEHD with PBF home visits compared with those areas with no home visits.

Methods: This was a cross sectional study carried out in the KEHD during the period February 1 to May 31, 2015. A multistage cluster sampling method was used to recruit 262 and 221 women aged 15–49 years in the intervention and nonintervention health areas, respectively. A structured, closed ended questionnaire was used.

Results: The average age of women was similar in both groups 30.40 (SD 8.57); median 30 years in the intervention group and 30.49 (SD 7.84); median 30 years in controls. Most participants in the intervention health area (60.3 %) used modern methods of contraception compared to 46.6 % of those in the control group (aOR: 1.75 %; 95 % CI: 1.212.53) and the most commonly used MMC was medroxyprogesterone in the intervention group and condoms in the control area.

Conclusion: Utilization of MMC was significantly higher in the area with PBF home visits than in areas without that service. While this indicates that the intervention has benefit, there may be other contributing factors.

Keywords: Performance based financing, Utilization, Modern methods of contraception, Women of childbearing age, Medroxyprogesterone acetate

Abbreviations: IHA, Intenvention health areas; KEHD, Kumbo east health district; MMC, Modern methods of contraception; NIHA, Non intervention health areas; PBF, Performance based financing; STD, Sexually transmitted diseases

* Correspondence: toegbe@gmail.com; tom.egbe@outloot.com; obinchemti@yahoo.com
[1]Department of Obstetrics and Gynecology, Faculty of Health Sciences, University of Buea, P.O. Box 63, Buea, Cameroon

Background

Over half of the 278,000 maternal deaths in 2010 occurred in Sub-Saharan Africa [1, 2]. Rates of unintended pregnancy in Cameroon in 2013 totaled 490,000 and was attributable in large part to low utilization of contraception, particularly modern methods [3–6]. These latter include combined hormonal contraceptives, progestin-only pills, contraceptive injections, intrauterine devices, implants, male and female condoms and permanent contraception for both men and women. On the other hand, non-modern methods (behavior methods) include fertility awareness and coitus interruptus [7]. Progress has been made in the use of contraception in Sub Saharan Africa overall and in Cameroon in particular. However, in 2011 only 23.4 % of the population of Cameroon used any contraception and 14.1 % used MMC [5].

In order to improve utilization of contraception, a performance based financing [PBF] pilot project was introduced in the Kumbo East Health District (KEHD) in 2012. The KEHD has a surface area of about 1,087 km^2, 20 health areas and a population of 179 789 inhabitants of which 43 689 are women of child bearing age. The KEHD has a hilly terrain with towns located on hills and valleys and there are fast flowing streams which render the district inaccessible all year round. Local community radios such as the Bui Community radio, Helenkris radio, City Community radio and radio Evangelium broadcast in the district, but many women in the study groups are farmers and do not have time to listen to radio-broadcast public health messages.

For this project, contracts were signed and nurses were trained to provide women education in their homes about contraception and prevention of sexually transmitted infections. They were taught about the reproductive cycle, mechanism of action for each of the methods. The training was designed to enable them to tell women about each method, including its effectiveness, medical eligibility, cost side effects and safety while appreciating the woman's preference, fertility desires and risks of STDs [8, 9].

The women then returned to their homes, in the intervention areas, in the District and went from house to house to educate women about their STD risks and their options and to refer them to the nearest hospital for counseling and method initiation [9].

In the Kumbo East health district, condoms are free and available at the pro-pharmacies in Government health facilities while the other methods are also subsidized at the Government health facilities. The average cost of contraceptives was 2.63 USD; range 0.17–8.62 USD. The majority of participants used male condoms and the injectable that cost 0.17 USD, respectively. The monthly income of the population ranged between 21.83 and 94.54 USD [10].

The aim of this study was to estimate the effect of home visits on the use of modern methods of contraception by women of childbearing age in the Kumbo East Health District, Cameroon by comparing the rates of use in KEHD in areas served by home visits compared to those areas without home visits. The distances between health facilities in both study groups were similar.

Methods

This cross sectional comparative study was approved by Faculty of Health Science Institute Review Board of the University of Buea, Cameroon and the Regional Delegation of Public Health of the North West. Women aged 15–20 years of age signed assent forms and agreement was obtained from their guardian/parent; women age 21–49 signed informed consents.

A 27-item questionnaire was developed and beta-tested on 10 sexually active women age 15–49, for comprehension and content validity. The questionnaire was designed to take 15 min to administer and covered the women's demographics (age, education, occupation, marital status, number of children and religion) and her knowledge of contraceptive options and her personal contraceptive use.

Women eligible to participate in the study had to live in the KEHD for at least twelve consecutive months and have been educated on the MMC; speak English or pidgin; be willing to give informed consent; and to be at-risk of pregnancy, defined as not being pregnant at enrollment, being fertile and of reproductive age (15–49 years of age). In addition, they needed to have had sex in the past month or be planning on having sex in the next month with at least one fertile male partner and not consistently using any birth control. We defined inconsistent use of birth control as not having used contraception during every sexual encounter within 3 months before enrollment. The surveyors were trained on all aspects of the study, including exclusion criteria.

Sample size determination

The sample size was calculated using the sample size formula for two proportions and confirmed with Epi info version 7. Based on the fact that we used cluster sampling in this study, a design effect of 2 was employed [11].

$$\mathrm{N} = \mathrm{DEFF\ X\ 2}\frac{\left| Zcrit\sqrt{2p(1-p) + Zpwr\sqrt{P1(1-P1) + P2(1-P2)}}\right| 2}{\mu^2} \qquad [12]$$

Where p1 and p2 are pre-study estimates of the two proportions to be compared, D = |p1-p2| or minimum expected difference, = (+)/2 N. was the total sample size (sum of the sizes of both comparison groups), was the desired significance criterion and was the desired statistical power. The values used for the calculation included a statistical power of 0.80, = 0.842, Significance criterion of 0.05, = 1.960 and DEFF = 2 was the design effect [12]. The p1 = 0.2 % was the proportion of women using modern methods of contraception in the KEHD in 2011 [13]. p2 =

7.1 % was an assumption. We assumed that through home visits the contraceptive use would have increased by 6.9 % as was observed in Rwanda [14]. = 3.6, D =6.9. This gave a sample size N of 460.

Assuming a 20 % non-response rate, we therefore had a sample size of 552 (276 in each study group). After data collection, the response rate was 87.5 % therefore giving a sample size of 483 participants. From this sample size 262 women were recruited in the intervention health areas (IHA-home visits) and 221 participants were enrolled in the nonintervention health areas (NIHA-no-home visits).

Sampling method

We used multistage cluster sampling method where a list of all the 20 health areas and their population of women of childbearing age was collected from the KEHD. The number of households per cluster was calculated from this population by dividing the total population by 6 (average size of a household in Cameroon was 6 persons per household) [15].

Next probability proportionate to size method was used to select the different clusters (communities) within the health areas. The representative sample of health areas within the district was done by calculating the sampling interval (the total number of households divided by the total number of clusters needed). A total of 25 clusters each was required for both the health areas implementing home visits and those with no home visits [13]. A random number between one and the sampling interval was chosen to represent our reference point. This random value was then added to the sampling interval to get the cluster positions. This was done continuously until we obtained the total number of clusters (communities) needed (25 clusters per group) (Table 1).

Finally, a simple random sampling of the groups was selected by balloting among the clusters in order to identify the communities to be used for the study in each health area. Then an equal number of participants (first 11 women per cluster or community) was selected and one woman of childbearing age was interviewed per household. Also, we had a briefing meeting with health personnel already in the pilot project at the beginning of our study to ensure that those staff also understood clearly the objectives of our study.

We entered data into Microsoft Excel and analyzed with the statistical package STATA. The analysis focused on the impact of home visit involving family planning counseling, without receipt of contraception, and no home visits. In computing the socio-demographic characteristics of study participants, measures of central tendencies: mean and standard deviation were used while frequencies were used to compute level of education, religion, marital status, occupation and number of children. The Chi squared, student *t*-test and Anova were used to test for significant associations when appropriate. Binary logistic regression was used to measure the level of association and multiple logistic regressions were computed to control for confounders. Statistical significance was set at $p < 0.05$.

Results

Data were collected from February 1 to May 31, 2015. Selected homes were visited and the questionnaire was administered to eligible participants who consented to be part in the study. Data was collected on traditional holidays, market days and after 4 pm when women were at home after their daily activities. We could not rely on telephone numbers because majority of our patients did not have phones and the telephone network was usually difficult to go through During that period 552 participants

Table 1 Cluster Characteristics

Health areas with Home visit intervention					Health areas with no home visit intervention						
Health area	No. of women age 15–49 years	No. of households	cumulative	No. of clusters per health area	percentage particiants per cluster	community	No. of women age 15–49 years	No. of households	cumulative	# of cluster	percentage participants per cluster
Shisong	4396	733	733	4	16 %	Mbah	1690	282	282	1	4 %
Jakiri CMA	2725	454	1187	3	12 %	Sop	3184	531	813	4	16 %
Jakiri IHC	2913	486	1673	3	12 %	Ngorin	1035	173	985	2	8 %
Mbam	3306	551	2224	3	12 %	Mbonso	1697	283	1268	2	8 %
Mbokam	1323	221	2444	2	8 %	Verkovi	3307	551	1819	4	16 %
Ndzeng	1912	319	2763	2	8 %	Wvem	1016	169	1989	1	4 %
Nkar	1348	225	2988	1	4 %	Nkwaso	1408	235	2223	3	12 %
Lip	607	101	3089	1	4 %	Wainamah	1433	239	2462	3	12 %
Tartum	3420	570	3659	3	12 %	Mbiame	5066	844	3306	5	20 %
Ngendzen	411	69	3727	1	4 %						
Wasiber	1492	249	397	2	8 %						
Total	23853	3976			100 %			3306			100 %

were enrolled, but only 483 (87.5 %) were interviewed and completed the survey. 262 were studied in health areas with home visits and 221 women in health areas with no home visits (Fig. 1). The mean age of women in each of the groups was similar 30.40 (SD 8.57); median 30 years; range 15–48 years versus 30.49 (SD 7.84); median 30 years; range 16–49 years ($p = 0.90$) (Table 1). Over half (52 %) of study participants were Catholics ($p < 0.03$) and 44.7 % had secondary education or less ($p < 0.06$). There were no statistical differences in participant characteristics between the intervention and no intervention groups, including marital status ($p < 0.25$), employment status ($p < 0.78$) and having parity of 2 or more children ($p = 0.54$) (Table 2).

Nearly 6 out of 10, (59.92 %) of the participants in health areas with home visits reported current use of MMC compared to 46.61 % participants in the control group used MMC, ($p = 0.003$). The odds ratio was 0.7 (95 % CI, 1.19–2.46.). After adjusting for differences in regions, the aOR was 1.8 (95 % CI, 1.21–2.53).

In both areas, the most frequently used methods were behavioral methods, but their use was much less common in the intervention group (25.9 vs 38.1 %). The most common MMC used in the intervention area was injections (24.1 %) whereas, the male condom was the most commonly used MMC in the nonintervention area (25.8 %). In the intervention group, use of other MMC was significantly more frequent; pill use was higher than implant use (7.7 vs 1.8 %) (Table 3).

Discussion

Our study has shown that MMC use was more common in areas served by PBF home visitors. The importance of PBF home visits to our study population stems from the fact that most women are farmers and are not readily at home to obtain information about MMC from local radio stations. This is consistent with other studies that have proved that use of social workers increase the use of MMC [16]. Mercer et al. in Bangladesh, did find that home visits increased the use of injectables from 5 to 10 % [17], as well as USAID report which found a significant increase in the use of injectables in programs that implemented home delivery of MMC [18]. The fundamental difference between our study and that in Bangladesh was that field workers in rural Bangladesh distributed injectables to women at home while in this study (KEHD) women had to go to health facilities to get the MMC.

However, our findings differ from a Rwandan study by Skile and colleagues; they found that home visit did not impact the use of MMC. It is possible that this may be due to the extreme equity gap seen between the two populations studied [14].

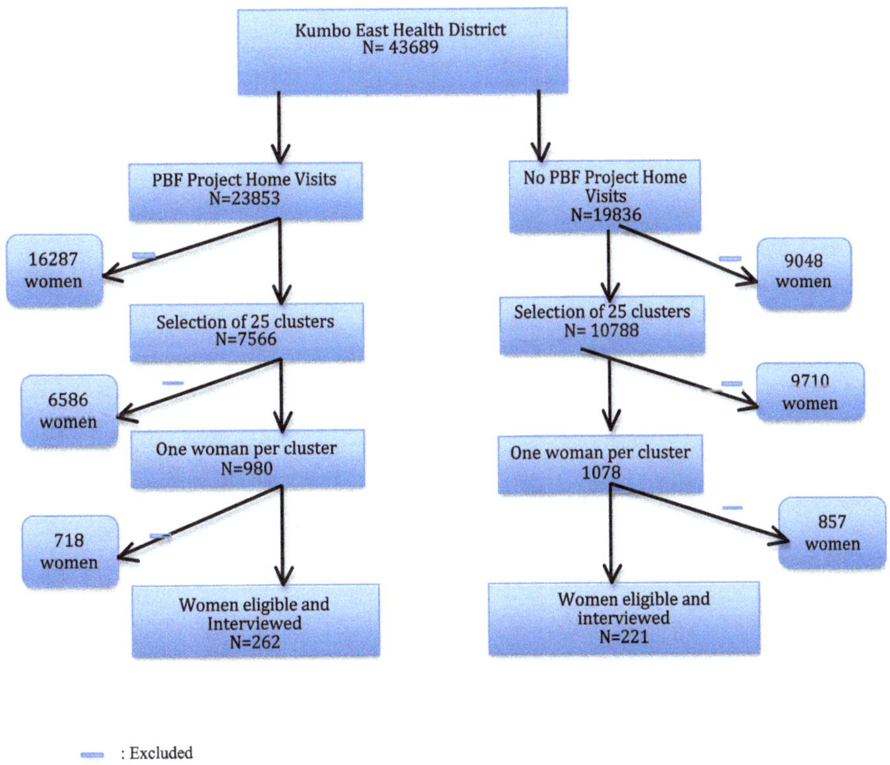

Fig. 1 Consort diagram

Table 2 Socio-demographic characteristics of study population

	Intervention (home visit)		
Variable	No ($N = 221$)	Yes ($N = 262$)	*P*-value
Age (years)			
Age (±SD)	30.40 ± 8.57	30.49 ± 7.84	0.90
Education (N, %)			
None	14 (6.33 %)	7 (2.67 %)	0.06
Primary level	94 (42.53 %)	98 (37.40 %)	
Secondary level	91 (41.18 %)	117 (44.66 %)	
Tertiary level	22 (9.95 %)	40 (15.27 %)	
Religion (N, %)			
Catholic	116 (52.49 %)	131 (50.00 %)	0.03
Baptist	35 (15.84 %)	22 (8.40 %)	
Presbyterian	32 (14.48 %)	53 (20.23 %)	
Pentecostal	0 %	3 (1.15 %)	
Muslim	38 (17.19 %)	53 (20.23 %)	
Marital status (N,%)			
Single	39 (17.65 %)	48 (18.32 %)	0.25
Married	164 (74.21 %)	195 (74.43 %)	
separated/divorced	15 (6.79 %)	10 (3.82 %)	
Widowed	3 (1.36 %)	9 (3.44 %)	
Occupation (N, %)			
Unemployed	80 (36.20 %)	98 (37.40 %)	0.78
Employed	141 (63.8 %)	164 (62.60 %)	
Number of children (N, %)			
0–2	95 (42.99 %)	126 (57.01 %)	0.54
3 > 5	120 (45.80 %)	142 (54.20 %)	

Melnick et al. in the USA did not find an association between the method of contraception used and home visits [19]. This difference could possibly be because our study recruited participants who were interested in delaying pregnancy using specific methods. In addition, we found that women in health areas with home visits were 3.6 times more likely to use implants compared to those without home visits. This was not consistent with the findings of Egede JO et al. in Nigeria who reported that the most commonly used forms of modern contraception were the barrier method (male condoms, 8.2 %, the oral contraceptive pill 3.0 %, injectables 2.5 %, and the intrauterine contraceptive device 2.0 % [20].

The use of MMC is responsible for improving maternal and infant health outcomes [7]. A global review of 172 studies by Ahmed and colleagues in 2012 calculated that the use of MMC prevented 272,040 maternal deaths, a 44 % reduction without which maternal deaths would have been 1.8 times higher than 2008 totals [21]. Cameroon has a maternal mortality rate of 680 women per 100,000 live births from pregnancy [6]. If all women with unmet needs of contraception were to use MMC, it is estimated that 373,000 unintended pregnancies could be prevented, and therefore, unplanned births, abortions and miscarriages could be reduced by $^3/_4$; maternal deaths would be reduced by 1,300 and infant deaths by 13,000 annually [6]. This would substantiate many of the older millennium development goals.

Table 3 Distribution of current use of MMC

intervention (home visit)								
Variable	no	yes	*p* value	OR	95 % CI	aOR	*p* value	95 % CI
Current use of MMC (N, %)								
No	118/221 (53.39 %)	105/262 (40.08 %)						
Yes	103/221 (46.61 %)	157/262 (59.92 %)	0.003	1.7 1	1.19–2.46	1.7 5	0.003	1.21–2.53
Current use of MMC by method (N, %)								
Natural	84/221 (38.01 %)	68/262 (25.95 %)						
Implant	4/221 (1.81 %)	12/262 (4.58 %)		3.71	1.14–12.01	3.56	0.029	1.08–11.73
IUD	7221 (3.17 %)	9/262 (3.44 %)		1.59	0.56–4.49	2.01	0.382	0.69–5.84
Tubal								
ligation	1/221 (0.45 %	2/262 (0.76 %)		2.47	0.22–27.83	2.82	0.464	0.23–34.77
Injectable	17/221 (7.69 %)	63/262 (24.05 %)		4.58	2.45–8.54	4.95	<0.001	2.63–9.34
Pills	17/221 (7.69 %)	26/262 (9.92 %)		1.89	0.95–3.77	2.04	0.071	1.01–9.34
male								
condoms	57/221 (25.79 %)	46/262 (17.56 %)		1.00	0.60–1.64	1.02	0.99	0.61–1.70
None	34/221 (15.38 %)	36262 (13.74 %)	<0.001	1.31	0.74–2.31	1.45	0.354	0.82–2.59
Frequency of use of MMC (N, %)								
Frequent	47/103 (45.63 %)	81/157 (51.59 %)						
Infrequent	56/103 (54.37 %)	76/157 (48.41 %)	0.35					

aOR adjusted odds ratio, *OR* odds ratio, *CI* Confidence Intervals

Our study was based on a self-reported use of MMC, therefore they may be a risk of recall bias and reporting bias. An additional limitation is potential selection bias. Because we could not obtain personal information on participants until they consented to participate in the study, we have no information on those who refused to participate, nor do we have information on potential participants who were difficult to reach.

Other confounders may have impacted on our findings. Some of the strategies from the intervention pilot project may have spread into the control area. Some women that were interviewed in the areas not served by the pilot project said they had heard of MMC from home-based counselors. Similarly, HIV prevention campaigns conducted in all health areas promoted both male and female condoms and may also have increased the use of the modern method in the control area. However, these confounders would have decreased the impact of the pilot project. The fact that we observed a 70 % higher utilization of MMC in the PBF pilot project despite these confounders supports the effectiveness of this initiative. Extension of this project into other regions may well yield important benefits to the health of reproductive age women and their families. Future research that explores the involvement of religious leaders in these regions may identify ways to magnify these benefits.

Conclusion

Utilization of MMC was significantly (1.7 times) higher in the area with PBF home visits than in areas without that service. While this indicates that the intervention has benefit, there may be other contributing factors.

Acknowledgements
We thank the health team of the KEHD specifically the District Medical Officer (Dr. Leuteu Petmi Landry) for being very supportive during proposal development and data collection. We also thank the women who comprised our study population in the KEHD for sharing their private experiences on sexuality and contraception. Special thanks to the Victory Outreach Ministries for their support. We also thank Dr Julius Che Tita for proof reading the manuscript. His suggestions have been valuable.

Authors' contributions
TOE and TE and MSBA designed the study. Data collection was done by TE. TOE, JA and TE conducted analysis and interpretation of study data. TOE and TE drafted the manuscript. All authors reviewed, edited and approved the final version of the manuscript.

Author details
[1]Department of Obstetrics and Gynecology, Faculty of Health Sciences, University of Buea, P.O. Box 63, Buea, Cameroon. [2]Department of Public Health, Faculty of Health Sciences, University of Buea, P.O.Box 63, Buea, Cameroon. [3]Delegation of Public Health, North West Region, Cameroon. [4]Department of Nursing and Midwifery, Faculty of Health Sciences, University of Bamenda, Bambili, Cameroon.

References
1. AfricaFiles | Sub-Saharan Africa's maternal death rate down 41 per cent [http://www.africafiles.org/article.asp?ID=26434] Accessed 17 May 2012.
2. Maternal Mortality in Sub-Saharan Africa: Steps Towards Millennium Developmental Goals - viewcontent.cgi [http://digitalcommons.hsc.unt.edu/cgi/viewcontent.cgi?article=1764&context=theses] by IU Eghieye - 2014.
3. Stephenson R, Baschieri A, Clements S, Hennink M, Madise N. Contextual influences on modern contraceptive use in sub-Saharan Africa. Am J Public Health. 2007;97:1233–40.
4. Gakidou E, Vayena E. Use of modern contraception by the poor is falling behind. PLoS Med. 2007;4:e31.
5. Kelodjouea S. Trends and Determinants of Unmet Need for Family Planning in Cameroon: The Role of Socio-Cultural Context. Sociology. 2015;5:39–52.
6. Vlassoff M, Beninguisse G, Kamgaing F, Jerman J and Zinvi F. The Costs and Benefits of Reproductive Health Interventions in Cameroon. PAA Annu Meet Boston MA 2014:20. [http://www.paa2014.princeton.edu/papers/142862].
7. WHO | Family planning/Contraception [http://www.who.int/mediacentre/factsheets/fs351/en/].
8. Contraception | Unintended Pregnancy | Reproductive Health | CDC [http://www.cdc.gov/reproductivehealth/contraception.htm].
9. Performance Based Financing Procedure Manual North West Region of Cameroon. 2012.
10. Cameroon map of Map of Cameroon: Average Monthly Rural Income by Region [2010 Data] by Province - TargetMap [www.targetmap.com/viewer.aspx?reportId=12773].
11. Reproductive Health Assessment Toolkit for Conflict-Affected Women - chapter-1_introduction_tag508.pdf [http://www.cdc.gov/reproductivehealth/global/tools/docs/pdf/chapter-1_introduction_tag508.pdf].
12. Eng J. Sample size estimation: how many individuals should be studied? Radiology. 2003;227:309–13.
13. Kumbo East Health Report.
14. Skiles MP, Curtis SL, Basinga P, Angeles G. An equity analysis of performance-based financing in Rwanda: are services reaching the poorest women? Health Policy Plan. 2013;28:825–37.
15. Report - IMC Cameroon - International Medical Corps. internationalmedicalcorps.org/document.doc?id=88.
16. Kincaid DL. Social networks, ideation, and contraceptive behavior in Bangladesh: a longitudinal analysis. Soc Sci Med. 2000;50:215–31.
17. Mercer A, Ashraf A, Huq NL, Haseen F, Uddin AHN, Reza M. Use of family planning services in the transition to a static clinic system in Bangladesh: 1998–2002. Int Fam Plan Perspect. 2005;31:115–23.
18. USAID Report; Home delivery of Injectable contraception - Google Scholar [http://pdf.usaid.gov/pdf_docs/PDACL615].
19. Melnick A: Nurse family partnership contraceptive study. In 141st APHA Annual Meeting and Exposition (November 2-November 6, 2013). APHA; 2013.
20. Egede JO, Onoh RC, Umeora OUJ, Iyoke CA, Dimejesi IBO, Lawani LO. Contraceptive prevalence and preference in a cohort of south-east Nigerian women. Patient Prefer Adherence. 2015;9:707–14.
21. Ahmed S, Li Q, Liu L, Tsui AO. Maternal deaths averted by contraceptive use: an analysis of 172 countries. Lancet. 2012;380:111–25.

Women's informed choice and satisfaction with immediate postpartum long-acting reversible contraception in Georgia

Carla L. DeSisto[1*], Arden Handler[1], Sadia Haider[2], Rachel Caskey[3], Nadine Peacock[1], Melissa Kottke[4] and Kristin Rankin[1]

Abstract

Background: Several state Medicaid agencies have recently started reimbursing for long-acting reversible contraception (LARC) placement immediately postpartum. Women's perspectives are critical for ensuring that this change increases access to LARC while empowering women to choose the method and timing of contraception that best meets their needs. We conducted a pilot study in Georgia, which recently changed its Medicaid reimbursement policy, to assess women's informed choice and satisfaction with immediate postpartum LARC.

Methods: We sampled all women with a live birth paid for by Georgia Medicaid during November 2015 through February 2017 who received an immediate postpartum LARC. We then used a one-to-one match to sample women who did not receive immediate postpartum LARC. Women were contacted via telephone for a 25–30 min interview regarding their knowledge, attitudes, and behaviors related to immediate postpartum LARC and their satisfaction with postpartum contraception. We calculated descriptive statistics and components of informed choice overall and by receipt of immediate postpartum LARC, using chi-square tests to calculate differences by group.

Results: We approached 470 women and completed interviews with 51; 25 (49%) received immediate postpartum LARC (24 implants, 1 intrauterine device). Two-thirds reported their provider discussed the option of receiving immediate postpartum LARC during prenatal care, with over 90% reporting they received all the information they needed to make a decision. Most women believed the ideal time to begin using birth control postpartum is in the hospital immediately after delivery, although this differed significantly by women's receipt of immediate postpartum LARC. Most women who received immediate postpartum LARC reported they are very or extremely happy with their device, although 40% also reported wanting their device removed at some point.

Conclusions: Women on Medicaid in Georgia report making informed choices regarding immediate postpartum LARC. Among those who received immediate postpartum LARC, women report high levels of satisfaction.

Keywords: Long-acting reversible contraception (LARC), Postpartum contraception, Informed choice, Medicaid policy

Background

Providing access to long-acting reversible contraception (LARC), which includes subdermal implants and intrauterine devices (IUDs), in the immediate postpartum period before hospital discharge has been recently promoted as a strategy for preventing unintended and rapid repeat pregnancies. This practice is considered safe by the Centers for Disease Control and Prevention [1] and the American Congress of Obstetricians and Gynecologists [2] and may be particularly convenient for women [3]. Several state Medicaid agencies have recently changed their policies to reimburse providers for LARC placement at the time of delivery [4], which may expand access given that Medicaid pays for approximately half of all deliveries across the nation [5] and Medicaid policies may later be adopted by private insurance plans.

There is much enthusiasm among providers and policy makers about the potential for immediate postpartum

* Correspondence: cdesis2@uic.edu
[1]University of Illinois at Chicago School of Public Health , 1603 W. Taylor St, Chicago, IL 60612, USA

LARC to decrease unintended pregnancies and reduce public expenditures [3, 6]. However, there is also some concern that this enthusiasm, while often well-meaning, could lead to coercion and a general disregard for women's informed choice and autonomy [7–9]. In light of past reproductive rights abuses against disadvantaged women in the U.S. [10], the recent documentation of women feeling coerced in their contraceptive decision making after undergoing abortion [11], and the fact that this initiative is specifically targeted to low-income women served by Medicaid, it is important to ensure that women's choice and reproductive justice are central when developing and implementing these policies.

There is a dearth of evidence about women's experiences with informed choice and satisfaction with immediate postpartum LARC. Women's perspectives are critical for informing protocols to implement immediate postpartum LARC in a way that ensures increased knowledge and access while empowering women to choose the method and timing of contraception that best meets their needs. Therefore, we conducted a small pilot study in Georgia, which officially changed its Medicaid reimbursement policy in April 2014 [12]. Our objective was to assess the extent to which women choosing or not choosing immediate postpartum LARC are acting in alignment with their own preferences ("informed choice") and in turn, whether or not they are satisfied with this decision.

Methods

First, we sampled all women who had a live birth paid for by Georgia Medicaid during November 2015 through February 2017 and who received immediate postpartum LARC. Live births were identified using International Classification of Diseases, Ninth Revision (ICD-9) codes 650, V27.0, V27.2, V27.5, or V27.9 and ICD-10 codes O60.x-O77.x, O80.x, O82.x, Z37.0, Z37.2, Z37.5, or Z37.9 from Medicaid claims. Immediate postpartum LARC was identified if women had one of the following Healthcare Common Procedure Coding System (HCPCS) codes for a date of service that fell within the delivery hospitalization begin and end dates: J7300, J7301, J7302, or J7307. Women who experienced an infant death or permanent sterilization were excluded [ICD-9 codes: V25.2, V26.51, 656.4, V27.1, V27.3, V27.4, V27.6, V27.7, 66.21–66.29; ICD-10 codes: Z30.2, Z98.51, O36.4XX0, Z37.1, Z37.3, Z37.4, Z37.69, Z37.7, 0UL74ZZ, 0UL78ZZ, 0U574ZZ, 0U578ZZ, 0UL74CZ, 0UL74DZ, 0UL78DZ; HCPCS code: A4264; Current Procedural Terminology (CPT) codes: 58565, 58,600, 58,605, 58,615, 58,611, 58,670, 58,671, 58,340, 74,740]. Then, for each woman who received immediate postpartum LARC, we used Medicaid claims to sample an additional woman who had a live birth paid for by Georgia Medicaid but who did not receive immediate postpartum LARC. We used a 1-to-1 match on delivery month, age category (18–19, 20–24, 25–29, 30–34, and 35+ years), and delivery hospital to sample the women who did not receive immediate postpartum LARC. The total number of women sampled was 470.

Sampled women were mailed study information by partners at the Georgia Department of Community Health (DCH). Women were informed that researchers from the University of Illinois at Chicago would contact them via telephone for a study about postpartum contraception and given the option to opt out of participation via email or telephone. Women were informed that upon completion of an interview, they would receive a $25 gift card to their choice of Target or Walmart as a thank you for their time and participation.

Research assistants (RAs) attempted to contact the sampled women via telephone up to six times and left voice messages when possible. When contact was made with a woman, the RA briefly explained the study. If the woman was interested in participating, the RA would ask for her verbal consent to begin the interview or schedule the interview for another time.

We used mixed methods to assess informed choice and satisfaction. The interview guide consisted of mostly close-ended questions. However, we included some open-ended questions to allow women to explain their experiences and decision-making in their own words. Interview questions asked women about their most recent pregnancy and focused on three previously published components of informed choice, modified to address immediate postpartum LARC: knowledge/information provided, attitudes, and behaviors [13, 14]:

- Measures of knowledge/information provided: We asked women if they knew whether Georgia Medicaid paid for immediate postpartum LARC and whether it was possible for women to receive IUDs and contraceptive implants immediately postpartum. We also asked women to reflect on discussions with their medical providers about postpartum contraception during pregnancy and at the time of delivery.
- Measures of attitudes: We asked women about their ideal time to begin using contraception postpartum, the importance of different characteristics of contraceptive methods, and their future pregnancy plans.
- Measures of contraceptive behaviors: We asked women about their postpartum contraceptive practices and experiences with breastfeeding and attending a postpartum visit. We also asked an open-ended question about her process in deciding whether or not to obtain LARC immediately postpartum.

Additionally, we asked women about their satisfaction with their postpartum contraception and collected general demographic information. We did not use the word "LARC" in the interviews; instead we explained what IUDs and contraceptive implants are and asked about each device. For example, we said, "An intrauterine device or IUD is a small, plastic T-shaped device that is inserted in the uterus. Mirena and Skyla IUDs work for 3-5 years and the copper IUD, called Paraguard, works for up to 12 years." Before asking questions related to IUDs or implants, we verified that the respondent understood what we were referring to and encouraged her to ask any clarifying questions she had.

All interviews were conducted in English. Interviews lasted approximately 25–30 min. Interviews were audio-recorded and the RAs entered data into a REDCap database [15]. Following completion of interviews, study data were transferred to a de-identified data set, which was analyzed in SAS version 9.4 (SAS Institute, Cary, NC). We calculated descriptive statistics of sample demographics and women's knowledge, attitudes, and behaviors overall and by receipt of immediate postpartum LARC. Chi-square tests were used to calculate differences by group and statistical significance was assessed as $p < .05$.

The Institutional Review Board at the University of Illinois at Chicago approved this study (protocol #2015–0155).

Results

Of the 470 women sampled, none emailed or called to opt out of participation. However, 12 were missing phone numbers and 163 phone numbers were disconnected or incorrect. Of the 295 women we were able to contact, 53 consented to participate (18.0% participation rate) and 51 completed interviews (96.2% completion rate). Three of the women who declined to participate did not speak English. The mean time from the infant's birth to the interview was 35.5 weeks (standard deviation: 17.7 weeks; range: 14–83 weeks). Participants were an average age of 24.2 years. The majority completed high school or a General Equivalency Degree (GED), were unmarried, black, and had unintended pregnancies (Table 1). Participants had a similar age and delivery hospital distribution to the overall sampled population ($p = 0.46$ and $p = 0.55$, respectively, data not shown).

About half the participants received immediate postpartum LARC ($n = 25$) and the other half did not ($n = 26$). Of those who received immediate postpartum LARC, one used an IUD and 24 used a contraceptive implant. Most demographic variables did not vary significantly by receipt of immediate postpartum LARC. However, women who received immediate postpartum LARC were more likely to be black and deliver preterm (< 37 weeks gestation) than women who did not receive immediate postpartum LARC. Women delivered at three different hospitals and lived in 12 different counties in Georgia, primarily representing the Atlanta and Savannah metropolitan areas (data not shown).

Knowledge/information provided

The majority of participants reported discussing ways to delay pregnancy after delivery with their prenatal care provider (Table 2). Two-thirds reported their provider discussed the option of receiving immediate postpartum LARC during prenatal care and 71% reported being offered immediate postpartum LARC at the time of delivery. The majority reported receiving all the information necessary to make a decision.

Among women who received immediate postpartum LARC, 92% reported signing a consent form at the hospital at the time of delivery, while 4% reported signing consent forms both during prenatal care and at the hospital during delivery; 4% did not remember when they signed a consent form.

The majority of women knew that Georgia Medicaid pays for immediate postpartum LARC (Table 2). Only about half knew it is possible to receive immediate postpartum IUDs, while the majority knew it is possible to receive immediate postpartum contraceptive implants.

Attitudes

Most participants believed that the ideal time to begin using birth control postpartum is in the hospital immediately after delivery, although this differed significantly by women's receipt of immediate postpartum LARC (Table 3). The majority reported that it was very important to have a birth control method they do not have to think about, they do not have to take every day, is very effective, is safe, and has very few side effects. About one-third reported not wanting to get pregnant again at any time in the future, while most others reported intention to be pregnant again in two or more years.

Behaviors

Women reported using a range of contraceptives between delivery and the interview, with the majority using condoms either alone or in combination with another method (Table 4). Most women reported initiating breastfeeding, and duration did not vary by receipt of immediate postpartum LARC. The majority of women reported attending a postpartum visit.

Decision-making

Few women reported feeling pressured to make a particular decision about immediate postpartum LARC. In response to our open-ended questions, women who received immediate postpartum LARC described the convenience of receiving contraception at the time of delivery, their desire for a long-acting method, and their past experiences

Table 1 Sample characteristics overall and by receipt of immediate postpartum long-acting reversible contraception

	Overall ($N = 51$) %	Received immediate postpartum LARC ($n = 25$) %	Did not receive immediate postpartum LARC (n = 26) %	Chi-square p-value
Maternal age (years)*				0.27
< 20	12.0	8.0	16.0	
20–24	44.0	56.0	32.0	
25–29	34.0	24.0	44.0	
≥ 30	10.0	12.0	8.0	
Race/Ethnicity				0.01
Black	66.7	88.0	46.2	
White	21.6	4.0	38.5	
Other	11.8	8.0	15.3	
Educational attainment				0.06
Less than high school diploma	11.8	16.0	7.7	
High school diploma or GED	49.0	32.0	65.4	
Some college or more	39.2	52.0	26.9	
Relationship status				0.14
Married	21.6	8.0	34.6	
Living with partner	33.3	40.0	26.9	
In a relationship not living with partner	11.8	12.0	11.6	
Single**	33.3	40.0	26.9	
Parity*				0.43
1	46.0	37.5	53.9	
2	28.0	29.2	26.9	
≥ 3	26.0	33.3	19.2	
Current health insurance				0.30
Medicaid	52.9	64.0	42.3	
Private insurance	5.9	4.0	7.7	
None	41.2	32.0	50.0	
Current employment status				0.20
Employed full-time	21.6	32.0	11.5	
Employed part-time	19.6	16.0	23.1	
Unemployed	58.8	42.0	65.4	
Pregnancy intention***				0.24
Intended	35.3	24.0	46.2	
Unintended	56.9	68.0	46.2	
Unsure	7.8	8.0	7.7	
Preterm birth (< 37 weeks gestation)	19.6	32.0	7.7	0.03
Delivery hospital				0.24
Hospital 1	68.6	80.0	57.7	
Hospital 2	25.5	16.0	34.6	
Hospital 3	5.9	4.0	7.7	

*1 missing
**"Single" includes women who reported being single and never married, separated, divorced, or widowed
***"Intended" includes women who reported that they wanted to be pregnant when they did or sooner; "unintended" includes women who reported that they wanted be pregnant later or that they did not want to be pregnant then or anytime in the future

Table 2 Knowledge provision and knowledge about availability of immediate postpartum long-acting reversible contraception, overall and by receipt

	Overall (N = 51) %	Received immediate postpartum LARC (n = 25) %	Did not receive immediate postpartum LARC (n = 26) %	Chi-square *p*-value
Discussed subsequent pregnancy prevention with provider during pregnancy?				0.67
Yes	90.2	92.0	88.5	
No	9.8	8.0	11.5	
During pregnancy, did provider offer option of immediate postpartum LARC?				0.12
Yes	66.7	76.0	57.7	
No	25.5	16.0	34.6	
Unsure	7.8	8.0	7.7	
During pregnancy, did provider give all the information needed to make a decision about immediate postpartum LARC?*				0.69
Yes	91.2	89.5	93.3	
No	8.8	10.5	6.7	
At time of delivery, did provider offer option of immediate postpartum LARC?				< .001
Yes	70.6	96.0	46.1	
No	29.4	4.0	53.9	
At time of delivery, did you have all the information needed to make a decision about immediate postpartum LARC?**				0.74
Yes	83.3	83.3	83.3	
No	13.9	12.5	16.7	
Unsure	2.8	4.2	0	
Does Medicaid in GA pay for immediate postpartum LARC?				0.32
Yes	86.3	92.0	80.8	
No	3.9	0	7.7	
Unsure	9.8	8.0	11.5	
Is it possible for a woman to receive IUD immediately postpartum?				0.10
Yes	51.0	60.0	42.3	
No	41.2	40.0	42.3	
Unsure	7.8	0	15.4	
Is it possible for a woman to receive implant immediately postpartum?				0.30
Yes	90.2	96.0	84.6	
No	5.9	4.0	7.7	
Unsure	3.9	0	7.7	

*$N = 34$; this question was only asked to women who said their provider offered them immediate postpartum LARC
**$N = 36$; this question was only asked to women who said they were offered immediate postpartum LARC at delivery

with other contraceptive methods. The exceptions were two women who felt like their doctor and father were pressuring them to receive immediate postpartum implants.

Most women who did not receive immediate postpartum LARC desired another contraceptive method instead. When given a list of possible reasons they did not want immediate postpartum LARC, the most common responses were concerns about side effects and disliking the idea of a foreign object in their bodies (Table 5). However, of the 26 women who did not receive immediate postpartum LARC, three reported wanting immediate postpartum IUD ($n = 1$) or implant ($n = 2$). These women

Table 3 Contraceptive attitudes overall and by receipt of immediate postpartum long-acting reversible contraception

	Overall (N = 51) %	Received immediate postpartum LARC (n = 25) %	Did not receive immediate postpartum LARC (n = 26) %	Chi-square *p*-value
Ideal time to begin using birth control postpartum				0.03
In the hospital after delivery	62.7	84.0	42.3	
After delivery hospitalization but before postpartum visit	2.0	0	3.9	
At the 4–6 week postpartum visit	21.6	8.0	34.6	
After the postpartum visit	9.8	8.0	11.5	
Unsure	3.9	0	7.7	
Importance of having birth control method you do not have to think about regularly				0.81
Very important	68.6	72.0	65.4	
Somewhat important	25.5	24.0	26.9	
Not important	5.9	4.0	7.7	
Importance of having birth control method you do not have to take every day				0.47
Very important	66.7	76.0	57.7	
Somewhat important	19.6	16.0	23.1	
Not important	11.8	8.0	15.4	
Unsure	2.0	0	3.8	
Importance of having very effective birth control method				0.17
Very important	84.3	92.0	76.9	
Somewhat important	9.8	4.0	15.4	
Not important	3.9	0	7.7	
Unsure	2.0	4.0	0	
Importance of having safe birth control method				0.61
Very important	94.1	96.0	92.3	
Somewhat important	3.9	4.0	3.9	
Not important	2.0	0	3.9	
Importance of birth control method having few side effects				0.22
Very important	94.1	92.0	96.1	
Somewhat important	3.9	8.0	0	
Not important	2.0	0	3.9	
Future pregnancy plans				0.02
Do not want to get pregnant at any time in the future	33.3	32.0	34.6	
Want to be pregnant again in 6 months to 2 years	17.6	4.0	30.8	
Want to be pregnant again in 2+ years	45.1	60.0	30.8	
Unsure	3.9	4.0	3.8	

were unable to receive their desired devices due to complications during delivery, lack of stocked device at the hospital, and not realizing it was an option until after hospital discharge, respectively.

Satisfaction

Most women who received immediate postpartum LARC reported they are very (40%) or extremely (32%) happy with their device. Of those who received immediate postpartum

Table 4 Contraceptive and postpartum behaviors overall and by receipt of immediate postpartum long-acting reversible contraception

	Overall (N = 51) %	Received immediate postpartum LARC (n = 25) %	Did not receive immediate postpartum LARC (n = 26) %	Chi-square *p*-value
Contraceptives used since delivery*				
Contraceptive implant	51.0	96.0	7.7	< .01
IUD	7.8	4.0	11.5	0.32
Sterilization	3.9	0	7.7	0.16
Oral contraceptive pill	13.7	4.0	23.1	0.05
Depo-Provera shot	17.6	4.0	30.8	0.01
Condoms	60.8	56.0	65.4	0.49
Emergency contraception	2.0	0	3.8	0.32
None	5.9	0	11.5	0.08
Other	5.9	4.0	7.7	0.58
Breastfeeding				0.29
Did not breastfeed	21.6	24.0	19.2	
≤ 1 month	27.5	20.0	34.6	
2–3 months	25.5	26.0	15.4	
≥ 4 months	25.5	20.0	30.8	
Postpartum visit attendance				0.57
Yes	80.4	80.0	80.8	
No	17.6	20.0	15.4	
Unsure	2.0	0	3.8	

*Women could select more than one option

Table 5 Reasons for not wanting/choosing immediate postpartum LARC (*n* = 20)

Reason	%
Had concerns about side effects	75.0
Did not like the idea of a foreign object	70.0
Did not like the idea of hormones in body	60.0
Did not like that it cannot be removed by self	50.0
Afraid it was going to hurt	40.0
Preferred another kind of birth control	40.0
Wanted to wait until postpartum visit	40.0
Worried that LARC would make breastfeeding harder	35.0
Partner did not want her to get LARC	30.0
Did not know could get one right after delivery, before leaving the hospital	30.0
Did not have the money to pay for it	25.0
Did not know enough about LARCs	20.0
Want to get pregnant again within a year	20.0
Other family members or friends did not want her to get LARC	15.0

LARC, 80% reported they would recommend it to a friend. None of the women using IUDs (1 immediately postpartum, 3 interval placements) experienced a device expulsion.

Of the 30 women who received a LARC (26 implants, 4 IUDs), either immediately postpartum or later in the postpartum period, 13 (43.3%) said they wanted the device removed at one point; 10 of these had immediate postpartum implants. Two women had their implants removed by the time of the interview (1 immediate postpartum placement and 1 interval placement). Among the remaining 11 women, three reported they were planning to have their immediate postpartum implants removed soon due to side effects. The other women said they were waiting to see if their side effects became more tolerable or they felt it was worth keeping their device to prevent pregnancy.

Discussion

To our knowledge, this is the first study to examine postpartum women's experiences with informed choice and satisfaction with immediate postpartum LARC. Our conceptual framework for informed choice focused on women's knowledge, attitudes, and behaviors, with the understanding that informed choice requires knowledge plus behaviors that are consistent with attitudes [13, 14].

We piloted the use of a novel population-based sampling technique in partnership with Georgia DCH to interview women who did and did not receive immediate postpartum LARC in two large metropolitan areas in Georgia. Women were well-informed about the fact that Georgia Medicaid reimburses for immediate postpartum LARC, reported receiving enough information to make a decision about using immediate postpartum LARC, and were generally satisfied with their experiences with LARC.

It was surprising that 90% of women in our study knew it was possible to receive an immediate postpartum implant, but about 41% did not think it was possible to receive an immediate postpartum IUD. While this aligns with the fact that the majority of women who received immediate postpartum LARC in our study obtained a contraceptive implant, it is contrary to other published studies reporting that IUDs are used more commonly than implants immediately postpartum [9, 16]. However, a Georgia study found that among early-adopting hospitals that placed immediate postpartum LARC, one was offering IUDs, one was offering implants, and two were offering both devices [17]. It is unclear if all three delivery hospitals represented in our study offered both IUDs and implants, but our results likely reflect the immediate postpartum LARC implementation process at the hospital level.

Most participants reported satisfaction with their devices, although more than two-thirds reported wanting the device removed at some point. Our results are consistent with previous studies about women's satisfaction and removal rates of immediate postpartum contraceptive implants [18]. A recently published study found that women had a high degree of satisfaction with immediate postpartum IUD insertion, but were unable to understand or recall the consent process [19]. In our study, we asked women if they recalled signing a consent form and if they received enough information to make a decision about immediate postpartum LARC. While our results are promising, the number of women desiring device removal at some point may reflect an ineffective informed consent process, specifically regarding potential side effects of implants. However, it is unclear if women attributed common postpartum symptoms, such as bleeding and cramping, to implants, which have been shown to produce these side effects in some women [20].

There has been concern that barriers to removal may inhibit uptake of LARC methods. Several women in our study reported that they did not want or choose immediate postpartum LARC because they did not like that they cannot remove the device themselves. Some women may encounter challenges to getting a LARC device removed when they desire, including resistance from providers and cost barriers [21]. Although Georgia Medicaid does not have any policies that may add barriers to LARC removal the way a few other states do [22], 41% of the women in our study were uninsured by the time of the interview. Additional examination of the data showed that of the 11 women who reported wanting their LARC removed but who had not had a removal by the time of the interview, 5 were uninsured and the other 6 remained on Medicaid. We did not specifically ask women if insurance affected their decision-making about LARC removal, but none of the women mentioned this in response to open-ended questions about their experiences. However, in order to ensure women's reproductive autonomy, it is important that providers and policy-makers do not impede women's decisions to have their LARC devices removed. Women receiving immediate postpartum LARC in our study were more likely to be black and to deliver preterm compared to women not receiving immediate postpartum LARC. Consistent with national data, black women were more likely to deliver preterm than other racial/ethnic groups in our study (data not shown). Further examination of the data revealed that the proportion of women reporting that immediate postpartum LARC was offered to them varied significantly by hospital of delivery. Since black women in our study more often delivered at the hospital most likely to offer immediate postpartum LARC (data not shown), the racial difference in receipt of immediate postpartum LARC is likely a result of the demographic distribution in Georgia and the uneven implementation of immediate postpartum LARC in hospitals around the state at the time.

Public health concerns about immediate postpartum LARC have included potential effects on breastfeeding and women's attendance at the 4–6 week postpartum visit [23]. In our study, neither of these outcomes varied by immediate postpartum LARC receipt. Similarly, there has been concern that women who use LARCs may be more prone to sexually transmitted infections because they may not feel the need to use barrier methods. However, more than half the women in our study, regardless of immediate postpartum LARC receipt, reported using condoms.

This study has several limitations. First, the low participation rate led to a relatively small sample with unknown generalizability. Women were notified about the study via mail and contacted via telephone based on information on file with Medicaid. Many women were uninsured by the time of the interview, which likely explains why Medicaid did not have their updated information. However, women we could not get in touch with may be particularly mobile or prone to changes in phone numbers, and may be different than the women we surveyed. Further, although we tried to contact women at various times, and asked women for a preferred time to call them back, nearly 60% of the women in our study were unemployed at the time of the interview, suggesting that our sample under-represents women in the workforce who may not have had time to participate. Few women in our study were Hispanic, Asian, or other races/ethnicities. Of all live births in Georgia during 2013–2015, 13.3% were Hispanic, 0.1% were American Indian/Alaska Native, and 4.4% were Asian/Pacific Islander [24]. However, the racial/ethnic breakdown of Medicaid-paid births in Georgia is unclear. We only interviewed women who spoke English. Although only three women are known to be excluded due to language, it is unknown how many women did not answer the phone or return our calls because they do not speak English. Also, due to the pattern of immediate postpartum LARC implementation in Georgia to date, women were only drawn from three hospitals. Therefore, despite the population-based sampling design, unevenness of implementation across the state and the low participation rate among women may have affected the generalizability of our results. Additionally, the time between delivery and interview ranged from 14 weeks to 20 months, which may have introduced recall issues, especially related to the counseling and decision-making process.

Conclusions

In conclusion, women on Medicaid in Georgia report making informed choices regarding immediate postpartum LARC. These findings about women's perspectives and desires for immediate postpartum LARC support continued efforts to increase immediate postpartum LARC access, while ensuring informed consent among all women. Ultimately, providing access to all methods of contraception at multiple time points during the postpartum period is the most effective approach to meeting women's contraceptive needs.

Abbreviations

CPT: Current Procedural Terminology; DCH: Department of Community Health; GED: General Equivalency Degree; HCPCS: Healthcare Common Procedure Coding System; ICD: International Classification of Diseases; IUD: Intrauterine device; LARC: Long-acting reversible contraception; RA: Research assistant

Acknowledgements

The authors would like to thank: Katrina Stumbras for her assistance in developing the questionnaire, Amanda Consigli and Paula Satariano for their interviewing assistance, Elizabeth Daubert for her assistance with data analysis, and Erica Baker, Heather Bond, Kris Covington, Daphanie Keit, and the Georgia Department of Community Health for their collaboration on this project.

Authors' contributions

KR, as the principal investigator, conceived of this study and acquired data from the Georgia Department of Community Health. AH, SH, RC, NP, and KR designed the questionnaire. CD led the data collection, data analysis, and writing of the manuscript. AH, SH, RC, NP, MK, and KR made substantial contributions to the interpretation of the data and critically revising the manuscript. All authors have given their final approval of the version to be published and are accountable for all aspects of the work.

Author details

[1]University of Illinois at Chicago School of Public Health , 1603 W. Taylor St, Chicago, IL 60612, USA. [2]Department of Obstetrics and Gynecology, University of Chicago, 5841 S. Maryland Ave, Chicago, IL 60637, USA. [3]College of Medicine, University of Illinois at Chicago, 840 S. Wood St, Chicago, IL 60612, USA. [4]Department of Gynecology and Obstetrics, Jane Fonda Center, Emory University School of Medicine, 49 Jesse Hill Jr. Drive SE, Atlanta, GA 30303, USA.

References

1. Curtis KM, Tepper NK, Jatlaoui TC, Berry-Bibee E, Horton LG, Zapata LB, et al. U.S. Medical Eligibility Criteria for Contraceptive Use, 2016. MMWR Recomm Rep. 2016;65(3):1–103.
2. American College of Obstetricians and Gynecologists. ACOG Practice Bulletin No. 121: long-acting reversible contraception: implants and intrauterine devices. Obstet Gynecol. 2011;118(1):184–96.
3. Rodriguez MI, Evans M, Espey E. Advocating for immediate postpartum LARC: increasing access, improving outcomes, and decreasing cost. Contraception. 2014;90(5):468–71.
4. Moniz MH, Dalton VK, Davis MM, Forman J, Iott B, Landgraf J, et al. Characterization of Medicaid policy for immediate postpartum contraception. Contraception. 2015;92(6):523–31.
5. Curtin SC, Osterman MJ, Uddin SF, Sutton SR, Reed PR. Source of payment for the delivery: births in a 33-state and District of Columbia reporting area, 2010. Natl Vital Stat Rep. 2013;62(5):1–20.
6. Washington CI, Jamshidi R, Thung SF, Nayeri UA, Caughey AB, Werner EF. Timing of postpartum intrauterine device placement: a cost-effectiveness analysis. Fertil Steril. 2015;103(1):131–7.
7. Gomez AM, Fuentes L, Allina A. Women or LARC first? Reproductive autonomy and the promotion of long-acting reversible contraceptive methods. Perspect Sex Reprod Health. 2014;46(3):171–5.
8. Higgins JA. Celebration meets caution: LARC's boons, potential busts, and the benefits of a reproductive justice approach. Contraception. 2014;89(4):237–41.
9. Moniz MH, Chang T, Heisler M, Admon L, Gebremariam A, Dalton VK, et al. Inpatient postpartum long-acting reversible contraception and sterilization in the United States, 2008-2013. Obstet Gynecol. 2017;129(6):1078–85.
10. Harris LH, Wolfe T. Stratified reproduction, family planning care and the double edge of history. Curr Opin Obstet Gynecol. 2014;26(6):539–44.
11. Brandi K, Woodhams E, White K, Mehta P. An exploration of perceived contraceptive coercion at the time of abortion. Contraception. 2018;97(4):329–34.
12. Georgia Department of Community Health. Long Acting Reversible Contraceptive (LARC) Procedure Codes. 2014. https://www.acog.org/-/media/Departments/LARC/GAPPLARCBannerMessage.pdf?la=en&hash=6BDC972985191678AE282C65651E9FBD0D4AA05A.
13. Marteau TM, Dormandy E, Michie S. A measure of informed choice. Health Expect. 2001;4(2):99–108.
14. O'Connor A, O'Brien-Pallas LL. Decisional conflict. In: Mcfarlane GK, Mcfarlane EA, editors. Nursing Diagnosis and Intervention. Toronto: Mosby; 1989. p. 486–96.
15. Harris PA, Taylor R, Thielke R, Payne J, Gonzalez N, Conde JG. Research electronic data capture (REDCap)--a metadata-driven methodology and workflow process for providing translational research informatics support. J Biomed Inform. 2009;42(2):377–81.
16. Eggebroten JL, Sanders JN, Turok DK. Immediate postpartum intrauterine device and implant program outcomes: a prospective analysis. Am J Obstet Gynecol. 2017;217(1):51.e7.
17. Hofler LG, Cordes S, Cwiak CA, Goedken P, Jamieson DJ, Kottke M. Implementing immediate postpartum long-acting reversible contraception programs. Obstet Gynecol. 2017;129(1):3–9.
18. Crockett AH, Pickell LB, Heberlein EC, Billings DL, Mills B. Six- and twelve-month documented removal rates among women electing postpartum inpatient compared to delayed or interval contraceptive implant insertions after Medicaid payment reform. Contraception. 2017;95(1):71–6.
19. Carr SL, Singh RH, Sussman AL, Rogers RG, Pereda B, Espey E. Women's experiences with immediate postpartum intrauterine device insertion: a mixed methods study. Contraception. 2017;97(3):219–26.
20. Diedrich JT, Desai S, Zhao Q, Secura G, Madden T, Peipert JF. Association of short-term bleeding and cramping patterns with long-acting reversible contraceptive method satisfaction. Am J Obstet Gynecol. 2015;212(1):50.e8.

21. Strasser J, Borkowski L, Couillard M, Allina A, Wood SF. Access to removal of long-acting reversible contraceptive methods is an essential component of high-quality contraceptive care. Womens Health Issues. 2017;27(3):253–5.
22. Walls J, Gifford K, Ranji U, Salganicoff A, Gomez I. Medicaid Coverage of Family Planning Benefits: Results from a State Survey. In: The Henry J. Washington: Kaiser Family Foundation; 2016.
23. American College of Obstetricians and Gynecologists' Committee on Obstetric Practice. Committee Opinion No. 670: Immediate Postpartum Long-Acting Reversible Contraception. Obstet Gynecol. 2016,128(2):32.
24. March of Dimes. Peristats: Georgia 2017. [https://www.marchofdimes.org/peristats/ViewSubtopic.aspx?reg=13&top=2&stop=10&lev=1&slev=4&obj=3].

Long-acting family planning method switching among revisit clients of public health facilities in Dire Dawa, Ethiopia

Meselu Atnafe[1], Nega Assefa[2*] and Tadesse Alemayehu[2]

Abstract

Background: "Contraceptive switching" from one method to another is a common phenomenon. Switching from a more effective long-acting method to a less effective method exposes women for unplanned pregnancy. The aim of this study was to assess the level and factors associated with long-acting family planning method switching to other methods.

Method: A facility-based cross-sectional study was conducted from January to March 2013 on 634 women attending public health facilities in Dire Dawa City Administration, Ethiopia. Participants of the study were revisit clients of family planning service and were interviewed as they appear in the clinics. Data were analyzed using crude and adjusted logistic regression, and results were reported using OR and corresponding 95 % CI.

Results: Long-acting family planning method switching among revisit clients was 40.4 %; switching from implant was 29.8 % and from IUCD, it was 10.6 %. The main reasons for methods switching were side effects of the methods such as bleeding, weight loss, and feeling of arm numbness. The tendency of switching was less among married women (AOR = 2.41, 95 % CI: 1.01, 5.74), women who had 2–4 and 5 and more children (AOR 3.00, 95 % CI: 1.59, 5.67) and (AOR 2.07, 95 % CI: 1.17, 3.66), respectively. It was also less among women who want to stop birth (AOR 5.11, 95 % CI: 1.15, 24.8), among those who mentioned health care providers as source of information for family planning (AOR 1.88, 95 % CI: 1.18, 3.01), and among women whose husbands were aware of their use of the methods (AOR 3.05, 95 % CI: 1.88, 4.94).

Conclusions: Method switching from long-acting contraceptives to less effective methods is high. Method switching was significant among unmarried women, who had one child, plan to postpone fertility, and whose husbands were not aware of their wive's use of the method. In the provision of family planning service, the health care providers should give adequate information about each method and risks of method switching. Appropriate family planning Information Education and Communication (IEC) and Behavioral Change Communication (BCC) strategies should be emphasized.

Keywords: Method switching, Long-acting contraceptives, Long-acting family planning method, Contraception

* Correspondence: negaassefa@yahoo.com
[2]College of Health and Medical Sciences, Haramaya University, Dire Dawa, Ethiopia

Background

The term "contraceptive switching" refers to the case where a person changes method of birth control [1]. Many family planning users switch from long-acting contraceptive to other methods. Long-acting contraceptives, such as implant and intrauterine contraceptive device are convenient for users and have high effectiveness in preventing pregnancy [2]. Despite the advantages, long-acting contraceptive methods remain not the primary choice among clients and the uptake of the method is minimal [3–6]. In many developing countries, majority of current contraceptive users had used at least one other method; such as oral contraceptives, injectable and other methods in the past. An exception is Cambodia, where only a quarter of current users have switched from other methods. Countries with the highest rates of contraceptive switching are Gabon and Colombia, where more than 80 % of current users have used another method before [7].

Switching from a more effective method to a less effective method (long-acting to short-acting contraceptives) creates a period for unplanned pregnancy. During the early period of use, as clients are still learning how to use the new method accurately and consistently, the risk of unplanned pregnancy is high [1]. Unplanned pregnancy increases the risk of unsafe abortion and STIs/HIV infection [8, 9]. Currently, more than 200 million women in developing countries want to avoid pregnancy but they cannot do it for many reasons. Some of the major obstacles are lack of access to proper information and proper health care services, contraceptive failure, contraceptive discontinuation, opposition from husbands, misperceptions about side effect and cost [10–14].

Though family planning enables couples to control their fertility, during method switching, the risk of adverse effects and failure to adapt the new method results in unplanned pregnancy [15]. So far method switching has received little attention from researchers and health executive bodies, hence, the size of the problem is not clearly known.

The aim of the study was to assess the level and factors contributing to method switching from long acting contraceptives to other methods in Dire Dawa city, Ethiopia. Identification of the levels of method switching and factors related to switching will help researchers and health executive bodies at national and regional level to guide programs, lead proper implementation and evaluate the outcomes of interventions.

Methods

The study was conducted in Dire Dawa City Administration, Eastern Ethiopia from January to March 2013. Dire Dawa is a city located about 525 km from Addis Ababa, the capital of Ethiopia. The total population of the city is 342,827 of which 233,224 (67.93 %) lives in urban and 108,610 (32.07 %) in the rural areas [16]. The city has five hospitals (1 public, 3 private and 1 company), 16 health centers (9 in urban and 7 in rural), 31 health post, 9 kebeles, 38 peasant associations, and two non-governmental clinics (Marie Stopes and FGAE). Family planning is given in all public and private health facilities integrated with the routine health system in maternal and child health (MCH) clinics [17].

A facility based cross-sectional study using quantitative and qualitative techniques was conducted. The sample size for the quantitative study was 634. In this study, data was generated from four health centers and one public hospital. Facility client registration was used as a sampling frame and systematic random sampling was used to identify specific women for interview. Only revisit women were invited for interview. To support and supplement the quantitative findings, four Focus Group Discussions (FGDs) consisting of 8–12 participants were conducted. Participants of the FGDs were selected on the basis of prior use of long-acting methods and their willingness to share their experiences.

The quantitative data was collected using pre-tested structured questionnaire adapted from Family Health International (FHI) 2009 questions. Open-ended discussion guide was used to lead the discussion of the focus groups. Female high school graduates collected the data and two nurses supervised the data collection process. A one-day training on the objective of the study, data collection tools and interview methods was given for the research team by the principal investigator.

Quality of data was maintained through adequate training of study tool, continuous follow-up during data collection, on-site supervision, and pre-test on one of the nearby health centers. In addition, data was carefully checked for completeness and consistency on daily basis. Each questionnaire was assigned a unique code to maintain its anonymity and facilitate data entry. Any confusion on the data collection procedure and/or responses was handled in a timely fashion.

Frequencies and odds ratios with 95 % confidence intervals (CI) were used to describe the results and show the presence of association between independent and dependent variable. Multiple logistic regression was used to control the effect of confounders. Qualitative data were tape recorded, transcribed verbatim and hand summarized using summary sheet. Notes taken during interviews also helped to complete the template.

The study was approved by the Institutional Research Ethical Review Committee (IRERC) of College of Health and Medical Sciences, Haramaya University. Official letter of cooperation was obtained from Dire Dawa Town Health Bureau. Participants were briefed about the purpose, procedures, potential risk, benefits, and right of participants to withdraw from the study at any time. Before the start of data collection, written informed consent was obtained from study participants. Confidentiality and privacy of information were maintained throughout the research process.

Results

A total of 634 women participated in the interview with a response rate of 100 %. These women were the ones who came for the second time to the family planning service. Among the 634 participants, the majority, 536 (84.5 %), were urban residents. The age of respondents ranged between 15 and 45 with mean age of 26.2 years (SD = ±5.7 years), the median age was 25 years. Regarding the educational status, 42.6 % had primary schooling and 32.6 % can read and write. By their occupation, the majority, 57.7 %, of respondents were housewives and 62.1 % were Muslims (Table 1).

The majority, 577 (91 %), of the respondents were married and 555(87.5%) had ever given birth. Among those who had ever given birth, 196 (30.9 %) had at least one child, 289(45.6 %) had 2 to 4 children, and 70(11 %) have 5 and more children. At the time of the interview, nearly 50 % of the respondents would like to have an additional child (Table 2).

Of the total participants, 498(78.5 %) were using injection and 136(21.5 %) were using oral contraceptive pills. Level of switching from long-acting family planning methods to other methods was 40.4 %. Switching from implants was reported by 189(29.8 %) respondents, while the rest 67(10.6 %) switched from Intrauterine Contraceptive Device (IUCD). Regarding the timing of method switching, 75(11.8 %) switched during the past 12 months and 143 (23.2 %) switched during 24–36 months (Figs. 1 and 2).

Regarding the reasons for method swiching; bleeding, weight loss and feeling of numbness were the major problems while using the previous long-acting family planning method. FGD participants responded that side effects of the methods were major reasons for shifting method (Fig. 3).

Regarding, sources of information of family planning, the majority, 305 (48.1 %) responded health care providers were the main source, followed by neighbors 89(14 %), and Health Extension Workers (HEWs) 83(13.1 %). Regarding the person who chose family planning method for the women, 474 (74.8 %) participants responded, they themselves chose the method (Table 3).

Marital status showed significant association with method switching; married women were three times less likely to switch method (COR = 2.96, 95 % CI: 1.27, 6.85). Women who had 2–4 children were less likely to change long-acting method to other method (COR = 1.63, 95 % CI: 1.12, 2.48), and women who had more than 5 children were 3.8 times less likely to switch long-acting method than those who had one child (COR = 3.8, 95 % CI: 2.14, 6.74). Women who want no more pregnancies were 5.2 times less likely to switch long-acting method compared to those women who need spacing (COR = 5.2, 95 % CI: 1.10, 24.9) (Table 4).

Results of multiple logistic regression showed that, married women were 2.4 times less likely to switch

Table 1 Socio-demographic characteristics of re-visit clients at family planning clinics in public health facilities, Dire Dawa City Administration, 2013 ($n = 634$)

Socio-demographic characteristics	Frequency	Percent
Age of the women		
15–19	62	9.8
20–24	189	29.8
25–29	181	28.5
30–34	127	20.0
35+	75	11.8
Educational status of the women		
Canot read and write	207	32.6
Primary (1–8 grade)	270	42.6
Secondary (9–12 grade)	117	18.5
Diploma and above	40	6.3
Educational status of husband		
Canot read and write	120	18.9
Primary (1–8 grade)	198	31.2
Secondary (9–12 grade)	213	33.6
Diploma and above	103	16.3
Religion of the women		
Muslim	394	62.1
Orthodox	208	32.8
Protestat	29	4.6
Catholic	3	0.5
Occupation of the women		
House wife	366	57.7
Government employee	77	12.1
House maid	11	1.7
Merchant	59	9.3
Student	42	6.6
Farmer	35	5.5
Daily laborer	39	6.1
Others	5	0.8
Marital Status of the women		
Single	36	5.7
Married	577	91.0
Divorced	14	2.2
Widowed	7	1.1

Table 2 Fertility characteristics of re-visit clients to family planning clinics in public health facilities, Dire Dawa City Administration, 2013

Fertility characteristics	Frequency	Percent
Ever given birth (*n* = 634)		
No	79	12,5
Yes	555	87,5
Number of children (*n* = 555)		
1	196	30,9
2–4	289	45,6
5+	70	11,0
Intention to have more children (*n* = 555)		
Yes	320	50,5
No	184	29,0
Depends on husband	22	3,5
Depends on God	18	2,8
I am not sure	11	1,7

method compared to unmarried women (AOR = 2.41, 95 % CI: 1.01, 5.74). Women who had 2–4 children were 3.0 times less likely to switch long-acting method than those who have one child (AOR = 3.00, 95 % CI: 1.59, 5.67). Similarly, women who had more than 5 children were 2.07 times less likely to switch long-acting method than those who have one child (AOR = 2.07, 95 % CI: 1.17, 3.66). Women who want no more pregnancies were 5.1 times less likely to switch method compared to those who wish to have more children (AOR = 5.11, 95 % CI: 1.15, 24.8). Women who got initial information about family planning from health care providers were 2 times less likely to switch compared to those women who received information from their husband (AOR = 1.88, 95 % CI = 1,18,3.01). On other hand, women whose husbands were aware about their use of long-acting family planning method were 3.05 times less likely to switch compared to those whose husbands were aware of their use of the method (AOR = 3.05, 95 % CI = 1.88–4.94) (Table 4).

Discussion

Long-acting Family Planning method switching among revisit clients was 40.4 %. The major determining factors for method switching were age of the respondent, educational status of husband/partner, marital status, number of children, and desire for having more children. The main reasons for method switching from long-acting method to other methods were bleeding, weight loss, and numbness in the arm.

Participants in this study were selected only from public health facilities, as majority of family planning users in the city are visiting public health facilities. Yet, there are some women who receive service from private and NGO clinics, the views of these women are not reflected in this report. Similarly, the perspectives of husband/partner and health care provider were not included. Hence readers are advised to read the paper taking these into account.

Method switching was 40.4 %, and switching from implant was 29.8 % and the rest, 10.6 %, switched from IUCD. This is relatively low compared to reports from other studies. For example, in Egypt method switching from IUCD and Norplant to another method was 45.9 % [18]. Similar study from 14 developing countries showed that there were high rates of switching in Peru (70.5 %) and Morocco (69.8 %). In Vietnam, two-thirds of women who had an IUCD reported to switch to other methods (n = 306/434) [19]. In contrast to our findings, method switching is low in Bolivia (16.7 %) and Kazakhstan (25.2 %). Reports of USAID in 2007, indicated that high method switching can be

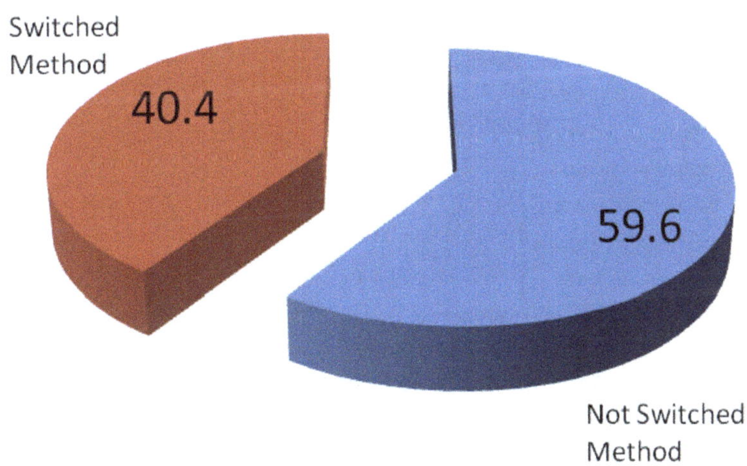

Fig. 1 Long-acting family planning method switching among revisit clients at public health facilities in Dire Dawa city Administration, 2013 (*n* = 634)

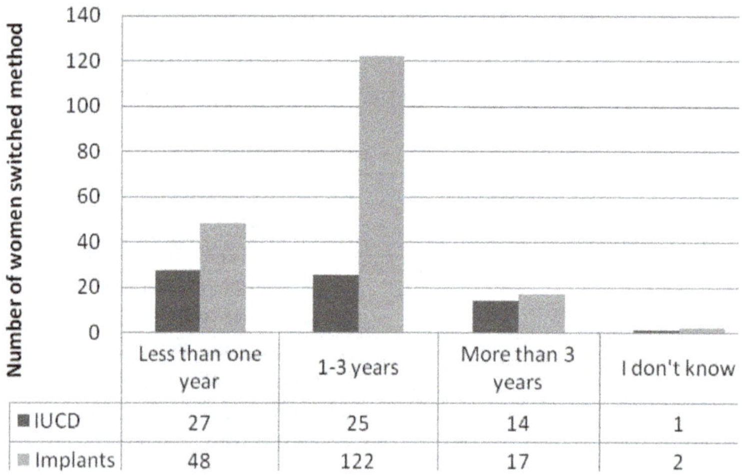

Fig. 2 Duration of use of long-acting family planning before switching to other method among revisit clients at public health facilities in Dire Dawa city Administration, 2013($n = 634$)

indicative of low satisfaction with the method used or poor service delivery. On the other hand, lower levels of method switching could mean user choices are limited [3].

The result from logistic regression analysis showed that women whose age ranged from 25–29 years were three to four fold less likely to switch method. Women who were 30–34 years of age were four times less likely to switch compared to those who were 15–19 years, and women who were 35 and above were six times less likely to switch compared to those women who were 15–19 years old. Similar study in Indonesia showed that as age increases, the probability of method switching decreases; those in the age group of 30–39 years had a low probability of switching method compared to their counterparts [20].

Married women were two times less likely to switch method compared to unmarried ones. In contrast to this study, studies in the Northern Africa indicated that method switching was common among married women than unmarried [21]. Women who had 2–4 children were three times less likely to switch long-acting method than those who had one child. In addition, women who had more than five children were two times less likely to switch long-acting method than those who had one child. Similar study from Indonesia in 2010 showed that women who want to stop birth were five times less likely to switch method compared to those who need additional children. This showed that women at higher parity were less likely to switch methods compared to women with no children [11, 12].

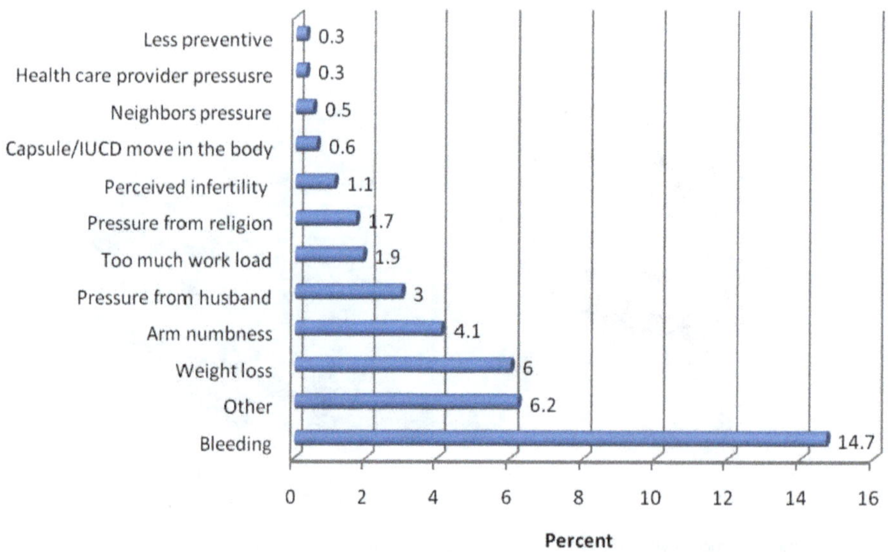

Fig. 3 Reasons for switching long-acting family planning methods at public health facilities in Dire Dawa city Administration, 2013 ($n = 634$)

Table 3 Family planning related characteristics of re-visit client at public health facilities in Dire Dawa City Administration, 2013($n = 634$)

Family planning related characteristics	Frequency	Percent
Where do you get information about family planning?		
Husband	32	5.0
Neighbors	89	14.0
Health care providers	305	48.1
Health Extension Workers	83	13.1
Others	125	19.7
Is your husband aware about your use of family planning?		
No	95	15.0
Yes	539	85.0
Who chooses family planning method for you?		
Myself	474	74.8
Husband	96	15.1
Neighbors	2	0.3
Health care provider	61	9.6
Other	1	0.2
Do religious leader in your area consider family planning?		
Yes	120	18.9
No	354	55.8
I donot know	160	25.2
Which family planning methods religious leaders considered? ($n = 120$)		
Pills	5	8
Injectable	22	3.5
Implant	1	0.2
IUCD	1	0.2
Calander method	11	1.7
Abstinence	6	0.9
All methods	52	8.2
Short methods only	22	3.5

Source of family planning information has significant role in the use long-acting methods. Yet, if the information provided is not sufficient, the probability of switching will be high. In this study, women who heard information about family planning from health care providers were less likely to switch method compared to women who received from other people. A health professional gives sufficient information on the methods, hence, continuity of its use is better [7].

Majority of FGD participants reported that side effects were the primarily reasons for shifting methods. *"I have four children and I decided to take family planning then the health care provider convinced me to take long term contraceptives and their advantages. But I couldn't tolerate excessive bleeding and and becoming weak and tired, that pushed me to change the method"———28 year old woman* [Sabian Health Center]

"After insertion of IUD, my menstruation became twice in a month and problem of stomachache became a common phenomenon, hence, it appeared very difficult to continue with it". —35year old [Melka health center].

"Since the time I put implant in my arm, I had seen no menstruation at all. I am afraid if blood accumulates in my abdomen, it can cause presser. So, I decided to take the implant out and shift to pills." ————22 year old woman - [Legeharie health center].

Women whose husbands were not aware of their use of long-acting family planning method were less likely to switch from long-acting to short-acting method compared to those whose husbands were aware. But once they learnt of that their wives use of the method, they created problems on the family life and beyond; this led to premature termination of family planning method.

One FGD participant said, *"I have been using implant in my arm without my husband knowing about it, I was comfortable with the method. After a year he came to know that I am using this method and he went to the health facility and quarreled with the nurses. I was afraid thought that he may leave me and I might be left alone, so I terminated the method"....... 30 year old woman* [Legeharie Health Center].

A qualitative study in Nigeria showed that, lack of support from the husband does not only hinder a woman's decision to use a long-acting contraceptive methods, but it also may lead to premature termination of its use [22]. Husbands/partners, who do not support women on the use of family planning, tend to have more children, and prevent their wives from using any family planning.

Some religious leaders discourage the use of family planning. This is true both in Christian and Muslim religions and fertility control discussions are not generally favored. In this study, few women reported that religious leaders advised them on the use of family planning. A study done in 2011 in Indonesia, where Islam is the dominant religion, method switching is not significantly associated with religion [23].

In this study, bleeding associated with the use of family planning and husband/partner not being aware of wife's use of long-acting fertility control methods were

Table 4 Predictors of long acting family planning method switching among re-visit clients in public health facilities, Dire Dawa City Administration, 2013($n = 634$)

Characteristics	Switched method			
	No (%)	Yes (%)	Crude OR (95 % CI)	Adjusted OR(95 % CI)
Age group				
15–19	50(80. 7)	12(19.3)	1.00	1.00
20–24	134(70.9)	55(29.1)	1.71(0.85,3.46)	0.38(0.73,2.01)
25–29	99(54.7)	82(45.3)	3.5(1.72, 6.91)*	0.68(0.13,3.56)
30–34	63(49.6)	64(50.4)	4.2 (2.06, 8.69)*	0.74(0.14,3.93)
35+	32(42.7)	43(57.3)	5.7(2.60,12.67)*	1.05(0.19,5.75)
Marital status				
Unmarried	29(80.6)	7(19.4)	1.00	1.00
Married	349(58.4)	249(41.6)	2.96(1.27,6.85)	2.41(1.01,5.74)*
Number of children				
1	133(67.8)	63(32.2)	1.00	1.00
2–4	163(56.4)	126(42.6)	1.63(1.12,2.48)*	3.00 (1.59, 5.67)*
5+	25(35.7)	45(64.3)	3.8(2.14, 6.74)*	2.07(1.17, 3.66)*
Future fertility control				
To space birth	207(64.7)	113(35.3)	1.00	1.00
To stop birth	85(46.2)	99(53.8)	5.2(1.10,24.92)*	5.11(1.15,24.79)*
Depends on husband	11(50.0)	11(50.0)	4.5(0.79,25.77)	3.48(0.59,20.48)
Depends on God	10(55.6)	8(44.4)	3.6(0.60,21.61)	3.95(0.64,24.34)
I am not sure	9(81.8)	2(18.2)	2.5(0.52, 11.66)	3.08(0.64,14,84)
Source of family planning information				
Husband	19(59.4)	13(40.6)	1.00	1.00
Neighbors	56(62.9)	33(37.1)	1.76(0.79, 3.94)	1.82(0.80,4.15)
Health Extension Workers	161(52.8)	144(47.2)	1.52(0.85, 2.71)	1.31(0.71,2.39)
Health care providers	52(62.6)	31(37.4)	2.30(1.56,3.61)*	1.88(1.18, 3.01)*
Others	90(72.0)	35(28.0)	1.53(0.85,2.86)	1.03(0.55,1.94
Husband is aware about use of Family planning				
Yes	345(64.0)	194(36.0)	1.00	1.00
No	33(34.7)	62(65.3)	3.34(2.11,5.28)*	3.05(1.88,4.94) *

N.B. where P-value < 0.05 and * Adjusted for all variables in the table

the main reasons for method switching. Similar studies from developing countries reported the same kind of result whereby two-fifths of the women switched due to side effects and the remaining switched because their husbands disliked the methods [24, 25].

Conclusion and Recommendation

Method switching from long-acting family planning to other method is high. Method switching is common among unmarried women, women who had one child, women who want to space children and women who were not sure of their future fertility, women who reported other than health care provider as a source of family planning information, and those who reported their husbands were not aware of their use of long-acting family planning methods. The main reason for method switching was adverse effects such as bleeding and numbness in the arm.

Authors would like to recommend, women should be advised properly at the start of family planning. The advice should focus on the method and its side effects, and intervention for problems related to the use. Health executive bodies should strengthen their effort in addressing the problems of women switching long-acting methods through effective IEC and BCC strategies.

Abbreviations
AOR, adjusted odds ration; BCC, behavioral change communication; CI, confidence interval; COR, crude odds ratio; FGAE, Family Guidance Association of Ethiopia; FGD, focus group discussion; FHI, Family Health International; HEW, Health Extension Worker; HIV, human immuno virus; IEC, information education and communication; IRERC, Institutional Research Ethical Review Committee; IUCD, intrauterine contraceptive devices; MCH, Maternal and Chile Health; NGO, Non-Governmental Organization; OR, odds ratio; SD, standard deviation; STIs, sexually transmitted illnesses; USAID, United States AID

Acknowledgement
Authors would like to thank Dire Dawa City Administration Health Office, health facilities and family planning service providers for facilitating data collection.

Authors' contributions
MA initiated the research, wrote the research proposal, conducted the field work, supervised data entry, analyzed the data and wrote the manuscript. NA and TA participated in refining the the proposal, supervised the field activity, analyzed the data, and wrote the report. All authors read and approved the final manuscript.

Author details
[1]Dire Dawa City Administration Health Bureau, Dire Dawa, Ethiopia. [2]College of Health and Medical Sciences, Haramaya University, Dire Dawa, Ethiopia.

References

1. Jaccard J. Unlocking the contraceptive conundrum Unplanned Pregnancy. Washington, DC <https://thenationalcampaign.org/> 2009, NW uite 200 1776 Massachusetts Ave.
2. FMOH-NPP. Federal Democratic Republic of Ethiopia Ministry of Health. Addis Ababa, Ethiopia: National Reproductive Health Strategy FMOH; 2006.
3. USAID. Long-Acting and Permanent Methods: AddressingUnmetNeedforFamilyPlanning in Africa. Calverton, Maryland, USA: Macro International Inc; 2007. Reports No. 16.
4. WHO. Maternal health, Health topics. Geneva: World Health Organization; 2011.
5. WHO. Trends in maternal mortality: 1990 to 2010, Estimates developed by WHO UNICEF, UNFPA and The World Bank. Geneva: World Health Organization; 2012.
6. WHO. Towards a monitoring framework with targets and indicators for the health goals of the post-2015 Sustainable Development Goals. Geneva, Swtzerland: World Helath Organization; 2015.
7. USAID. Agency for International Development- Long-term contraceptive protection, discontinuation and switching behavior -IUD use dynamics developing countries. Washington Calverton, Maryland, USA: Macro International Inc; 2011. Reports No. 18.
8. Lawrence B. Use of Highly Effective Contraceptive Methods Increases Substantially, but Remains Low Among Women at Highest Risk of Unplanned Pregnancy. ≤https://www.guttmacher.org/news-release/2012/use-highly-effective-contraceptive-methodsincreases-substantially-remains-low≥ Guttmacher Institute July 2012.
9. Jacqueline C. The rising proportion of repeat teenage pregnancies in young women presenting for termination of pregnancy from 1991 to 2007. Contraception. 2009;79(5):393–6.
10. WPRB. World_population. Wikipedia the free encyclopedia 2012.
11. Bongaarts J. Human population growth and the demographic transition. The Impact of Population Growth on Tomorrow's World. Philosophical Transactions: Biological Sciences. 2009;364(1532):2985–90.
12. Bongaarts J, Casterline J. Fertility transition: Is sub-saharan africa different? Population and Development Review. 2013;38:153–68.
13. Cleland J, Mohamed M. Reproductive Consequences of Contraceptive Failure in 19 Developing Countries. Volume 104. New York, USA: The American College of Obstetricians and Gynecologists; 2004.
14. Becker D, Koenig M, Kim Y, Cardona K, Sonenstein F. The Quality of Family Planning Services in the United States: Findings from a Literature Review. Perspectives on Sexual and Reproductive Health. 2007;39(4):206–15.
15. Stephen G. Family planning-use of contraception to control number of children. Gale Encyclopedia of Public Health: 2010(Random House Word Menu© 2010 Inc.).
16. EDHS. Ethiopia Demographia Health survey. Addis Ababa, Ethiopia and Calverton (MD), USA: Central Statistical Agency ORCMACRO statistical Abstract; 2011.
17. Dire Dawa city administration profile book. Dire Dawa; 2011
18. Etemad A, Gamal H. Contraceptive use dynamics and effect of counseling on use continuation of contraception in assiut Governorate Upper Egypt. J Am Sci. 2011;**7**(6).
19. Park M, Nguyen T, Ngo T. Dynamics of IUD use in Vietnam: implications for family planning services at primary Health care level. International Journal of Women's Health. 2011:3429–434.
20. Desy NF. Factors affecting the reasons for discontinuation among modern contraceptive users in Indonesia. Asia Pac Popul J. 2010(122B)
21. Sedgh, G., Hussain, R., Bankole, A., & Singh, S. Women with an unmet need for contraception in developing countries and their reasons for not using a method. In Occasional Report. New York, USA: New York Guttmacher Institute; 2007.
22. Stella B. Factors Underlying the Use of Long-acting and Permanent Family Planning Methods in Nigeria. Baltimore, USA: Johns Hopkins Bloomberg School of Public Health Center for Communication Programs; 2011.
23. Rina G. Factors Associated with contraceptive discontinuation in Indonesia. Mahidol Univ MA (Pop & Repro H Res). 2007
24. USAID. Agency for International Development- Long-term contraceptive protection, discontinuation and switching behavior -IUD use dynamics *developing countries* 2011, No.18.
25. Janine B, Ilene S. Contraceptive Discontinuation and Switching Among Honduran Women. Int Perspect Sex Reprod Health. 2011;37(Number 1).

27

Knowledge, attitude and practice GAP in family planning usage: An analysis of selected cities of Uttar Pradesh

Anjali Singh*, K. K. Singh and Prashant Verma

Abstract

Background: The GAP between the knowledge of contraception and its actual practice is well recognized in the literature of family welfare studies. The present study assessed the relation between the level of knowledge and practice of contraception among the women and sought to explore the reasons behind the Knowledge, Attitude, and Practice - GAP (KAP GAP) regarding contraceptive users in six cities of Uttar Pradesh.

Method: Present analysis based on 17,643 currently married women aged 15 to 49. A Bivariate analysis ($\chi2$ test) and a multivariable logistic regression were performed for the study.

Result: The highest percentages of respondents (women) were in the age group 35–49 (40–45 %) in all the districts considered. Knowledge of contraceptives was almost universal; tubal ligation and pill were the commonly known methods. Information about the contraceptive methods was mostly obtained through the husband. In the present study, there was a highly significant association ($p < 0.01$) of age group, educational status of respondents, the number of living children, the wealth of the respondent, media exposure and husband's education with the variable KAP GAP for all six cities. Health concern issues in all the districts were the most prominent reason for not using contraception.

Conclusion: There differences in the socioeconomic and demographic factors exist, which lead to KAP GAP in the family planning (FP) usages. Therefore, in designing effective family planning programme, there is a need to understand the various factors which influence the practice of contraception.

Keywords: Contraceptives, Family Planning, Knowledge Attitude and Practice, Chi-Square

Background

India became the pioneer nation in the world to launch a nationwide family planning programme in the year 1952, with an intention to reduce fertility and thereby to stabilize the population growth in the near future, even though India is the second most populous country in the world. The family planning programme was initiated with a very cautious approach in India, after the independence (1952) natural method of family planning was considered to be the most appropriate technique for limiting births but a major breakthrough in contraceptive technology occurred, when intrauterine device known as the '*Lippes Loop*' was accepted in India in 1965, the government started promoting the device through intensive campaigns.

In 1977 the programme was renamed as *Family Welfare Programme*. The Family Welfare Programme has relaxed its compulsive approaches in the modification of family planning at various nodes so as to make the programme more educational and wholly voluntary. Desired family size and timing of births are two primary objectives that are fulfilled by the family planning through contraception.

Although the family planning programme was not as successful as was expected, it has succeeded in generating universal knowledge of family planning methods among the masses [1]. But, even with this high awareness of contraception there exists a large gap between the knowledge and Practice of these methods due to the existing variations in the socioeconomic and geographical characteristics within its territory [2].

* Correspondence: anjali.chhaya28@gmail.com
Department of Statistics, Banaras Hindu University, Varanasi, India

For measuring the success of Family Planning Programmes there exists one method suggested by a WHO expert in 1975 which is the evaluation of knowledge, attitude, and behavior among people regarding the family planning methods. The concept of KAP - GAP theory was postulated by Bongaarts in 1991, "*The proportion of currently married women who want no more children and are not practicing birth control referred to as the conventional KAP-GAP or unmet need. That is a discrepancy between the practice of contraception and reproductive intentions. This GAP is then assumed to be an indication of unmet need for contraception. Estimates of this measure are readily obtained from most fertility surveys because information on only two items is required: the desire for more children and the current practice of contraception.*" [3]

The concept of KAP-GAP given by Bongaarts and Bruce utilized for understanding the causal factors of contraceptive behavior in Pakistan (Punjab province) [4]. The usage of contraceptive methods has increased over a period but there still exists a KAP- GAP i.e. a GAP between knowledge, attitude, and practices for contraception [5].

Considering the above literature as the base of study, the present research carried out in six major urban districts of Uttar Pradesh, with an objective to assess the knowledge of various family planning methods and also to explore the current trends in usage of contraceptive methods by the women of reproductive age group (15–49), so that the KAP GAP of family planning can be targeted. The most populous state of India, Uttar Pradesh, is the focus state of this study for several reasons. It is the most populated state in India with approximately 16.4 % (more than 19 billion population as of 2011 census) of the total population. Among the high fertility states, Uttar Pradesh with the total fertility rate (TFR) 3.82 is the one that has shown a near stall in fertility decline in the past period. The low contraceptive prevalence rate (47.4) and high level of fertility in Uttar Pradesh are of considerable concern to the Indian Government (NFHS-III (2005–2006)) [6]. This study attempts to explore the reasons for this KAP GAP and the factors affecting the outcome of family planning programme and to have a better understanding of the situation to help the government in the formulation of policies and modify its approach in Uttar Pradesh.

Methods

Data source

The data use for the present study was collected by Measurement, Learning & Evaluation (MLE) Project as the part of data collection for the evaluation of Urban Reproductive Health Initiatives, implemented by FHI360 with funding from the Bill & Melinda Gates Foundation. Data collection took place between January and July 2010 in six cities of Uttar Pradesh: Agra (3007), Aligarh (3112), Allahabad (2670), Gorakhpur (3022), Moradabad (2817), and Varanasi (3015). MLE collected information from the representative sample of 17,643 currently married women aged 15–49 years. It is designed to improve family planning and reproductive health services for urban residents and to provide estimates of fertility, mortality, family planning, and health care for urban (slum and non-slum) Uttar Pradesh. The present analysis is based on 17,643 currently married women who were in the reproductive age group 15–49 years (See reference [7] for details of the sampling frame and study design).

Dependent and explanatory variables

The primary variables of interest (dependent variables) are knowledge, attitude, practice of family planning methods and KAP GAP. The explanatory variables used in the study are age group of women, education level, place of residence, number of living children, religion, caste, economic status, media exposure and husband education. In the present study age of the currently married women has been classified into five groups which are (15–19), (20–24), (25–29), (30–34) and (35–49) years. Education of women has been categorized into four parts namely no education, primary education, secondary education and higher education. Place of residence has been classified into two groups (non-slum and slum). A number of living children have been classified into five groups as no children, one child, two children, three children and four & above children. The religion variable has been classified into two categories as Non-Muslim and Muslim; in the Non-Muslim religion category Hindu, Christian, Sikh, Buddhist/Neo-Buddhist, Jain, and others have been used.

In this study, caste has been taken into three components, namely scheduled caste/scheduled tribe, other backward caste, and others. The description of these caste categories is given as follows The Scheduled Caste (SC) and Scheduled Tribe (ST) are official designations given to various groups of historically disadvantaged indigenous people in India, the second one is Other Backward Caste (OBC) which is a collective term used by the Government of India to classify castes which are socially and educationally disadvantaged and the last one is Others category also known as Forward Class, denote groups of people who do not qualify for any of the positive discrimination schemes operated by the government of India. Wealth has been categories into three parts (Poor, Medium and Rich) Women who fall under the 'poorest' and 'poorer' wealth index groups are put into the category of 'poor' while women who are observed to be in the 'richer' and 'richest' wealth index groups are considered to be of 'rich' in the present study. Media exposure classified into two categories, namely no exposure and media exposure to at least one form of media (newspaper/magazine, listing radio and watching television). Husband's education level is classified into two categories not educated and educated.

Statistical methods

Descriptive analysis has been done to explore the levels of knowledge (on different types of contraceptive and knowledge level), attitude and practice among currently married women living in six cities of Uttar Pradesh. To examine the degree and pattern of KAP GAP among

Table 1 Percentage distribution of women according to different characteristics

Background characteristics	Agra	Aligarh	Allahabad	Gorakhpur	Moradabad	Varanasi	Total
Age group							
15–19	3.5	3.6	1.7	2.1	2.2	1.8	2.5
20–24	17.2	15.1	13.7	14.9	12.9	13.7	14.8
25–29	21.6	20.2	20.3	19.3	18.7	21.7	20.6
30–34	18.0	20.0	21.1	19.3	21.0	19.0	19.5
35–49	39.7	41.1	43.2	44.3	45.2	43.9	42.6
Educational status							
No education	38.0	42.3	22.0	26.9	36.0	32.1	32.3
Primary education	9.8	9.2	9.5	8.3	9.3	12.6	9.8
Secondary education	33.9	28.8	35.7	39.3	33.9	38.3	34.9
Higher education	18.2	19.7	32.8	25.5	20.8	16.9	22.8
Place of residence							
Non Slum	75.0	81.3	89.2	90.3	86.8	73.9	81.7
Slum	25.0	18.7	10.8	9.7	13.2	26.1	18.3
No of living children							
No child	8.5	9.1	8.8	10.2	10.1	8.4	9.0
One child	16.7	12.4	17.8	16.2	13.7	15.7	15.8
Two children	24.9	21.1	30.0	25.8	23.3	25.4	25.5
Three children	18.6	19.7	19.2	20.9	20.0	18.4	19.3
Four & more than 4 children	31.1	37.8	24.3	26.9	32.5	32.2	30.3
Religion							
Non muslim	87.2	66.6	81.0	81.5	62.6	77.8	78.5
Muslim	12.8	33.4	19.0	18.5	37.4	22.2	21.5
Caste							
Sc/St	30.8	20.7	15.3	12.7	13.5	12.3	18.5
OBC	32.2	39.3	40.0	47.2	48.8	54.2	42.9
Others	37.0	40.0	44.7	40.0	37.6	33.5	38.6
Wealth index							
Poor	37.5	36.9	32.9	38.4	36.6	38.1	36.7
Medium	19.9	20.5	21.9	19.9	20.0	20.2	20.4
Rich	42.6	42.5	45.2	41.6	43.2	41.7	42.8
Media exposure							
No exposure	19.4	21.4	10.3	11.0	22.1	19.9	27.9
Exposure to at least one form of media	80.6	78.6	89.7	89.0	77.9	80.1	72.1
Husband education							
Not educated	27.1	42.1	27.0	22.8	33.4	22.9	17.0
Educated	72.9	57.9	73.0	77.2	66.6	77.1	83.0

women of six cities, a bivariate technique was used and the association between the variables was determined using $\chi 2$ test. For investigating the important socioeconomic and demographic determinants of KAP GAP univariable and multivariable logistic regression technique was employed. Data was analyzed using SPSS software (version 19).

Results

Before going into the detailed analysis of the study that how KAP GAP is operating in six cities of Uttar Pradesh, one must have knowledge of the demographic and socioeconomic characteristics of the sample involved under study.

Table 1 corresponds to the percentage distribution of women involved in the study by their different socio-demographic and economic characteristics. It was observed that the highest percentage of respondents were in the age group of 35–49, which corresponded to 40 to 45 % of respondents in the entire city. Nearly 32.3 % of women had received no schooling; 9.8, 34.9 and 22.8 % of respondents have enrolled in primary, secondary and higher education respectively. Further, the percentage of illiterate women was found to be the highest in Aligarh city (42.3 %). About 81.7 % of respondents live in non-slum area, and maximum slum population (26.1 %) lived in Varanasi city. Among the respondents, 30.3 % had parity four or higher than four while 25.5 % had parity two at the time of the survey. Moradabad and Aligarh are predominantly Muslim majority cities whereas, the smallest percentage Muslims were found in Agra (12.8 %). The 42.9 % of the study subjects belonged to other backward class. About 42.8 % of the entire samples of women belonged to rich wealth group, and 36.7 % of women belonged to poor wealth group. Further, the percentage distribution of women in all cities according to the wealth was almost uniform in the entire sample. Around three-quarters of respondents had exposure of at least one form of media; media exposure is highest around 90 % in Allahabad. The educational composition of respondent's husband comprised that 17 % of the husband had no education.

Knowledge of contraceptives

The underlying section deals with the methods, the source of information and source of services availed by the respondents in six major cities of Uttar Pradesh. The knowledge of contraceptives refers to the number of contraceptive methods known to the women, sources of information for family planning known, and the sources of family planning services known by respondents.

From Table 2, it is clear that knowledge of contraceptives was almost universal in all six urban cities of Uttar Pradesh, where every woman has heard about at least one of the contraceptive methods regardless of educational background and socioeconomic status. All except two women in Varanasi city (more than 99 %) have heard about contraceptives and knew at least one method. Though this study reveals the higher prevalence of knowledge of contraceptives among respondents, the knowledge varied from one method to another also from one city to another. In Moradabad condom (male) was the most popular method known by the respondents, while pill was the most commonly known method in Aligarh and Allahabad, and for rest of the three cities, tubal ligation was the commonly known method. The IUCD is another most popular method cited by respondents, followed by the Vasectomy. However, female condom was the least known method for respondents. Among permanent methods, the knowledge percentage

Table 2 Percentages of different contraceptive methods known by respondents

Method	Agra	Aligarh	Allahabad	Gorakhpur	Moradabad	Varanasi	Total
At least one method	100.0	100.0	100.0	100.0	100.0	99.9	100.0
Modern method							
Pill	63.1	62.0	67.5	54.0	66.9	62.6	63.1
Injectables	16.9	9.6	13.8	16.6	14.9	21.6	16.3
IUCD	32.3	23.6	39.3	26.6	32.0	45.8	35.0
Condom (Male)	59.8	61.3	63.4	62.2	73.1	58.5	62.5
Condom (Female)	0.6	0.2	0.4	0.2	1.6	2.0	0.8
Tubal ligation	69.4	48.1	57.0	68.1	59.8	70.7	64.5
Vasectomy	28.3	6.0	11.1	14.2	10.0	32.7	19.6
Traditional method							
Rhythm	19.8	6.4	9.6	15.4	11.8	15.2	14.1
Withdrawal	13.2	1.8	3.0	5.5	5.3	9.3	7.1
Lam	2.5	0.1	0.1	0.8	0.3	3.3	1.2

Table 3 Percentage of sources of family planning information

Source	Agra	Aligarh	Allahabad	Gorakhpur	Moradabad	Varanasi	Total
Health personal	9.6	5.1	8.3	13.1	6.0	13.3	9.2
Partner	62.8	27.5	27.2	51.8	44.1	48.3	43.5
Friend/Peer educator	7.5	11.8	12.4	7.9	10.7	7.4	9.7
Relatives	12.3	13.5	7.3	9.9	11.3	11.2	11
Media	18.7	14.9	21.4	22.7	16.0	21.6	18.9

of tubal ligation was much higher than vasectomy in all cities, which indicates that tubal ligation is a well-known family planning method than that of the male sterilization. The analysis shows that Rhythm was a most known method among traditional methods followed by withdrawal method. The knowledge of traditional methods was highest in Agra (rhythm (19.8 %), withdrawal (13.2 %)) and lowest in Aligarh (rhythm (6.4 %), withdrawal (1.8 %)).

The distribution of the source of the knowledge of family planning methods is shown in Table 3. The study suggests that information about the contraceptive methods was mostly obtained through Spousal (husband) communication which was consistent in all six cities of Uttar Pradesh. Media was the second most popular source of information followed by relatives. But in two cities Gorakhpur and Varanasi health personnel were the third most popular source of information in place of relatives, and Allahabad friends/peer educator was the third popular source of information.

Table 4 shows that the percentage distribution of knowledge about the places from where the respondents get family planning. The result indicates that about 90.7 % of respondents knew at least one place, where from family planning services can be made available. The pharmacy/drugstore was the most cited source of family planning services in all six cities. Private clinics and public medical sectors were other options from which respondents said that they could receive family planning services.

Practice of family planning method

Figure 1 presents the CPR of currently married women using any family planning method for all six cities. To obtain a true contraceptive use rate, the denominator should reflect the population at risk (of pregnancy), i.e., sexually active women who are not infecund, pregnant, or amenorrheic. The numerator should indicate the number of contraceptive users from that population. The Figure shows that the CPR is highest among currently married women in Moradabad (79.3 %) and lowest in Varanasi (66.0 %), while in all other four cities Agra, Aligarh, Allahabad, and Gorakhpur the practice of family planning methods are figured were nearly comparable to 71.1, 70.0, 75.5 and 71.8 % respectively.

Table 5 represents the percentage distribution of all users according to the method they choose for family planning. Among all available contraceptive methods, tubal ligation was the most commonly used method in four cities Agra (34.5 %), Allahabad (36.4 %), Gorakhpur (38.9 %), and Varanasi (45.5 %) while in Aligarh and Moradabad male condom was the most adopted method of contraception. Respondents also preferred the natural methods and this method was most commonly used in Aligarh (32.8 %) and least often employed in Varanasi (14.8 %). The analysis shows that among permanent methods of contraception, the percentage of using tubal ligation was much higher than male sterilization. The other available modern family planning methods such as combining pill and IUD were the least used methods by the respondents in all six cities.

Knowledge attitude practice gap

Table 6 represents the percentage distribution of KAP GAP among the women according to the socioeconomic and demographic characteristics of all six urban cities of Uttar Pradesh. The highest percentage of KAP GAP was found in Varanasi (34 %) and lowest percentage was found in Moradabad (20.7 %). It observed from the table that the KAP GAP was affected by the socioeconomic and demographic differential. In age group (15–19 years) KAP GAP was highest for all cities except Allahabad and it decreased in age group (20–24) (25–29) and (30–34) years except for city Agra (where

Table 4 Percentage distribution of source of family planning services known by respondents

Knowledge	Agra	Aligarh	Allahabad	Gorakhpur	Moradabad	Varanasi	Total
Any place	89.0	93.7	90.6	89.5	93.8	91.6	90.7
Public medical sector	4.4	13.5	9.7	6.7	12.9	6.5	9.2
Private medical sector	7.7	10.8	9.8	6.7	11.5	8.7	9
Pharmacy/Drug store	67.6	25.7	45.2	55.6	39.9	62.6	48.7

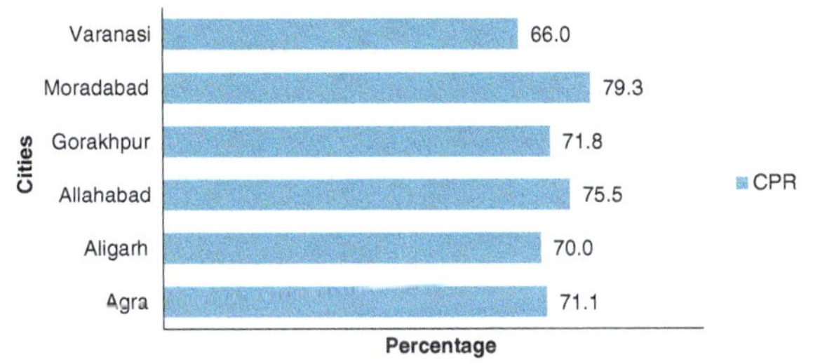

Fig. 1 Represent the percentage of Contraceptive Prevalence Rate for all selected cities of Uttar Pradesh (2010)

the KAP GAP again increase in 30–34 age group) and again increases in the 35–49 years age groups in all cities except Allahabad. The association of KAP GAP and education of the women was negative. Not educated women have the greater percentage of KAP GAP while the percentage of KAP GAP was decreasing as the level of education increases, and this result held true for all five cities except Gorakhpur where the second highest percentage of KAP GAP (24.6 %) found in the women of higher education group. KAP GAP is greater in the women who live in a slum area in comparison to the women live in non-slum area. As the number of living children increased KAP GAP decreases up to two children but it again increases for three and more living children, this pattern was followed by all four cities except Gorakhpur and Moradabad. The percentage of KAP GAP was higher in Muslims as compared to non-Muslims (Hindu, Christian, Buddhist and others). Scheduled caste/scheduled tribe women have a higher percentage of KAP GAP followed by others backward class in all four cities except Agra and Aligarh where the highest percentage of KAP GAP found in other backward class. The association of KAP GAP and wealth of the women was also negative, and the scenario was same for all cities. Among the women who had at least one form of media exposure, the percentage of KAP GAP was low in comparison to those who had no exposure to family planning message. For the background variable husband's education KAP GAP was highest in the no education group in all six selected cities.

Chi-square analysis

In the present study, there was a highly significant association ($p < 0.01$) among age group, educational status of respondents, the number of living children, the wealth of the respondent, media exposure, and husband's education with the variable KAP GAP for all six cities. But for the religion variable the association was highly significant ($p < 0.01$) for three cities Aligarh, Allahabad and Varanasi and significant ($p < 0.05$) only for Agra. Similarly, an association of the variable place of residence with KAP GAP was not significant only for Aligarh. The relationship between caste and KAP GAP variable was highly significant for all five cities except Moradabad where the significance level was less than 0.05. The value of chi-square with its level of significance (p-value) for all the variable shown in Table 6.

Logistic regression analysis

To estimate the degree of effect of each independent variable on the study variable and to verify whether the differences provided by the different categories of the various explanatory variables considered in our study are statistically significant or not, we have applied logistic regression technique and obtained crude as well as adjusted odds ratios.

Table 7 depicts the crude and adjusted odds ratios with their confidence interval of KAP GAP among women for different socio-economic and demographic characteristics, obtained from logistic regression analysis. From the figures of crude odds ratio of KAP GAP one can conclude that place of residence, religion, the caste of women and husband education were highly significant but as soon as the procedure controlled for all explanatory variables the differences arises from these variables remain no more significant.

Taking 15–19 years age group as a reference category, the odds for KAP GAP for the women with increasing age was decreased up to age 34 and again increased in the age group 35–49. Media exposure significantly affects the KAP GAP among the women. The odds for women who were exposed to at least one form of media were lower as compared to the women who had no exposure to any type of media. In the logistic regression model, one more covariate education level of the women

Table 5 Pattern of family planning method usage

Method	Agra	Aligarh	Allahabad	Gorakhpur	Moradabad	Varanasi	Total
Tubal ligation	34.5	22.2	36.4	38.9	28.7	45.5	34.7
Male sterilization	0.1	0.2	0.2	0.2	0.1	0.5	0.2
Natural methods	23.7	32.8	26.4	27.8	21.6	14.8	24.4
Male condom	30.9	33.3	25.9	24.3	42.7	26.6	31
Combined pill	3.2	2.5	1.8	2.5	2.0	3.3	2.4
IUD/loop	2.7	4.3	5.0	2.2	3.3	7.1	4.1

Table 6 Percentage of KAP GAP according to different characteristics

Background characteristics	Agra	Aligarh	Allahabad	Gorakhpur	Moradabad	Varanasi
Total	28.9	30.4	24.5	28.2	20.7	34.0
Age group						
15–19	47.5	54.5	28.4	54.3	51.9	50.2
20–24	35.5	44.4	37.6	33.2	34.4	44.3
25–29	20.5	29.6	26.6	31.4	19.7	31.5
30–34	27.1	25.7	21.2	17.7	10.5	26.7
35–49	31.8	25.8	18.7	29.2	22.7	35.5
	($\chi2 = 44.37$, $p = 0.000$)	($\chi2 = 35.83$, $p = 0.000$)	($\chi2 = 42.42$, $p = 0.000$)	($\chi2 = 31.10$, $p = 0.000$)	($\chi2 = 39.92$, $p = 0.000$)	($\chi2 = 28.49$, $p = 0.000$)
Educational status						
No education	39.7	41.3	49.4	36.9	29.6	45.6
Primary education	34.3	30.6	20.6	23.8	21.9	36.1
Secondary education	23.6	26.6	19.6	21.2	16.9	33.5
Higher education	18.1	14.5	15.5	24.6	13.6	18.3
	($\chi2 = 63.51$, $p = 0.000$)	($\chi2 = 100.10$, $p = 0.000$)	($\chi2 = 107.74$, $p = 0.000$)	($\chi2 = 17.45$, $p = 0.001$)	($\chi2 = 43.01$, $p = 0.000$)	($\chi2 = 60.30$, $p = 0.000$)
Place of residence						
Non-slum	27.6	29.4	23.3	27.5	19.3	32.6
Slum	33.1	32.3	34.9	35.2	30.2	37.5
	($\chi2 = 6.35$, $p = 0.007$)	($\chi2 = 0.70$, $p = 0.223$)	($\chi2 = 12.06$, $p = 0.001$)	($\chi2 = 3.64$, $p = 0.037$)	($\chi2 = 7.34$, $p = 0.006$)	($\chi2 = 3.88$, $p = 0.028$)
No of living children						
No child	58.6	54.9	45.9	83	66.3	57.2
One child	29.4	32.7	23.1	23.7	22.1	35.6
Two children	24.1	21.4	16.6	24	17.9	25.5
Three children	27.5	27.2	26.3	22.5	15.6	31.9
Four & more than 4 children	33	34.7	37.7	36.8	22.6	40.8
	($\chi2 = 19.02$, $p = 0.001$)	($\chi2 = 26.39$, $p = 0.000$)	($\chi2 = 52.31$, $p = 0.000$)	($\chi2 = 56.21$, $p = 0.000$)	($\chi2 = 49.73$, $p = 0.000$)	($\chi2 = 48.38$, $p = 0.000$)
Religion						
Non muslim	28.1	26.1	22.1	27.3	20.2	29.7
Muslim	33.6	37.5	33.4	31.6	21.4	45.8
	($\chi2 = 4.06$, $p = 0.044$)	($\chi2 = 11.54$, $p = 0.001$)	($\chi2 = 18.84$, $p = 0.000$)	($\chi2 = 0.25$, $p = 0.613$)	($\chi2 = 1.03$, $p = 0.308$)	($\chi2 = 26.11$, $p = 0.000$)
Caste						
Sc/St	32.6	31.9	35.5	31.9	25	42.2
OBC	32.7	35.7	24.3	31.1	22.3	35.8
Others	22.8	23.9	21.4	24	17.4	28.2
	($\chi2 = 16.95$, $p = 0.000$)	($\chi2 = 15.38$, $p = 0.000$)	($\chi2 = 22.86$, $p = 0.000$)	($\chi2 = 11.91$, $p = 0.003$)	($\chi2 = 8.29$, $p = 0.016$)	($\chi2 = 11.42$, $p = 0.003$)
Wealth index						
Poor	35.9	43.5	38.4	34.1	29.2	42.1
Medium	32.7	27.6	27	27.8	23.2	36.6
Rich	21.4	20.3	16.6	24.1	13.4	26
	($\chi2 = 29.16$, $p = 0.000$)	($\chi2 = 63.13$, $p = 0.000$)	($\chi2 = 69.96$, $p = 0.000$)	($\chi2 = 38.61$, $p = 0.000$)	($\chi2 = 51.16$, $p = 0.000$)	($\chi2 = 42.91$, $p = 0.000$)

Table 6 Percentage of KAP GAP according to different characteristics *(Continued)*

Media exposure						
No exposure	39.8	42.7	33.7	37	29.1	44.6
Exposure to at least one form of media	25.4	22.1	21.8	25.8	17	31.1
	(χ2 = 29.32, p = 0.000)	(χ2 = 74.44, p = 0.000)	(χ2 = 28.72, p = 0.000)	(χ2 = 37.59, p = 0.000)	(χ2 = 21.78, p = 0.000)	(χ2 = 32.02, p = 0.000)
Husband education						
Not educated	41.7	42.8	45.5	36.8	29.4	43.1
Educated	26.1	27	22.7	27.3	18.5	31.8
	(χ2 = 26.26, p = 0.000)	(χ2 = 21.98, p = 0.000)	(χ2 = 52.58, p = 0.000)	(χ2 = 17.48, p = 0.000)	(χ2 = 26.35, p = 0.000)	(χ2 = 19.30, p = 0.000)

was also included. Keeping no education group as a reference category primary and secondary education groups had similar odds which were lower than reference category.

Further considering the no of living children, as the no of living children increased adjusted odds for KAP GAP decreased up to parity two and again increases for three and higher parity these results were highly significant. This study also indicates that Wealth index significantly influenced the KAP GAP with raising the level of wealth index there was a rapid decline in the odds ratio.

Reasons for KAP GAP

Table 8 shows that decision for adopting any family planning method was influenced by health concern issues (20.7 %); this is one of the primary reasons for the KAP GAP. Evidently for Agra and Varanasi, the same reason accounted for 28.9 %, and 27.9 % women were not using any contraceptive method. The study show that some of the respondents had not planned their fertility and leave it up to God, so this is also a second important reason for KAP GAP in all cities except Varanasi where fear of side effects was a second important reason for not using contraception. The KAP GAP due to the reason of disapproval of husband and other relatives was subtle (3.2 %) in this study.

Discussion

Finding and interpretation

The above study reveals that knowledge among married women about at least one family planning method was universal, and it was independent of their socioeconomic characteristic [8, 9]. Substantial variation in the knowledge of usages of one contraceptive method over another was clearly visible in the study and is well supported by the existing literature. Among permanent method knowledge about tubal ligation was far better than vasectomy [10, 11]. The variation of knowledge was also visible for cities like in Aligarh and Allahabad pill was the most known method and it was not same for all other cities. The analysis shows that spouse communication was the major source of knowledge carrier regarding family planning usage. The role of health personals in the awareness programme of family planning was not found to be satisfactory in our results. Knowledge about the source to get family planning was also excellent, and a medical store was the most prominent source for getting family planning services.

The present analysis shows that more than half of the respondents use family planning methods in all cities. Tubal ligation and male condom were most used methods in our study. The reasons for adoption of tubal ligation may be because of its permanent nature, physical safety and comfort and no fear of failure [10].

The Majority of women have the knowledge of family planning in spite of only one-third of study population not practicing any method. This difference shows that there exists KAP GAP in the population among these urban districts of Uttar Pradesh. KAP GAP was found to be affected by the socioeconomic differentials; maximum KAP GAP was discovered in the females of the younger age group (15–19) years [12] and it was negatively associated with respondent education, it means uneducated women had higher KAP GAP as compared to educated women. Media exposure was also an important factor in shaping the decision of women to use family planning [2, 13–15] this may be a reason that media exposure affects KAP GAP. Instead of these covariates total no of children and women's wealth index were also an important factors which influences the KAP GAP but husband education was not significantly associated with KAP GAP after adjusting the regression for other background characteristics. A decision to adopt family planning was influenced by issues of health concerns [10, 11, 16].

Strength and weakness

The MLE survey is the recent study that covers Family planning issues in a comprehensive manner in Uttar

Table 7 Logistic regression results of KAP GAP by different background characteristics

Background characteristics	Crude odds ratio	Confidence interval (95 %)		Adjusted odds ratio	Confidence interval (95 %)	
		Lower	Upper		Lower	Upper
Age group						
15–19	Ref			Ref		
20–24	0.627**	0.463	0.848	0.989*	0.767	1.47
25–29	0.368**	0.273	0.497	0.734*	0.526	1.023
30–34	0.273**	0.202	0.369	0.573**	0.406	0.809
35–49	0.379**	0.282	0.509	0.766*	0.542	1.082
Educational status						
No education	Ref			Ref		
Primary education	0.614**	0.521	0.724	0.683**	0.575	0.812
Secondary education	0.529**	0.475	0.588	0.688**	0.602	0.788
Higher education	0.324**	0.286	0.367	0.499**	0.417	0.597
Place of residence						
Non Slum	Ref			Ref		
Slum	1.435**	1.283	1.606	1.134	1.007	1.276
No of living children						
No child	Ref			Ref		
One child	0.247**	0.191	0.32	0.247**	0.188	0.323
Two children	0.178**	0.138	0.229	0.205**	0.155	0.269
Three children	0.214**	0.165	0.279	0.206**	0.153	0.277
Four & more than 4 children	0.328**	0.255	0.422	0.231**	0.171	0.314
Religion						
Non Muslim	Ref			Ref		
Muslim	1.415**	1.285	1.559	1.106	0.986	1.239
Caste						
Sc/St	Ref			Ref		
OBC	0.906**	0.801	1.023	0.972	0.847	1.115
Others	0.608**	0.536	0.691	0.967	0.834	1.121
Wealth index						
Poor	Ref			Ref		
Medium	0.688**	0.611	0.776	0.900**	0.79	1.024
Rich	0.425**	0.384	0.469	0.680**	0.597	0.774
Media exposure						
No Exposure	Ref			Ref		
Exposure to atleast one form of Media	0.514**	0.467	0.565	0.725**	0.652	0.807
Husband education						
Not educated	Ref			Ref		
Educated	0.531**	0.474	0.594	1.051	0.919	1.202

* $p < 0.05$
** $p < 0.01$

Pradesh, the most populous state in India. KAP GAP in six major districts in Uttar Pradesh gives an indication of a universal presence of knowledge but differences in the actual practices of family planning methods based on recent data from the year 2010. The studied population did not reflect the whole population of Uttar Pradesh it covered only urban part of the state which is the biggest limitation of the study.

Table 8 Reason given for not using any contraceptive methods

Reasons	Agra	Aligarh	Allahabad	Gorakhpur	Moradabad	Varanasi	Total
Fear of side effect	18.5	9.4	6.7	11.2	9.8	23.4	14.7
Health concern issue	28.9	11.2	10.3	22.1	9.4	27.9	20.7
Up to god	24.1	14.3	9.5	17.6	22.1	19.7	18.2
Disapproval of husband/ relatives	2.5	3.8	2.1	2.3	2.6	6.0	3.2

Unanswered question and future research

Every study forms a basis for further research and in the line of a survey carried out; we have witnessed differences in knowledge and practice regarding usage of family planning methods leading to KAP GAP in six major cities including slum and non-slum population of Uttar Pradesh. Contraceptive method generally divides into two groups, modern and traditional contraception the above study address the GAP but the strength or magnitude of KAP GAP according to the type of contraceptive method and its corresponding differentials have not been dealt with in the study because of limitation of the survey, also the factors that are encouraging women to use family planning were not analyzed in the paper which needs to be addressed in further research.

Conclusion

The analysis explicitly mentioned that there exist differences in the socioeconomic and demographic factors, which in turn affects contraceptive usages, leading to KAP GAP in the family planning. The research clearly brings out the reason according to the region specific primary correlates for KAP GAP. Therefore, in designing effective family planning programmes, policy makers must understand the various factors which influence the practice of family planning methods according to regions. It comes from the study that method related issues are also a major reason for not using the contraceptive, so family planning programme should have to focus on giving the correct information and knowledge for the different methods to improve the family planning practices.

Abbreviations

CPR: Contraceptive prevalence rate; FP: Family planning; KAP: Knowledge attitude and practice; MLE: Measurement learning & evaluation; OBC: Other backward caste; Sc/St: Scheduled caste/Scheduled tribe

Acknowledgment

The authors are grateful to Measurement Learning and Evaluation (MLE) Project for providing the data set.

Authors' contribution

AS conceived of the study, and performed the quantitative analysis. Prof KKS and PV made substantial contributions to drafting the manuscript. All authors read and approved the final manuscript.

References

1. International Institute for Population Science (IIPS) and Macro International. National Family Health Survey (NFHS-2), Mumbai,India.1998–1999.
2. Kulkarni MS. Exposure to mass media and its impact on the use of family planning methods by women in Goa. Health Popul Perspect Issues. 2003;26: 87–93.
3. Bongaarts J. The KAP-GAP and the Unmet Need for Contraception. Popul Dev Rev. 1991;17:293–313.
4. Bongaarts J, Bruce J. The causes of unmet need for contraception and the social content of services. Stud Fam Plan. 1995;26:57–75.
5. Ashoke S, John S, Jayanti MT. The KAP-GAP in Nepal: reasons for non-use of contraception among couples with an unmet need for family planning. Asia-Pac Popul J. 2000;6(1):25–38.
6. International Institute for Population Science (IIPS) and Macro International. National Family Health Survey (NFHS III). (2005–06): India Volume I. Mumbai: IIPS; 2007.
7. Nanda P, Achyut P, Mishra A, Calhoun L. Measurement, learning & evaluation of the urban health initiative: Uttar Pradesh, India, baseline survey 2010. Chapel Hill: Measurement, Learning & Evaluation Project; 2011. Available from: https://www.urbanreproductivehealth.org/sites/mle/files/MLE_TWP_%20INDIA_2011_7Oct_nh.pdf.
8. Kaushal SK, Saxena SC, Srivastva VK, et al. Kap study on contraceptive method in Kanpur district of UP. Indian J Community Health. 2010;21(2):33–8.
9. Santanu G, Samanta A, Mukharjee S. Knowledge and practice of family planning in married women of reproductive age group in a slum of Kolkata, US National Library of Medicine enlisted journal. 2013.
10. Kumar R, Singh MM, Manmeet K. Dynamics of contracetive use in rural community of Hryana. Indian J Med Sci. 1999;43:201–11.
11. Tilahun T, Coene G, Luchters S, et al. Family planning knowledge, attitude and practice among married couples in Jimma Zone, Ethiopia. Pone J. 2013; 8:e61335.
12. Mahavar P, Anand S, Ragunath D, et al. Contraceptive knowledge attitude and practice in mothers of infant: a cross sectional study. Natl J Community Med. 2011;2:105–7.
13. Retherford RD, Mishra V. Media exposure increase contraceptive use. Natl Fam Health Surv Bull. 1997;7:1–4.
14. Sahoo H. Determinants of contraceptive use in Orissa: an analysis from National Family Health Survey III. Health Popul Perspect Issues. 2007;30:208–21.
15. Singh KK, Verma S, Tanti S. Contraceptive use among postpartum women in India. Asian Popul Stud. 2013;10(1):23–39.
16. Tuladhar H, Marahtta R. Awareness and practice of family planning methods in women attending Gyne OPD at Nepal Medical College Teaching Hospital. Nepal Med Coll J. 2008;10(3):184–91.

28

State of emergency contraception in the U.S., 2018

Kristin O. Haeger[1*], Jacqueline Lamme[2] and Kelly Cleland[3]

Abstract

Emergency contraception is indicated in instances of unprotected sexual intercourse, including reproductive coercion, sexual assault, and contraceptive failure. It plays a role in averting unintended pregnancies due to inconsistent use or non-use of contraception. Options for emergency contraception vary by efficacy as well as accessibility within the U.S. This paper provides an overview of levonorgestrel (Plan B One-Step and generic counterparts), ulipristal acetate (sold as ella), and the copper intrauterine device (IUD, sold as ParaGard), including the mechanisms of action, administration, efficacy, drug interactions, safety, side effects, advantages, and drawbacks. It will also review current misconceptions about emergency contraception and access for subpopulations, including adolescents, immigrants, survivors of sexual assault, rural populations, and military/veteran women. This paper will address barriers such as gaps in knowledge, and financial, health systems, and practice barriers. Continuing areas of research, including the impact of body weight on the efficacy of emergency contraceptive pills and potential interactions between ulipristal acetate and ongoing hormonal contraceptives, are also addressed.

Keywords: Emergency contraception, Levonorgestrel, Plan B One-Step, Ulipristal acetate, Ella, Copper IUD

Background

In the US, 45% of pregnancies were unintended in 2011, dropping from 51% in 2008 [1]. Although 68% of women at risk for unintended pregnancy consistently used contraception, these women account for only 5% of unintended pregnancies [2]. The vast majority of unintended pregnancy is due to inconsistent use or non-use of contraception, and this is where emergency contraception has a potentially important role [2]. Indications for emergency contraception include any situation in which sexual intercourse is unprotected, including reproductive coercion, sexual assault, and contraceptive failure.

Since 1995, ever-use of emergency contraception has increased among women age 15–44 from 0.8% in 1995 to 20.0% from 2011 to 2015 (see Fig. 1) [3]. Multiple options for emergency contraception exist; however, the options vary in efficacy. Among both medical providers and the general population, there is a gap in knowledge as well as persistent misperceptions about the options for emergency contraception, the timing, side effects, and mechanism of action [4–10]. Our intent is to give an overview of the options for emergency contraception currently available in the United States; address misconceptions about emergency contraception and issues of access and barriers; review emergency contraception in special populations; and touch on future research.

Levonorgestrel

Levonorgestrel (LNG) is a progestin-only emergency contraception pill (ECP) that should be taken orally as soon as possible, within a 72-h window following sexual intercourse, although some studies suggest moderate efficacy up to 120 h post-coitus [11–14]. It is sold in the United States as Plan B One-Step® (1.5 mg) as a single dose and is sold under several generic labels, including Take Action, My Way, AfterPill (available only online), Aftera, and Option 2. It sometimes referred to colloquially as "the morning-after pill" and was originally sold as Plan B, which included two doses (0.75 mg) to be administered 12 h apart before studies showed the single dose to be as effective as the staggered doses. The two-dose version is no longer sold in the United States.

* Correspondence: kristin.haeger@va.gov
[1]Department of Veterans Affairs, Veterans Health Administration, Office of Patient Care Services, Women's Health Services, 810 Vermont Ave., NW, Washington, DC 20420, USA

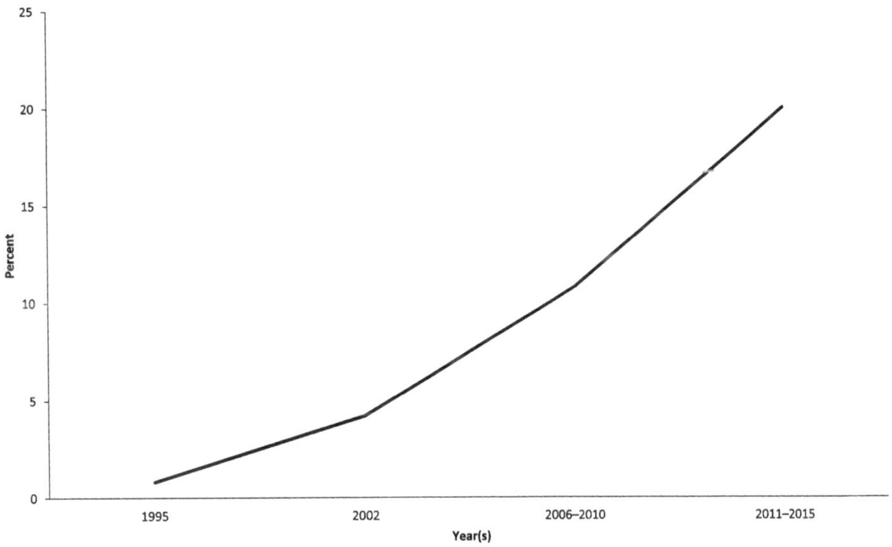

Fig. 1 Ever-use of emergency contraception among women aged 15–44 who have ever had sexual intercourse. Based on National Center for Health Statistics using National Survey of Family Growth, 2013 and 2017 [3, 104]

Mechanism of action

The primary mechanism of action of LNG is suppression of luteinizing hormone, which delays or inhibits ovulation [15–22]. Studies are inconclusive in showing whether it may also interfere with fertilization by thickening cervical mucus and impairing tubal transport of sperm or the egg [19, 22–27]. The best available evidence suggests that progestin-only ECPs work only before ovulation has occurred and do not inhibit implantation of a fertilized egg [15, 28]. Progestin-only ECPs are ineffective after an embryo has implanted in the uterus and thus cannot work as an abortifacient [15, 29].

Administration: Timing and importance of long-term contraception plans

No physical exams, laboratory tests, or pregnancy tests are required before taking LNG [30]. It can be administered regardless of timing of a patient's menstrual cycle [14]. When post-coital emergency contraception is needed, when feasible and welcome, it is recommended that providers offer counseling on long-term contraception plans for patients as well as physical and psychological assessments in instances of sexual assault/rape, while being sensitive to women who are not emotionally ready to talk [14, 30]. In the case that the patient vomits within 3 h of consumption of LNG, the patient should take a second dose [13, 14]. Subsequent to taking LNG, it is safe to start or resume ongoing contraception methods immediately, sometimes referred to as quick-starting [13, 14].

Efficacy

Plan B One-Step (1.5 mg) has a half-life of approximately 27.5 ± 5.6 h [31]. A series of randomized trials examining the efficacy of LNG have demonstrated that for the single-dose regimen (1.5 mg), the failure rate ranges from 0.3–2.6% [11, 32, 33].

LNG may be used after a single episode of unprotected intercourse (UPI) [14]. If a patient has UPI again after taking LNG, she will need to use a backup method of contraception because LNG does not prevent against future acts of intercourse (although it is not necessary to take it more than once within 24 h) [14]. It is safe to use a second dose of LNG within the same menstrual cycle for a subsequent episode of UPI [14, 30]. A study of the use of 1.5 mg of LNG as a primary method of contraception found that the method was about as effective as other coitus-dependent methods, and was highly acceptable to women. Side effects were generally mild and transient, although some women experienced changes in menstrual patterns [34].

Recently, studies have investigated the attenuation of the efficacy of LNG for post-coital emergency contraception across weight and body mass index (BMI). Evidence suggests that the efficacy of 1.5 mg of LNG may decrease among patients weighing more than 75 kg or with a BMI greater than 26 kg/m^2 [35–37]. Recent pharmacokinetic studies of 1.5 mg LNG show that the blood serum level in women with an obese BMI (greater than or equal to 30) was 50% that of women with a normal BMI (between 18.5 and 25 kg/m^2), and that doubling the dose to 3.0 mg in women with an obese BMI resulted in equal serum concentrations of LNG as the 1.5 mg dose in normal-BMI women [38]. Therefore, if other EC options are not available, providing a double dose of LNG may be a reasonable recommendation for women with an obese BMI [38, 39].

Drug interactions

Drugs that may reduce LNG plasma levels include barbiturates, bosentan, carbamazepine, felbamate, griseofulvin, oxacarbazepine, phenytoin, rifampin, St. John's wort, topiramate, and certain anti-retroviral therapies [14, 40]. Because the efficacy of LNG EC for women using enzyme-inducing drugs may be compromised, a double dose of LNG (3.0 mg) is recommended, although the effectiveness of this approach is unproven [14].

Safety/contraindications

There are no risks of LNG EC that outweigh the benefits of preventing an unintended pregnancy and no deaths attributed to its use [30, 40, 41]. Contraindications in instances of ongoing levonorgestrel-containing contraception (e.g., cardiovascular disease, migraines, liver diseases, breastfeeding, and thromboembolic complications) are mediated for EC users by the short-term exposure and relatively low quantity of hormones consumed [14]. Therefore, women with these contraindications to hormonal birth control use may still use LNG EC [40]. Known or suspected pregnancy is the only contraindication for LNG EC; this is not because LNG EC would harm an existing pregnancy, but because it will not be effective. Studies show that it has no documented teratogenic effects on fetuses or subsequent indications of birth defects [30, 40]. For patients who use LNG EC and experience a treatment failure, there is no heightened risk of ectopic pregnancy [42]. Breastfeeding is not a contraindication to using LNG EC [14, 40].

Side effects

Documented side effects include the following: nausea (13–23%), vomiting (5.6%), abdominal pain (13–18%), fatigue (13–17%), dizziness (9–11%), headaches, and breast tenderness [11, 32, 43]. Most symptoms subside within 24 h of administration of the pill [29]. In instances when LNG is taken in the preovulatory stage of menses, the length of the cycle may be abbreviated; in the peri- and postovulatory phases, cycle length is unaffected, but the duration of bleeding is elongated in the subsequent cycle [44–46].

Pros/cons

The potential ease of access of LNG EC is beneficial for many patients. Within the U.S., LNG EC 1.5 mg (Plan B One-Step and generics including Take Action, My Way, and Aftera) is available over the counter without restrictions by age or gender; additionally, no identification is required for purchase [7]. Typically it costs \$50 for the brand name and \$40 for a generic version. Individuals can purchase lower-cost LNG EC online for \$20 plus \$5 shipping online for advanced provision. However, LNG EC is less effective than other EC options (ulipristal acetate or the copper IUD), particularly for women who are obese or overweight [14].

Ulipristal acetate

Ulipristal acetate (UPA) is an antiprogestin sold in the U.S. as ella® (30 mg). It should be taken as soon as possible post-coitus and remains effective for 120 h following intercourse [14, 40].

Mechanisms of action

Like LNG, ulipristal acetate delays ovulation [14]. It does not appear to impair sperm function [47]. Some studies have shown that UPA may alter certain endometrial parameters, although in-vitro studies show no difference in the ability of embryos to implant when exposed or not exposed to UPA [48]. The best available evidence suggests that the primary mechanism of UPA in doses used for EC is interference with ovulation [16, 49]. Because UPA works primarily by delaying ovulation, it may only be used for a single episode of UPI. For subsequent episodes of intercourse within that menstrual cycle, additional contraception methods will be required to prevent an unintended pregnancy.

Administration: Timing and importance of long-term planning

Since both UPA and progestin-based contraceptives bind to progesterone receptors, patients are advised to wait for at least 5 days between the administration of UPA and starting/resuming a hormonal contraceptive [13, 14]. The packaging on ella further recommends the use of barrier protection (e.g., a condom) until the patient's next menstrual cycle.

One study evaluated repeated use of ulipristal acetate within the same cycle; women took UPA either once every 5 days or once every 7 days for 8 weeks [50]. No safety concerns emerged, although most women ovulated at some point during the study. This suggests that while repeated use of UPA within the same cycle is safe, it may not be suitable for use as an ongoing, regular method because users are likely to ovulate at some point and therefore be at risk for pregnancy [50].

Efficacy

Overall, ulipristal acetate is more effective than LNG in the first 72 h post-coitus and is the only US Food and Drug Administration (FDA)-approved ECP for use between 72 and 120 h post-coitus with a half-life of 32.4 ± 6.3 h [11, 51]. Randomized trials evaluating the efficacy of UPA (30 mg) have documented failure rates ranging from 0.0–1.8% with no decrease in efficacy over the 120 h period unlike LNG, which does decrease in efficacy over that timeframe [11, 43, 49].

A meta-analysis of two randomized trials directly found that UPA to be more effective than LNG; the odds of pregnancy for UPA compared with LNG were 42% lower up to 72 h and 65% lower in the first 24 h [11].

A randomized pharmacokinetic study compared LNG and UPA in women with a normal BMI in the control group with those with an obese BMI [38]. Relative to control subjects, those with a BMI greater than 30 using UPA had similar serum levels, while those using LNG had serum levels about half of the control group [38].

Drug interactions

Hepatic enzyme-inducing medication ingested in the previous month may reduce the efficacy of ulipristal acetate [14, 40]. Furthermore, drugs intended to increase levels of gastric pH, including antacids, histamine H2 antagonists, and proton pump inhibitors, are also contraindicated [14, 40]. Doubling the dose of UPA in women using these medications has not been studied and is not recommended at this time [14]. Because UPA is an antiprogestin, it is likely to compete with ongoing progestin-based contraceptive methods, which is why it is recommended that patients wait 5 days prior to starting a hormonal method of contraception after UPA use [14].

Safety

As with LNG, there are no risks of UPA that outweigh the benefits of preventing an unintended pregnancy and no deaths have been attributed to it [13]. It is well-tolerated in studies evaluating its repeated use over time [41, 50], although the FDA label for ella currently indicates that is not intended for this purpose [52].

No teratogenic effects or birth defects have been associated with UPA taken during pregnancy in the case it is inadvertently taken by a woman who does not realize she is already pregnant [14, 40]. Though there are no adverse outcomes associated with breastfeeding after taking UPA [40], the ella label discourages it. U.S. guidelines recommend mothers avoid giving breastmilk in the 24 h following consumption of UPA [40], while European guidelines suggest a 7-day window before resuming breastfeeding an infant following the ingestion of UPA [14].

Side effects

Side effects of ulipristal acetate include delayed menses by 2.1 days (standard deviation ± 8.2 days), headache (19%), dysmenorrhea (13%), nausea (13%), fatigue (6%), dizziness (5%), abdominal pain (5%), upper abdominal pain (3%), and back pain (3%) [11, 49].

Pros/cons

The primary advantage of ulipristal acetate is that it has greater efficacy than LNG and is the only ECP labeled for use 72–120 h after UPI [11, 13, 30]. Additionally, it is more efficacious for overweight and obese women than LNG [38]. However, unlike the LNG ECP at this time, UPA is only available by prescription, and it is not immediately available in many pharmacies in the United States [53]. In some states, pharmacists are authorized to directly prescribe ulipristal, but in most states, a patient must get a prescription from a provider [54]. UPA can be purchased through online pharmacies for $67, including consultation with a physician and shipping.

Copper IUD

The most effective form of emergency contraception is the copper intrauterine device (IUD) (see Table 1) [16, 40]. Most guidelines recommend insertion within 5 days of ovulation following an episode of UPI, although one study showed that the copper IUD is effective for emergency contraception at any point in the menstrual cycle, as long as pregnancy has been ruled out [55]. For the sake of parsimony and clarity, World Health Organization (WHO) guidelines recommend insertion within 5 day post-coitus [56]. In the U.S., it is sold as ParaGard® T 380A Intrauterine Copper Contraceptive.

Mechanism of action

The T-shaped device is wrapped in copper coil that releases copper ions. While the mechanisms of action are not fully understood [57], it is known that the copper ions reduce sperm motility in passing through cervical mucus and create a hostile environment for the sperm [57]. Copper can also alter the uterine and tubal environment and increase prostaglandins, enzymes, and white blood cells, although this is not believed to disrupt an already-implanted blastocyst [16].

Administration

A clinician should first reasonably rule out pregnancy and assess for medical contraindications, including active infection with gonorrhea or chlamydia, which may put the patient at risk for a pelvic inflammatory disease [13]. A copper IUD may be inserted into the uterus by a trained medical provider at any point during a menstrual cycle as long as pregnancy has been ruled out [40]. Upon insertion of the IUD, the patient may resume all activities, including sex and exercise, as soon as the patient feels ready.

Upon insertion, the IUD will prevent a pregnancy for that episode of UPI as well as subsequent episodes for at least 12 years as long as the IUD remains in place, and no other method of birth control is needed [29]. The provider should still discuss risks of sexually transmitted

Table 1 Comparison of methods of emergency contraception

	Copper IUD	UPA	LNG
Efficacy[a, b, c, d]	1 Most effective overall	2 Not as effective as copper IUD; most effective ECP	2 Less effective than copper IUD or UPA
Timing of use[b, c, d, e, f]	Typically 5 days after UPI (120 h), but may be effective at any point in the cycle	5 days after UPI (120 h)	3 days after UPI (72 h), although may have efficacy up to 120 h
Available OTC[c, g]	No	No	Yes
Timing of long-term birth control after use[b, c]	Leave in for continued use for up to 12 years	Wait 5 days	Immediately (quick-start)
Dosage[b, g]	N/A, insertion by medical provider	30 mg, one dose	1.5 mg, one dose
BMI[g, h]	1 No decrease in efficacy by BMI	2 Decrease in efficacy for BMI ≥ 30	2 Decrease in efficacy for BMI ≥ 25
Breastfeeding[e]	1	1	1
Hx of severe cardiovascular disease[e]	1	2	2
Migraine[e]	1	1	1
Severe liver disease[e]	1	2	2
CYP3A4 inducers[e]	1	2	2

IUD intrauterine device, *UPA* ulipristal acetate, *LNG* levonorgestrel, *ECP* emergency contraception pill, *UPI* unprotected intercourse, *OTC* over-the-counter, *N/A* not applicable, *mg* milligrams, *BMI* body mass index, *Hx* history. CDC MEC Categories for classifying emergency contraception: "1 = A condition for which there is no restriction for the use of the contraceptive method; 2 = A condition for which the advantages of using the method generally outweigh the theoretical or proven risks" [b]

[a]ACOG Committee Opinion [68],
[b]Curtis, Jatlaoui, Tepper, et al. [13],
[c]Trussel, Raymond, Cleland [29],
[d]FSRH, 2017 [14]
[e]Curtis, Tepper, Jatlaoui, et al. [40],
[f]Emergency contraception should be taken as soon as possible following UPI
[g]ACOG Practice Bulletin [30],
[h]Glasier, Cameron, Blithe, et al. [35],

infections, including HIV, which copper IUDs do not protect against [13]. If menses does not start on time following insertion of the copper IUD, a urine pregnancy test is recommended [14].

Efficacy

The copper IUD is the most effective form of emergency contraception available [13, 14, 30]. Failure rates are less than 0.1% with only 10 pregnancies documented for over 7000 post-coital insertions [29, 58]. Copper IUDs do not vary in efficacy by BMI, and are therefore the best option for patients without other contraindications with a BMI above 25 [14, 40].

Drug interactions

There are no known drug interactions [14].

Safety/contraindications

Contraindications to the copper IUD placement for emergency contraception are the same as at any other time of IUD placement. Contraindications in which the risks outweigh the benefits include pregnancy; untreated cancer of the uterus, cervix, or genital tract; unexplained vaginal bleeding; malignant gestational trophoblastic disease; current pelvic inflammatory disease; Wilson's disease; uterine malformation preventing insertion; pelvic tuberculosis; a copper allergy; or active gonorrhea or chlamydia [56]. WHO guidelines indicate the following conditions are contraindications to use unless an unsuitable alternative is found, in which case it may be considered under close medical supervision: benign gestational trophoblastic disease; ovarian cancer; HIV/AIDS which is not virally suppressed; or being 48 h to 4 weeks postpartum, when risk of IUD expulsion and uterine perforation is heightened [56]. Relative to women not using any form of contraception, the absolute risk of ectopic pregnancy is lower among women using copper IUDs, with 3.0–4.5 ectopic pregnancies per 1000 person-years without contraception versus 0.2 with a copper IUD [57]. The risks of insertion of the copper IUD for EC are the same as they are for placement of the copper IUD in a patient switching from another contraceptive method. There is no evidence of increased birth defects due to use of a copper IUD [40]. There are no contraindications for breastfeeding with a copper IUD as there are no hormones present to alter breastmilk [40].

Side effects

Insertion of copper IUDs is associated with increased risk of menstrual cramping, heavier periods, irregular menses, anemia, back pain, and fainting immediately following insertion [14]. Some patients may also experience discomfort at the time of insertion.

Pros/cons

Pros of copper IUDs are the long-term efficacy for the subsequent 12 years following an episode of UPI as well as consistent efficacy regardless of the patient's BMI [40]. A limitation to access is that copper IUDs must be inserted by a trained medical provider. Patients in the U.S. who have coverage through a private provider or the Affordable Care Act (ACA) may be able to acquire a copper IUD for little or no cost as long as the ACA remains in effect [6, 58]. Otherwise, the cost may be prohibitively expensive, costing up to $1300 out-of-pocket in the U.S. including both the device and the cost of insertion [59]; however, if the IUD is kept in place, over the course of the following decade it is highly cost-effective [14, 29]. An IUD still costs less than carrying a pregnancy to term for most women when collateral costs, healthcare expenses, leave from work for prenatal checkups, expenses related to giving birth, and other incidentals are factored in. A further limitation is lack of awareness on the part of both patients and providers about the utility of copper IUDs as a form of emergency contraception [60]. Additionally, some healthcare providers adhere to unnecessary protocols requiring two visits for insertion, adding dual burdens of cost and inconvenience for the patient [61].

Other options

Although not marketed specifically for emergency contraception, a precursor to current methods was a combination of oral contraceptive pills, referred to as the "Yuzpe regimen." Historically, women would combine pills containing ethinyl estradiol (100 mcg) and LNG (0.50 mg) with a second dose 12 h later. This method lacks the efficacy of more modern interventions [56], has more severe side effects, and is no longer recommended unless other options for EC are not available.

Mifepristone, previously known as RU-486, is an antiprogestin that is highly effective as emergency contraception, with an excellent safety and side-effect profile [62]. It is sold as EC in doses of 10 to 25 mg in several countries, including Armenia, Moldova, Ukraine, China, Russia, and Vietnam [29]. Mifepristone is also used, at much higher doses, to induce abortion.

Currently, studies of LNG IUD alone as a form of emergency contraception are underway [14]. A small prospective cohort study among 188 EC users examining simultaneous use of a LNG IUD and oral LNG EC pills showed that women were twice as likely to choose a combination of oral LNG (1.5 mg) and a LNG IUD compared to a copper IUD [63]; with the exception of one woman who had multiple episodes of UPI, there were no pregnancies in either group. Alternative forms of EC are currently under investigation. However, little data is available on their efficacy at this time.

Misconceptions about EC

Myths and misconceptions persist regarding emergency contraception that may interfere with its use, including perceptions that emergency contraception acts as an abortifacient [64–66]. Another persistent myth is that patients on other forms of birth control would have no reason to take emergency contraception or that patients would not be able to follow the directions to take an advanced provision of EC [67, 68]. There are many reasons why a person using another form of birth control could require EC, for example, if a condom breaks, a patient forgets to consistently take ongoing hormonal contraceptives, or an IUD is expelled. Women, and even some providers, believe that because they are nulliparous, they are not able to get an IUD [69]. Finally, there is an unfounded belief that the availability of EC could lead to increased risk-taking behavior among teens [70–72]. One of the biggest hurdles to increasing uptake of EC is dispelling myths and increasing knowledge among providers, pharmacists, and individuals of reproductive age who have sex with opposite-sex partners and are thus at risk of unintended pregnancy.

Access

The U.S. has several forms of emergency contraception available with varying degrees of accessibility. Since August of 2013, Plan B One-Step has been available over-the-counter (OTC) without restriction by age or gender (and all generic forms have been available OTC since 2014), while ella is available by prescription only, and IUDs must be inserted by medical providers [7, 73]. Studies show that, within pharmacies, barriers to access include consumers being able speak to a human on the phone; misinformation from employees (e.g., age restrictions, ID requirements); keeping OTC medication in a locked cabinet or behind the counter; stock-outs; choosing not to carry ella due to low consumer demand; and barriers to pharmacists' ability to dispense ella without a physician prescription in 43 states [7, 53, 54, 74–76]. Out-of-pocket costs quoted for ella varied widely, ranging from $2.59–$1200.99 with a median cost of $50

[53]. In spite of advances since Plan B One-Step was made available OTC without restriction, systematic barriers still exist that restrict access to emergency contraception [68].

Gaps in knowledge

Patients often do not realize or appreciate the full range of emergency contraception options that are available [30]. This problem spans across sociodemographic characteristics and neighborhood, although certain groups are less likely to be well-versed and knowledgeable about contraceptive choices [68]. Surveys show there are gaps in knowledge related to age-restrictions, parental consent, confidentiality, what methods are available, efficacy, side effects, and timing [5, 7, 77]. A problem exacerbating lack of knowledge among women at risk of unintended pregnancy is that patients have fewer and more abbreviated opportunities to receive counseling from providers about the most effective forms of emergency contraceptives as well as longer-term contraceptives now that they can acquire EC over-the-counter [10, 78].

Patients are not the only ones with gaps of knowledge around emergency contraceptives; providers are often ill-informed about the options available as well [77]. For providers who do not specialize in reproductive health, there is much less familiarity with ulipristal acetate or IUDs for emergency contraception relative to LNG [6]. In a survey of clinicians in a range of hospital specialties, provider knowledge ranged from 95% knowing of LNG and 62% offering it to only 29% knowing about ulipristal acetate and just 7% providing it [6]. A survey among emergency department providers in Georgia found that only 3% of providers knew the maximum window of efficacy for EC [8].

Financial barriers

Financial barriers disproportionately impact individuals closer to the federal poverty line, which is also a risk factor for unintended pregnancy [68]. Relative to higher-income neighborhoods, pharmacies in low-income neighborhoods are 50% more likely to have permanent stock-outs of ECPs (odds ratio (OR) 1.5, 95% confidence interval (CI): 1.20–1.94) [74]. Out-of-pocket costs for EC can range from $0–1300 in the U.S. depending on if a woman has insurance or not [59]; the device itself costs $778 [79]. Changes to the Affordable Care Act could potentially impact whether birth control and emergency contraception would be covered in the future [7], but at the time of writing, EC should be covered under the ACA with the caveat that there may be a lack of coverage for employees who work for religious employers or religious nonprofits [80].

In terms of economics, because of the lack of awareness of copper IUDs and ulipristal acetate as the most effective forms of emergency contraception, there is less demand for them [6]. This depresses the supply, as well, feeding into a vicious cycle, as exemplified in Hawaii, where only 2.6% of pharmacies had ulipristal acetate on hand in a phone survey [81]. Providers may also be disincentivized to keep IUDs on hand due to the high upfront costs and concerns about not being fully reimbursed [82].

Health systems barriers

Several health systems barriers impede a patient's ability to access emergency contraception. In instances of rape and sexual assault, only 17 states and the District of Columbia (D.C.) have laws in place requiring emergency departments to inform patients about emergency contraception [54]. Thirteen states and D.C. stipulate that EC must be dispensed upon request, although in Pennsylvania, providers may refuse for moral or religious reasons, provided that they transport the patient to the nearest medical facility willing to dispense EC [54]. Religiously affiliated hospitals may restrict access to care relative to secular facilities [83]. In the US, one in ten hospitals beds falls under the purview of the Catholic Directives, a set of guidelines that restricts access to reproductive healthcare, among other services [84].

On the grounds that it impinges on religious freedoms, some pharmacists and pharmacy-owners take issue with stocking and dispensing EC [85–87]. Among those who cite conscientious objection, a reason that is raised is that individuals believe dispensing EC is tantamount to facilitating an abortion, despite evidence to the contrary [87, 88]. In 2015, in *Stormans, Inc. v Wiesman*, the US Ninth Court of Appeals found that pharmacies must fill prescriptions regardless of conscientious objection [87]. A consensus was established by the international human rights community, comprised of the United Nations (UN) Committee on Economic, Social, and Cultural Rights; the UN Committee on the Elimination of Discrimination against Women; the UN Human Rights Committee; the European Court of Human Rights, as well as the American College of Obstetrics and Gynecology and the World Health Organization: "The Primary conscientious duty of healthcare providers is to treat, or to provide benefit and prevent harm to patients; conscientious objection is secondary to this primary duty." In spite of this, there are 7 states in the U.S. that explicitly allow either pharmacies or pharmacists to refuse EC to a patient and another 4 states that are worded more loosely but permit pharmacies and/or pharmacists to refuse dispensing EC for religious or moral reasons [54].

Practice barriers

Many providers believe that if they mention advanced provision of emergency contraception, this may lead to risk-taking behaviors among patients, not realizing the utility of it as a backup method in an instance when a long-term method fails [68]. There are no risks of unintended pregnancy that outweigh the benefits achieved by use of emergency contraception according to the Centers for Disease Control and Prevention's *US Medical Eligibility Criteria for Contraceptive Use, 2016* [40]. This includes women with a history of ectopic pregnancy, cardiovascular or liver disease, thromboembolism, migraines, as well as women who are currently breastfeeding. Neither physical exams nor pregnancy tests need to be performed before administering emergency contraceptive pills [68]. Many providers surveyed are unaware of the most efficacious forms of emergency contraception [6]. Another barrier is lack of training on IUD insertion, which may lead to fewer patients accessing them [68].

Special populations

While studies show improvements in some areas of access to and knowledge of EC among adolescents, barriers persist among systematically disenfranchised segments of the population.

Adolescents

Providers have been addressing gaps in access among some groups through counseling those at greatest risk, in particular, adolescents. When adjusting for confounders, providers were 88% more likely to talk about EC to black non-Hispanic patients than white ones (95% CI: 1.05–3.39); 90% more likely to talk to a girl whose mother did not get a high school diploma relative to one whose mother had at least some college education (95% CI: 1.05–3.45), 95% more likely to talk to a girl with two or more sexual partners in the previous 12 months compared to one (95% CI: 1.25–3.05), and 84% more likely to talk to a girl at a Non-Title X public clinic than at a private clinic [10].

Concerns expressed by adolescents related to accessing EC include confidentiality, transportation, and embarrassment [68, 89]. Some providers are conflicted in striking a balance between maintaining confidentiality and adhering to policies and/or legal rulings [89–91]. Using the National Survey of Family Growth, 2011–2015, researchers found differences by race/ethnicity, mother's level of education, number of partners in the previous 12 months, and source of care in the levels of communication regarding emergency contraception by providers during Pap smears [10]. In a survey of adolescent males, only 42% were aware what emergency contraception was [92]. One study found that among a racially heterogeneous group of adolescents, 44% interpreted the "morning after pill" literally, believing Plan B was only effective for 1 day following an episode of UPI [93].

Immigrants/non-English speaking patients

When patients are able to access healthcare in their native language or at least one they have attained basic proficiency in, they are more likely to seek timely treatment [68]. Within the US, more than half of all pharmacies offer Spanish language services [68]. Online, the Princeton website not-2-late.com is available in both Spanish and Arabic. Increasing language options improves timeliness of access to emergency contraception [67].

Sexual assault survivors

Among adult women who are raped or sexually assaulted, it is estimated that 5% become pregnant [94]. Women presenting to a medical provider subsequent to a rape/sexual assault should be offered EC, including a copper IUD, as well as the option of collecting forensic evidence [14]. In instances when a woman chooses to have forensic evidence collected, the provider should conduct a forensic examination prior to insertion of an IUD if that option is selected [14]. In spite of guidelines, only 13 states and DC require emergency departments to dispense EC upon request [54].

Rural populations

Women in rural areas have higher overall, unintended, and teenage pregnancy rates relative to women in urban and suburban areas in the US [95]. Gaining timely access to emergency contraception is paramount for patients who are not located in major urban centers; Bigbee et al. (2007) found that lack of training and demand were the biggest barriers to stocking EC [96].

Military/veterans

Both women veterans and active duty servicewomen are at heightened risk of unintended pregnancy relative to the general US population: among active duty women, the rate of unintended pregnancy is 34 per 1000 among officers and 80 per 1000 among enlisted women (OR 2.71, 95% CI 1.99–3.69, $p < 0.001$) [97]. Risk factors for unintended pregnancy include lack of use of contraception [98, 99]; history of military sexual trauma; and inconsistent contraceptive use among women veterans with mental illness with/out a substance use disorder [100].

Women veterans are able to access an advanced provision of emergency contraception through the Veterans Health Administration (VHA) for a $9 copay; there is no copay for those with a service-connected disability or a discharge from Iraq or Afghanistan within the past 5 years [98]. Through TRICARE, active duty servicewomen have coverage for all forms of EC, including LNG, ella, and IUDs. However, like at many civilian locations, the availability may be limited and misconceptions and limited provider availability may reduce access [101]. This can be especially challenging for women stationed overseas as alternative services are not available. Active servicewomen surveyed indicate that it is harder to adhere to a daily oral contraceptive regimen across time zones/long shifts on active duty while deployed [102].

Continuing areas of research

Timing of restarting hormonal contraception after Ulipristal acetate

Because ulipristal acetate is an anti-progestin, there is concern that immediate start of a progestin-containing contraceptive could counteract the effect of ulipristal acetate [14]. In one pharmacodynamic study, women took ulipristal acetate and then were given either a placebo or started a desogestrel-containing contraceptive pill the next day [103]. Among women who used the progestin-containing pill, 45% of women ovulated within the next 5 days, compared with 3% in the placebo group [103]. It is of significant clinical concern that hormonal contraceptives could render ulipristal acetate EC ineffective and put the woman at risk for unintended pregnancy, given that previous standard clinical practice was to quick-start an ongoing contraceptive immediately for all women using EC pills who wanted a longer-term method. Desogestrel progestin-only pills are not available in the United States and have a different mechanism of action than other progestin-containing hormones, so it is unclear whether these results apply to all progestin-containing hormones. Until more research is available, it is recommended that women wait 5 days after taking ulipristal acetate to start a hormonal contraceptive method.

Appropriate dosing based on body weight

Research is ongoing; at this point, evidence suggests that for a person who is overweight or obese, a copper IUD is the best option for emergency contraception. Barring that, ulipristal acetate is more effective than LNG, which is only marginally more effective than no form of EC at all among obese women [13, 14, 30]. Double-dosing of LNG is being investigated at this time [38, 39].

Conclusion

Given the risks for unintended pregnancy among women of reproductive age who have sex with an opposite-sex partner or partners or are subject to rape or sexual assault, emergency contraception is an important last chance to prevent pregnancy. EC pills should be taken as soon as possible after sex. The most effective EC option is the copper IUD, followed by ulipristal acetate, and lastly LNG. Patients using ulipristal acetate EC should wait 5 days before starting an ongoing progestin-containing hormonal contraceptive subsequent to taking EC. Barriers to accessing EC persist, including lack of awareness among providers and low levels of stocking of EC in many stores and pharmacies. Finally, all EC methods are contraceptives–they prevent pregnancy rather than ending an established pregnancy.

Abbreviations

ACA: Affordable Care Act; BMI: Body mass index; CI: Confidence interval; DC: District of Columbia; EC: Emergency contraception; ECP: Emergency contraception pill; FDA: Food and Drug Administration; Hx: History; IUD: Intrauterine device; kg/m: Kilograms/meter; LNG: Levonorgestrel; mcg: Microgram; mg: Milligrams; N/A: Not applicable; OR: Odds ratio; OTC: Over-the-counter; UN: United Nations; UPA: Ulipristal acetate; UPI: Unprotected intercourse; VHA: Veterans Health Administration; WHO: World Health Organization

Authors' contributions

All authors read and approved the final manuscript.

Disclaimer

Author details

[1]Department of Veterans Affairs, Veterans Health Administration, Office of Patient Care Services, Women's Health Services, 810 Vermont Ave., NW, Washington, DC 20420, USA. [2]Department of Obstetrics & Gynecology, U.S. Naval Hospital Okinawa, Okinawa, Japan. [3]Office of Population Research, Princeton University, 218 Wallace Hall, Princeton, NJ 08544, USA.

References

1. Finer LB, Zolna MR. Declines in unintended pregnancy in the United States, 2008-2011. N Engl J Med. 2016;374(9):843–52.
2. Sonfield A, Hasstedt K, Gold RB. Moving forward: family planning in the era of health reform. New York: Guttmacher Institute; 2014. p. 1–56.
3. Key statistics from the National Survey of Family Growth. Centers for disease control and prevention. Atlanta: National Center for Health Statistics; 2017. Available from: https://www.cdc.gov/nchs/nsfg/key_statistics.htm. Accessed 13 Oct 2017
4. Lopez-del Burgo C, Mikolajczyk RT, Osorio A, Carlos S, Errasti T, de Irala J. Knowledge and beliefs about mechanism of action of birth control methods among European women. Contraception. 2012;85(1):69–77.
5. Hickey MT, White J. Female college students' experiences with and perceptions of over-the-counter emergency contraception in the United States. Sex Reprod Healthc. 2015;6(1):28–32.
6. Batur P, Cleland K, McNamara M, Wu J, Pickle S, E.C.S. Group. Emergency contraception: a multispecialty survey of clinician knowledge and practices. Contraception. 2016;93(2):145–52.
7. Cleland K, Bass J, Doci F, Foster AM. Access to emergency contraception in the over-the-counter era. Womens Health Issues. 2016;26(6):622–7.
8. Liles I, Haddad LB, Lathrop E, Hankin A. Contraception initiation in the emergency department: a pilot study on providers' knowledge, attitudes, and practices. South Med J. 2016;109(5):300–4.
9. Hickey MT, Shedlin MG. Emergency contraceptive pill users' risk perceptions for sexually transmitted infections and future unintended pregnancy. J Am Assoc Nurse Pract. 2017;29(9):527–34.
10. Liddon N, Steiner RJ, Martinez GM. Provider communication with adolescent and young females during sexual and reproductive health visits: findings from the 2011-2015 national survey of family growth. Contraception. 2018;97(1):22–8.
11. Glasier AF, Cameron ST, Fine PM, Logan SJS, Casale W, Van Horn J, Sogor L, Blithe DL, Scherrer B, Mathe H, Jaspart A, Ulmann A, Gainer E. Ulipristal acetate versus levonorgestrel for emergency contraception: a randomised non-inferiority trial and meta-analysis. Lancet. 2010; 375(9714):555–62.

12. Piaggio G, Kapp N, von Hertzen H. Effect on pregnancy rates of the delay in the administration of levonorgestrel for emergency contraception: a combined analysis of four WHO trials. Contraception. 2011;84(1):35–9.
13. Curtis KM, Jatlaoui TC, Tepper NK, Zapata LB, Horton LG, Jamieson DJ, Whiteman MK. U.S. selected practice recommendations for contraceptive use, 2016. MMWR Recomm Rep. 2016;65(4):1–66.
14. Faculty of Sexual & Reproductive Healthcare. Emergency contraception March 2017 (Updated December 2017). London: Faculty of Sexual & Reproductive Healthcare; 2017. p. 1–52.
15. Noe G, Croxatto HB, Salvatierra AM, Reyes V, Villarroel C, Munoz C, Morales G, Retamales A. Contraceptive efficacy of emergency contraception with levonorgestrel given before or after ovulation. Contraception. 2011;84(5):486–92.
16. Gemzell-Danielsson K, Berger C, GLL. P. Emergency contraception–mechanisms of action. Contraception. 2013;87(3):300–8.
17. Marions L, Hultenby K, Lindell I, Sun X, Stabi B, Gemzell Danielsson K. Emergency contraception with mifepristone and levonorgestrel: mechanism of action. Obstet Gynecol. 2002;100(1):65–71.
18. Hapangama D, Glasier AF, Baird DT. The effects of peri-ovulatory administration of levonorgestrel on the menstrual cycle☆. Contraception. 2001;63(3):123–9.
19. Durand M, del Carmen Cravioto M, Raymond EG, Durán-Sánchez O, De la Luz Cruz-Hinojosa M, Castell-Rodríguez A, Schiavon R, Larrea F. On the mechanisms of action of short-term levonorgestrel administration in emergency contraception. Contraception. 2001;64(4):227–34.
20. Marions L, Cekan SZ, Bygdeman M, Gemzell-Danielsson K. Effect of emergency contraception with levonorgestrel or mifepristone on ovarian function. Contraception. 2004;69(5):373–7.
21. Croxatto HB, Brache V, Pavez M, Cochon L, Forcelledo ML, Alvarez F, Massai R, Faundes A, Salvatierra AM. Pituitary-ovarian function following the standard levonorgestrel emergency contraceptive dose or a single 0.75-mg dose given on the days preceding ovulation. Contraception. 2004;70(6):442–50.
22. Okewole IA, Arowojolu AO, Odusoga OL, Oloyede OA, Adeleye OA, Salu J, Dada OA. Effect of single administration of levonorgestrel on the menstrual cycle. Contraception. 2007;75(5):372–7.
23. Kesserü E, Camacho-Ortega P, Laudahn G, Schopflin G. In vitro action of progestogens on sperm migration in human cervical mucus. Fertil Steril. 1975;26(1):57–61.
24. Kesserü E, Garmendia F, Westphal N, Parada J. The hormonal and peripheral effects of -norgestrel in postcoital contraception. Contraception. 1974;10(4): 411–24.
25. Durand M, Seppala M, Cravioto Mdel C, Koistinen H, Koistinen R, Gonzalez-Macedo J, Larrea F. Late follicular phase administration of levonorgestrel as an emergency contraceptive changes the secretory pattern of glycodelin in serum and endometrium during the luteal phase of the menstrual cycle. Contraception. 2005;71(6):451–7.
26. do Nascimento JA, Seppala M, Perdigao A, Espejo-Arce X, Munuce MJ, Hautala L, Koistinen R, Andrade L, Bahamondes L. In vivo assessment of the human sperm acrosome reaction and the expression of glycodelin-A in human endometrium after levonorgestrel-emergency contraceptive pill administration. Hum Reprod. 2007;22(8):2190–5.
27. Palomino WA, Kohen P, Devoto L. A single midcycle dose of levonorgestrel similar to emergency contraceptive does not alter the expression of the L-selectin ligand or molecular markers of endometrial receptivity. Fertil Steril. 2010;94(5):1589–94.
28. Novikova N, Weisberg E, Stanczyk FZ, Croxatto HB, Fraser IS. Effectiveness of levonorgestrel emergency contraception given before or after ovulation–a pilot study. Contraception. 2007;75(2):112–8.
29. Trussell J, Raymond EG, Cleland K. Emergency contraception: A last chance to prevent unintended pregnancy. Princeton: Princeton University: Office of Population Research; 2017. p. 1–38.
30. Practice bulletin No. 152. Emergency contraception. Obstet Gynecol. 2015; 126(3):e1–11.
31. Highlights of prescribing information: Plan B® One-Step. Health and Human Services: U.S. Food and Drug Administration, Silver Spring, MD. 2009. Available from: https://www.accessdata.fda.gov/drugsatfda_docs/label/2009/021998lbl.pdf. Accessed 13 Oct 2017.
32. von Hertzen H, Piaggio G, Peregoudov A, Ding J, Chen J, Song S, Bártfai G, Ng E, Gemzell-Danielsson K, Oyunbileg A, Wu S, Cheng W, Lüdicke F, Pretnar-Darovec A, Kirkman R, Mittal S, Khomassuridze A, Apter D. Low dose mifepristone and two regimens of levonorgestrel for emergency contraception: a WHO multicentre randomised trial. Lancet. 2002; 360(9348):1803–10.
33. Dada OA, Godfrey EM, Piaggio G, von Hertzen H, R. Nigerian Network for Reproductive Health, and Training. A randomized, double-blind, noninferiority study to compare two regimens of levonorgestrel for emergency contraception in Nigeria. Contraception. 2010;82(4):373–8.
34. Festin MP, Bahamondes L, Nguyen TM, Habib N, Thamkhantho M, Singh K, Gosavi A, Bartfai G, Bito T, Bahamondes MV, Kapp N. A prospective, open-label, single arm, multicentre study to evaluate efficacy, safety and acceptability of pericoital oral contraception using levonorgestrel 1.5 mg. Hum Reprod. 2016;31(3):530–40.
35. Glasier A, Cameron ST, Blithe D, Scherrer B, Mathe H, Levy D, Gainer E, Ulmann A. Can we identify women at risk of pregnancy despite using emergency contraception? Data from randomized trials of ulipristal acetate and levonorgestrel. Contraception. 2011;84(4):363–7.
36. Kapp N, Abitbol JL, Mathe H, Scherrer B, Guillard H, Gainer E, Ulmann A. Effect of body weight and BMI on the efficacy of levonorgestrel emergency contraception. Contraception. 2015;91(2):97–104.
37. Festin MP, Peregoudov A, Seuc A, Kiarie J, Temmerman M. Effect of BMI and body weight on pregnancy rates with LNG as emergency contraception: analysis of four WHO HRP studies. Contraception. 2017;95(1):50–4.
38. Praditpan P, Hamouie A, Basaraba CN, Nandakumar R, Cremers S, Davis AR, Westhoff CL. Pharmacokinetics of levonorgestrel and ulipristal acetate emergency contraception in women with normal and obese body mass index. Contraception. 2017;95(5):464–9.
39. Edelman AB, Cherala G, Blue SW, Erikson DW, Jensen JT. Impact of obesity on the pharmacokinetics of levonorgestrel-based emergency contraception: single and double dosing. Contraception. 2016;94(1):52–7.
40. Curtis KM, Tepper NK, Jatlaoui TC, Berry-Bibee E, Horton LG, Zapata LB, Simmons KB, Pagano HP, Jamieson DJ, Whiteman MK. U.S. Medical eligibility criteria for contraceptive use, 2016. MMWR Recomm Rep. 2016; 65(3):1–103.
41. Jatlaoui TC, Curtis KM. Safety and effectiveness data for emergency contraceptive pills among women with obesity: a systematic review. Contraception. 2016;94(6):605–11.
42. Cleland K, Raymond E, Trussell J, Cheng L, Zhu H. Ectopic pregnancy and emergency contraceptive pills: a systematic review. Obstet Gynecol. 2010; 115(6):1263–6.
43. Creinin MD, Schlaff W, Archer DF, Wan L, Frezieres R, Thomas M, Rosenberg M, Higgins J. Progesterone receptor modulator for emergency contraception. Obstet Gynecol. 2006;108(5):9.
44. Tirelli A, Cagnacci A, Volpe A. Levonorgestrel administration in emergency contraception: bleeding pattern and pituitary-ovarian function. Contraception. 2008;77(5):328–32.
45. Gainer E, Kenfack B, Mboudou E, Doh AS, Bouyer J. Menstrual bleeding patterns following levonorgestrel emergency contraception. Contraception. 2006;74(2):118–24.
46. Raymond EG, Trussell J, Polis CB. Population effect of increased access to emergency contraceptive pills: a systematic review. Obstet Gynecol. 2007; 109(1):181–8.
47. Zumoffen C, Gomez-Elias MD, Caille AM, Bahamondes L, Cuasnicu PS, Cohen DJ, Munuce MJ. Study of the effect of ulipristal acetate on human sperm ability to interact with tubal tissue and cumulus-oocyte-complexes. Contraception. 2017;95(6):586–91.
48. Berger C, Boggavarapu NR, Menezes J, Lalitkumar PG, Gemzell-Danielsson K. Effects of ulipristal acetate on human embryo attachment and endometrial cell gene expression in an in vitro co-culture system. Hum Reprod. 2015; 30(4):800–11.
49. Li HW, Lo SS, Ng EH, Ho PC. Efficacy of ulipristal acetate for emergency contraception and its effect on the subsequent bleeding pattern when administered before or after ovulation. Hum Reprod. 2016;31(6):1200–7.
50. Jesam C, Cochon L, Salvatierra AM, Williams A, Kapp N, Levy-Gompel D, Brache V. A prospective, open-label, multicenter study to assess the pharmacodynamics and safety of repeated use of 30 mg ulipristal acetate. Contraception. 2016;93(4):310–6.
51. Highlights of prescribing information: ella (ulipristal acetate) tablet. Silver Spring: Health and Human Services: U.S. Food and Drug Administration; 2014. Available from: www.accessdata.fda.gov/drugsatfda_docs/label/2014/022474s004lbl.pdf. Accessed 13 Oct 2017.

52. FDA communication on levonorgestrel emergency contraceptive effectiveness and weight. Silver Spring: U.S. Department of Health and Human Services; 2016. Available from: https://www.fda.gov/Drugs/DrugSafety/PostmarketDrugSafetyInformationforPatientsandProviders/ucm109775.htm. Accessed 13 Dec 2017.
53. Shigesato M, Elia J, Tschann M, Bullock H, Hurwitz E, Wu YY, Salcedo J. Pharmacy access to Ulipristal acetate in major cities throughout the United States. Contraception. 2017; Article in Press(6)
54. Emergency Contraception: State Laws and Policies. New York: Guttmacher Institute; 2017. Available from: https://www.guttmacher.org/state-policy/explore/emergency-contraception. Accessed 1 Dec 2017.
55. Turok DK, Godfrey EM, Wojdyla D, Dermish A, Torres L, Wu SC. Copper T380 intrauterine device for emergency contraception: highly effective at any time in the menstrual cycle. Hum Reprod. 2013;28(10):2672–6.
56. WHO. Medical eligibility criteria for contraceptive use. 5th ed. Geneva: World Health Organization; 2015.
57. Kaneshiro B, Aeby T. Long-term safety, efficacy, and patient acceptability of the intrauterine copper T-380A contraceptive device. Int J Womens Health. 2010;2:211–20.
58. Cleland K, Raymond EG, Westley E, Trussell J. Emergency contraception review: evidence-based recommendations for clinicians. Clin Obstet Gynecol. 2014;57(4):741–50.
59. How can I get an IUD? New York: Planned Parenthood Federation of America Inc.; 2018; Available from: https://www.plannedparenthood.org/learn/birth-control/iud/how-can-i-get-an-iud. Accessed 15 Jan 2018.
60. Harper CC, Speidel JJ, Drey EA, Trussell J, Blum M, Darney PD. Copper intrauterine device for emergency contraception: clinical practice among contraceptive providers. Obstet Gynecol. 2012;119(2 Pt 1):220–6.
61. Bergin A, Tristan S, Terplan M, Gilliam ML, Whitaker AK. A missed opportunity for care: two-visit IUD insertion protocols inhibit placement. Contraception. 2012;86(6):694–7.
62. Hamoda H, Ashok PW, Stalder C, Flett GM, Kennedy E, Templeton A. A randomized trial of mifepristone (10 mg) and levonorgestrel for emergency contraception. Obstet Gynecol. 2004;104(6):1307–13.
63. Turok DK, Sanders JN, Thompson IS, Royer PA, Eggebroten J, Gawron LM. Preference for and efficacy of oral levonorgestrel for emergency contraception with concomitant placement of a levonorgestrel IUD: a prospective cohort study. Contraception. 2016;93(6):526–32.
64. Corbett PO, Mitchell CP, Taylor JS, Kemppainen J. Emergency contraception: knowledge and perceptions in a university population. J Am Acad Nurse Pract. 2006;18(4):161–8.
65. Whittaker PG, Armstrong KA, Adams J. Implementing an advance emergency contraception policy: what happens in the real world? Perspect Sex Reprod Health. 2008;40(3):162–70.
66. Johnson R, Nshom M, Nye AM, Cohall AT. There's always plan B: adolescent knowledge, attitudes and intention to use emergency contraception. Contraception. 2010;81(2):128–32.
67. Sampson O, Navarro SK, Khan A, Hearst N, Raine TR, Gold M, Miller S, de Bocanegra HT. Barriers to adolescents' getting emergency contraception through pharmacy access in California: differences by language and region. Perspect Sex Reprod Health. 2009;41(2):110–8.
68. Access to emergency contraception. Committee opinion no. 707. Obstet Gynecol. 2017;130(1):5.
69. Grindlay K, Grossman D. Contraception access and use among U.S. servicewomen during deployment. Contraception. 2013;87(2):162–9.
70. Karasz A. The visit before the morning after: barriers to preprescribing emergency contraception. Ann Fam Med. 2004;2(4):345–50.
71. Polis CB, Schaffer K, Blanchard K, Glasier A, Harper CC, Grimes DA. Advance provision of emergency contraception for pregnancy prevention: a meta-analysis. Obstet Gynecol. 2007;110(6):1379–88.
72. Cameron ST, Li H, Gemzell-Danielsson K. Current controversies with oral emergency contraception. BJOG. 2017;124(13):1948–56.
73. Chau VM, Stamm CA, Borgelt L, Gaffaney M, Moore A, Blumhagen RZ, Rupp L, Topp D, Gilroy C. Barriers to single-dose levonorgestrel-only emergency contraception access in retail pharmacies. Womens Health Issues. 2017;27(5):518–22.
74. Wilkinson TA, Fahey N, Shields C, Suther E, Cabral HJ, Silverstein M. Pharmacy communication to adolescents and their physicians regarding access to emergency contraception. Pediatrics. 2012;129(4):624–9.
75. Ritter AH, Isaacs CR, Lee SM, Lee AJ. Single-dose levonorgestrel emergency contraception and silent barriers to its access: is it really just one step? J Women's Health (Larchmt). 2017;27(5):646-50.
76. Wilkinson TA, Clark P, Rafie S, Carroll AE, Miller E. Access to emergency contraception after removal of age restrictions. Pediatrics. 2017;140(1). https://doi.org/10.1542/peds.2016-4262.
77. Fok WK, Blumenthal PD. Update on emergency contraception. Curr Opin Obstet Gynecol. 2016;28(6):522–9.
78. Upadhya KK, Santelli JS, Raine-Bennett TR, Kottke MJ, Grossman D. Over-the-counter access to oral contraceptives for adolescents. J Adolesc Health. 2017;60(6):634–40.
79. How much does a Paragard IUD cost? San Francisco: Amino, Inc.; 2018. Available from: https://amino.com/blog/paragard-iud-cost/. Accessed 15 Jan 2018.
80. Health benefits & coverage–birth control benefits. Baltimore: U.S. Centers for Medicare & Medicaid Services; 2018. Available from: https://www.healthcare.gov/coverage/birth-control-benefits/. Accessed 15 Jan 2018.
81. Bullock H, Steele S, Kurata N, Tschann M, Elia J, Kaneshiro B, Salcedo J. Pharmacy access to ulipristal acetate in Hawaii: is a prescription enough? Contraception. 2016;93(5):452–4.
82. Beeson T, Wood S, Bruen B, Goldberg DG, Mead H, Rosenbaum S. Accessibility of long-acting reversible contraceptives (LARCs) in federally qualified health centers (FQHCs). Contraception. 2014;89(2):91–6.
83. Guiahi M, Sheeder J, Teal S. Are women aware of religious restrictions on reproductive health at Catholic hospitals? A survey of women's expectations and preferences for family planning care. Contraception. 2014;90(4):429–34.
84. Uttley L, Reynertson S, Kenny L, Melling L. Miscarriage of medicine: the growth of Catholic hospitals and the threat of reproductive health care. New York: The MergerWatch Project and the American Civil Liberties Union; 2013. p. 38.
85. Card RF, Williams KG. Emergency contraception, institutional conscience, and pharmacy practice. J Pharm Pract. 2014;27(2):174–7.
86. Morrell KM, Chavkin W. Conscientious objection to abortion and reproductive healthcare: a review of recent literature and implications for adolescents. Curr Opin Obstet Gynecol. 2015;27(5):333–8.
87. Yang YT, Sawicki NN. Pharmacies' duty to dispense emergency contraception: a discussion of religious liberty. Obstet Gynecol. 2017;129(3):551–3.
88. Montanari Vergallo G, Zaami S, Di Luca NM, Marinelli E. The conscientious objection: debate on emergency contraception. Clin Ter. 2017;168(2):e113–9.
89. Miller MK, Mollen CJ. Critical access to care: bringing contraception to adolescents in nontraditional settings. J Adolesc Health. 2017;61(6):667–8.
90. Reddy DM, Flemming R, Swain C. Effect of mandatory parental notification on adolescent girls' use of sexual health care services. JAMA. 2002;288(6):5.
91. Ford C, English A, Sigman G. Confidential health care for adolescents: position paper of the society for adolescent medicine. J Adolesc Health. 2004;35(2):160–7.
92. Richards MJ, Peters M, Sheeder J, Kaul P. Contraception and adolescent males: an opportunity for providers. J Adolesc Health. 2016;58(3):366–8.
93. Yen S, Parmar DD, Lin EL, Ammerman S. Emergency contraception pill awareness and knowledge in uninsured adolescents: high rates of misconceptions concerning indications for use, side effects, and access. J Pediatr Adolesc Gynecol. 2015;28(5):337–42.
94. Holmes MM, Resnick HS, Kilpatrick DG, Best CL. Rape-related pregnancy: estimates and descriptive characteristics from a national sample of women. Am J Obstet Gynecol. 1996;175(6):320-5.
95. Mulder PL, Shellenberger S, Streiegel R, Jumper-Thurman P, Danda CE, Kenkel MB, Constantine MG, Sears SF, Kalodner M, Hager A. Behavioral health care needs of rural women. Washington, D.C: Rural Task Force of the American Psychological Association and the American Psychological Association's Committee on Rural Health; 2006. p. 51.
96. Bigbee JL, Abood R, Landau SC, Maderas NM, Foster DG, Ravnan S. Pharmacy access to emergency contraception in rural and frontier communities. J Rural Health. 2007;23(4):294–8.
97. Grindlay K, Grossman D. Unintended pregnancy among active-duty women in the United States military, 2011. Contraception. 2015;92(6):589–95.
98. Borrero S, Callegari LS, Zhao X, Mor MK, Sileanu FE, Switzer G, Zickmund S, Washington DL, Zephyrin LC, Schwarz EB. Unintended pregnancy and contraceptive use among women veterans: the ECUUN study. J Gen Intern Med. 2017;32(8):900–8.

99. Witkop CT, Webber BJ, Chu KM, Clark LL. Contraceptive prescriptions for US servicewomen, 2008-2013. Contraception. 2017;96(1):47–53.
100. Callegari LS, Zhao X, Nelson KM, Borrero S. Contraceptive adherence among women veterans with mental illness and substance use disorder. Contraception. 2015;91(5):386–92.
101. Chung-Park M. Emergency contraception knowledge, attitudes, practices, and barriers among providers at a military treatment facility. Mil Med. 2008; 173(3):8.
102. Duke MR, Ames GM. Challenges of contraceptive use and pregnancy prevention among women in the U.S. Navy. Qual Health Res. 2008;18(2): 244–53.
103. Brache V, Cochon L, Duijkers IJ, Levy DP, Kapp N, Monteil C, Abitbol JL, Klipping C. A prospective, randomized, pharmacodynamic study of quick-starting a desogestrel progestin-only pill following ulipristal acetate for emergency contraception. Hum Reprod. 2015;30(12):2785–93.
104. Daniels K, Mosher WD, Jones J. Contraceptive methods women have ever used: United States, 1982–2010. Atlanta: Centers for disease control and prevention: National Center for Health Statistics; 2013. p. 1–16.

Permissions

All chapters in this book were first published by BioMed Central; hereby published with permission under the Creative Commons Attribution License or equivalent. Every chapter published in this book has been scrutinized by our experts. Their significance has been extensively debated. The topics covered herein carry significant findings which will fuel the growth of the discipline. They may even be implemented as practical applications or may be referred to as a beginning point for another development.

The contributors of this book come from diverse backgrounds, making this book a truly international effort. This book will bring forth new frontiers with its revolutionizing research information and detailed analysis of the nascent developments around the world.

We would like to thank all the contributing authors for lending their expertise to make the book truly unique. They have played a crucial role in the development of this book. Without their invaluable contributions this book wouldn't have been possible. They have made vital efforts to compile up to date information on the varied aspects of this subject to make this book a valuable addition to the collection of many professionals and students.

This book was conceptualized with the vision of imparting up-to-date information and advanced data in this field. To ensure the same, a matchless editorial board was set up. Every individual on the board went through rigorous rounds of assessment to prove their worth. After which they invested a large part of their time researching and compiling the most relevant data for our readers.

The editorial board has been involved in producing this book since its inception. They have spent rigorous hours researching and exploring the diverse topics which have resulted in the successful publishing of this book. They have passed on their knowledge of decades through this book. To expedite this challenging task, the publisher supported the team at every step. A small team of assistant editors was also appointed to further simplify the editing procedure and attain best results for the readers.

Apart from the editorial board, the designing team has also invested a significant amount of their time in understanding the subject and creating the most relevant covers. They scrutinized every image to scout for the most suitable representation of the subject and create an appropriate cover for the book.

The publishing team has been an ardent support to the editorial, designing and production team. Their endless efforts to recruit the best for this project, has resulted in the accomplishment of this book. They are a veteran in the field of academics and their pool of knowledge is as vast as their experience in printing. Their expertise and guidance has proved useful at every step. Their uncompromising quality standards have made this book an exceptional effort. Their encouragement from time to time has been an inspiration for everyone.

The publisher and the editorial board hope that this book will prove to be a valuable piece of knowledge for researchers, students, practitioners and scholars across the globe.

List of Contributors

Rebecca L. Fischbein
Department of Family and Community Medicine, Northeast Ohio Medical University, 4209 St. Rt. 44, Rootstown, OH 44272, USA

Bethany G. Lanese, Lynn Falletta, Kelsey Hamilton and Deric R. Kenne
College of Public Health, Department of Health Policy and Management, Kent State University, 750 Hilltop Drive, 322 Lowry Hall, Kent, OH 44242, USA

Jennifer A. King
Old Brooklyn Community Development Corporation, Cleveland, OH, USA

Justin E. Hellwinkel, Matthew W. Konigsberg and R. Kumar Kadiyala
Department of Orthopedics, Columbia University Irving Medical Center, 622 W 168th St PH 11 - Center, NY 10032 New York, USA

Johana Oviedo
Department of Obstetrics and Gynecology, New York University Langone Health, 550 First Avenue, NY 10016 New York, USA

Paula M. Castaño
Department of Obstetrics and Gynecology, Columbia University Irving Medical Center, 622 W 168th St, NY 10032 New York, USA

Mulugeta Mekuria and Teka Girma
Department of Public health, Ambo University College of Medicine and Health Science, Ambo, Ethiopia

Dechasa Daba
West Shoa Health office, West Shewa, Ethiopia

Adamu Birhanu
Department of Psychiatry, Ambo University College of Medicine and Health Science, Ambo, Ethiopia

Tadese Ejigu Tafere
School of Public Health (SPH), College of Health Sciences, Addis Ababa University, Addis Ababa, Ethiopia
School of Public Health, College of Medicine and Health Sciences, Bahir Dar University, Bahir Dar, Ethiopia

Mesganaw Fanthahun Afework and Alemayehu Worku Yalew
School of Public Health, College of Health Sciences, Addis Ababa University, Addis Ababa, Ethiopia

Rachel Lefebvre and Milan Stevanovic
Department of Orthopaedic Surgery, Division of Hand Surgery, University of Southern California, 1200 N State Street A7-CT, Los Angeles, CA 90033, USA

Marianne Hom
Department of Obstetrics and Gynecology, University of Southern California, 2020 Zonal Ave., IRD Room 512, Los Angeles, CA 90033, USA

Hyuma Leland
Department of Plastic and Reconstructive Surgery, University of Southern California, 1510 San Pablo St., Suite 415, Los Angeles, CA 90033, USA

Ifeyinwa Chizoba Akamike, Ugochukwu Chinyem Madubueze, Ijeoma Nkem Okedo-Alex, Chika Julius Anyigor and Chukwuma David Umeokonkwo
Department of Community Medicine, Alex Ekwueme Federal University Teaching Hospital, Abakaliki, Ebonyi State, Nigeria

Benedict Ndubueze Azuogu
Department of Community Medicine, Alex Ekwueme Federal University Teaching Hospital, Abakaliki, Ebonyi State, Nigeria
Department of Community Medicine, Ebonyi State University, Abakaliki, Nigeria

Chinyere Ojiugo Mbachu
Department of Community Medicine, College of Medicine, University of Nigeria, Nsukka, Nigeria

Enyew Abate and Walelign Kindie
College of Medicine and Health Sciences, Department of Obstetrics and Gynecology, Bahir Dar University, Bahir Dar, Ethiopia

Yolanda R. Smith
Department of Obstetrics and Gynecology, University of Michigan and Centers for International Reproductive Health Training (CIRHT), Ann Arbor, Michigan, USA

Addisu Girma
Debre Birhan Referral Hospital, Debre Birhan, Ethiopia

Yonas Girma
Centers for International Reproductive Health Training (CIRHT), Addis Ababa, Ethiopia

Shana M. Miles
Second Medical Group, 243 Curtiss Rd, Barksdale AFB, Louisiana 71110, USA

Katerina Shvartsman
Department of Obstetrics and Gynecology, Uniformed Services University, 4301 Jones Bridge Rd, Bethesda, MD 20814, USA

Susan Dunlow
Department of Obstetrics and Gynecology, Walter Reed National Military Medical Center, 8901 Wisconsin Ave, Bethesda, MD 20889, USA

Mesele Damte Argaw, Hailemariam Segni Abawollo, Binyam Fekadu Desta, Zergu Taffesse Tsegaye and Melkamu Getu Abebe
USAID Transform: Primary Health Care, JSI Research & Training Institute, Inc., Addis Ababa, Ethiopia

Dejene Mengistu Belete
Mekoy Health Center, Mekoy, Antsokiya Gemza District, Ethiopia

Ashley Wiltshire, Kiwita Phillips, Roland Matthews and Desiree McCarthy-Keith
Morehouse School of Medicine, Department of Obstetrics and Gynecology, 720 Westview Drive, Atlanta, GA 30310, USA

Lynae M Brayboy
Department of Obstetrics and Gynecology Division of Reproductive Endocrinology and Infertility Women & Infants Hospital, Alpert Medical School of Brown University, 101 Dudley Fl 1, Providence, RI 02905, USA

Fengxia Yan
Morehouse School of Medicine Department of Community Health & Preventive Medicine, 720 Westview Drive, Atlanta, GA 30310, USA

Gebremaryam Temesgen Birgoda
Department of Midwifery, College of Medicine & Health Sciences, Arba Minch University, Arba Minch, Ethiopia

Haftom Gebrehiwot
Department of Midwifery, College of Health Sciences, Mekele University, Mekele, Ethiopia

Sultan Hussen Hebo, Negussie Boti Sidamo and Mulugeta Shegaze Shembri
Department of Public Health, College of Medicine & Health Sciences, Arba Minch University, Arba Minch, Ethiopia

Birhane Hagos
Department of Midwifery, College of Medicine & Health Sciences, Dilla Minch University, Arba Minch, Ethiopia

Genet Assefa
Department of Midwifery, College of Medicine & Health Sciences, Wolkite University, Wolkite, Ethiopia

Alemayehu Gonie Mekonnen, Alebachew Demelash Bayleyegn, Yared Asmare Aynalem and Tigist Demssew Adane
Department of Nursing, College of Health Science, Debre Berhan University, Debre Berhan, Ethiopia

Mikyas Arega Muluneh
Department of Midwifery, College of Health Science, Debre Berhan University, Debre Berhan, Ethiopia

Meaza Asefa
Department of Medical Laboratory, College of Medicine, Debre Berhan University, Debre Berhan, Ethiopia

Kiondo Solomon Kiondo and Sophia Kiwango
Kilimanjaro Christian Medical University College, Moshi, Tanzania

Julius Pius Alloyce
Department of Obstetrics and Gynecology, Kilimanjaro Christian Medical Centre, Moshi, Tanzania

Eusebious Maro and Benjamin C. Shayo
Kilimanjaro Christian Medical University College, Moshi, Tanzania
Department of Obstetrics and Gynecology, Kilimanjaro Christian Medical Centre, Moshi, Tanzania

Michael Johnson Mahande
Kilimanjaro Christian Medical University College, Moshi, Tanzania
Department of Epidemiology and Biostatistics, Institute of Public Health, Kilimanjaro Christian Medical University College, Moshi, Tanzania

Fred Yao Gbagbo
University of Education Winneba, Winneba, Ghana

Esinam Afi Kayi
Regional Institute for Population Studies, University of Ghana, Accra, Ghana

Glenmarie Matthews, Jessica Atrio and Nerys Benfield
Department of Obstetrics and Gynecology, Montefiore Hospital & Albert Einstein College of Medicine, 1695 Eastchester Road, Bronx 10461, NY, USA

Horace Fletcher, Nathalie Medley and Leo Walker
University of West Indies - Mona Campus, Kingston, West Indies, Jamaica

Girma Alemayehu Beyene
Department of Public Health, College of Health Science and Medicine, Wolkite University, Wolkite, Ethiopia

Laxmi Tamang
APS Prasuti Tatha Prajanan Swasthya Kendra, Link Marg 1045, Kuleshwor, Kathmandu, Nepal

Camille Raynes-Greenow and Kevin McGeechan
School of Public Health, Faculty of Medicine, The University of Sydney, Camperdown, NSW 2006, Australia

Kirsten Black
Discipline of Obstetrics, Gynaecology and Neonatology, Faculty of Medicine, The University of Sydney, Camperdown, NSW 2006, Australia

Chisato Masuda and Michelle Helena van Velthoven
School of Tropical Medicine and Global Health, Nagasaki University, Sakamoto 1-12-4, Nagasaki 852-8523, Japan

Elisa Oreglia
Kings College London, London, UK

Sokhey Ly, Camille Tijamo, Amra Ou and Amy Williamson
Marie Stopes International Cambodia, Phnom Penh, Cambodia

Megan McLaren
Marie Stopes International, London, UK

Chris Smith
School of Tropical Medicine and Global Health, Nagasaki University, Sakamoto 1-12-4, Nagasaki 852-8523, Japan
Clinical Research Department, London School of Hygiene and Tropical Medicine, Keppel Street, London WC1E7HT, UK
Room 150, Department of Population Health, London School of Hygiene and Tropical Medicine, Keppel Street, London WC1E 7HT, UK

Dylane N. Davis, Clara Lemani, Nenani Kamtuwanje, Billy Phiri, Prisca Masepuka and Sally Kuchawo
UNC Project-Malawi, c/o Kamuzu Central Hospital, 100 Mzimba Road, Lilongwe, Malawi

Jennifer H. Tang
UNC Project-Malawi, c/o Kamuzu Central Hospital, 100 Mzimba Road, Lilongwe, Malawi
Department of Obstetrics & Gynecology, University of North Carolina at Chapel Hill, 100 Manning Drive, Chapel Hill, North Carolina, 27599-7570 CB-7570, USA

Nivedita L. Bhushan
UNC Project-Malawi, c/o Kamuzu Central Hospital, 100 Mzimba Road, Lilongwe, Malawi
Department of Health Behavior, University of North Carolina at Chapel Hill, Rosenau Hall, CB #7440, Chapel Hill, North Carolina, 27599-7570 27599, USA

Girma Bacha Ayane
Department of Nursing, College of Medicine and Health Science, Jimma University, Jimma, Ethiopia

Kalkidan Wondwossen Desta and Emebet Berhane Woldemariam
School of Nursing and Midwifery, College of Health Science, Addis Ababa University, Addis Ababa, Ethiopia

Birhanu Wondimeneh Demissie and Netsanet Abera Assefa
School of Nursing, College of Health Sciences and Medicine, Wolaita Sodo University, Sodo, Ethiopia

Phil Edwards and Caroline Free
Department of Population Health, London School of Hygiene and Tropical Medicine, Keppel Street, London WC1E 7HT, UK

Vannak Uk
Marie Stopes International, Phnom Penh, Cambodia

Ruby Warnock
Department of Obstetrics, Gynecology and Reproductive Sciences, University of California, San Francisco, USA

Bola Lukman Solanke, Funmilola Folasade Oyinlola and Benjamin Bukky Ilesanmi
Department of Demography and Social Statistics, Obafemi Awolowo University, Ile-Ife, Nigeria

Olaoye James Oyeleye
Department of Demography and Social Statistics, Obafemi Awolowo University, Ile-Ife, Nigeria
Action Against Hunger, ACF-International, Damaturu, Yobe State, Nigeria

Tadele Girum and Abebaw Wasie
Department of Public Health, College of Medicine and Health Sciences, Wolkite University, Wolkite City, Ethiopia

Thomas Obinchemti Egbe
Department of Obstetrics and Gynecology, Faculty of Health Sciences, University of Buea, Buea, Cameroon

Julius Atashili
Department of Public Health, Faculty of Health Sciences, University of Buea, Buea, Cameroon

Emmanuella Talla
Delegation of Public Health, North West Region, Cameroon

Mary Bih Suh Atanga
Department of Nursing and Midwifery, Faculty of Health Sciences, University of Bamenda, Bambili, Cameroon

Carla L. DeSisto, Arden Handler, Nadine Peacock and Kristin Rankin
University of Illinois at Chicago School of Public Health, 1603 W. Taylor St, Chicago, IL 60612, USA

Sadia Haider
Department of Obstetrics and Gynecology, University of Chicago, 5841 S. Maryland Ave, Chicago, IL 60637, USA

Rachel Caskey
College of Medicine, University of Illinois at Chicago, 840 S. Wood St, Chicago, IL 60612, USA

Melissa Kottke
Department of Gynecology and Obstetrics, Jane Fonda Center, Emory University School of Medicine, 49 Jesse Hill Jr. Drive SE, Atlanta, GA 30303, USA

Meselu Atnafe
Dire Dawa City Administration Health Bureau, Dire Dawa, Ethiopia

Nega Assefa and Tadesse Alemayehu
College of Health and Medical Sciences, Haramaya University, Dire Dawa, Ethiopia

Anjali Singh, K. K. Singh and Prashant Verma
Department of Statistics, Banaras Hindu University, Varanasi, India

Kristin O. Haeger
Department of Veterans Affairs, Veterans Health Administration, Office of Patient Care Services, Women's Health Services, 810 Vermont Ave., NW, Washington, DC 20420, USA

Jacqueline Lamme
Department of Obstetrics & Gynecology, U.S. Naval Hospital Okinawa, Okinawa, Japan

Kelly Cleland
Office of Population Research, Princeton University, 218 Wallace Hall, Princeton, NJ 08544, USA

Index

www.ingramcontent.com/pod-product-compliance
Lightning Source LLC
LaVergne TN
LVHW082139200926
848484LV00008B/2078
* 9 7 9 8 8 8 7 4 0 0 2 2 8 *